Dental Ultrasound in Periodontology and Implantology

Hsun-Liang (Albert) Chan •
Oliver D. Kripfgans
Editors

Dental Ultrasound in Periodontology and Implantology

Examination, Diagnosis and Treatment Outcome Evaluation

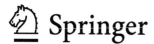 Springer

Editors
Hsun-Liang (Albert) Chan
Department of Periodontics and Oral
Medicine, School of Dentistry
University of Michigan–Ann Arbor
Ann Arbor, MI, USA

Oliver D. Kripfgans
Department of Radiology, Medical School
University of Michigan–Ann Arbor
Ann Arbor, MI, USA

ISBN 978-3-030-51290-3   ISBN 978-3-030-51288-0   (eBook)
https://doi.org/10.1007/978-3-030-51288-0

This Springer imprint is published by the registered company Springer Nature Switzerland AG.
The registered company address is: Gewerbestrasse 11, 6330 Cham, Switzerland

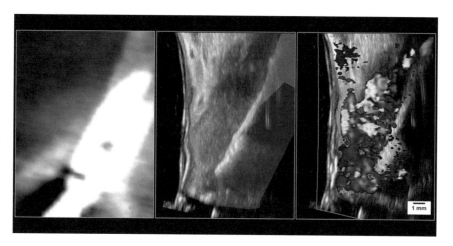

An implant clinically diagnosed with peri implantitis, shown on CBCT (right), B-mode ultrasound (center), and color-mode ultrasound (left). B-mode ultrasound delineated mucosa, thin facial bone, and implant surface well. The pixel brightness in soft tissue may indicate the degree of inflammation and tissue loss. The color-mode shows the blood velocity, which may be an indicator for the severity of inflammation. The shades were added to the B-mode image for illustration of different structures

This book is dedicated to all who break through existing mindsets and look for the future.
We would also like to dedicate this book to Eric, who left us too early. You will always be remembered.

Foreword

The visualization of soft and hard tissues in the dental, oral, and craniofacial complex is critically important in the diagnosis of disease, congenital deficiencies, or following traumatic injury. In the development of this book, *Dental Ultrasound in Periodontology and Implantology: Examination, Diagnosis, and Treatment Outcome Evaluation*, Drs. Hsun-Liang (Albert) Chan and Oliver D. Kripfgans have assembled an excellent and first-of-its-kind text that comprehensively describes the many advances of the dynamic and rapidly evolving field of oral and dental ultrasonography. The discipline of biomedical imaging is moving at a fast pace and this landmark book makes available information on key facets of dental ultrasonography ranging from the physics and mechanism of action on nonionizing imaging for oral and dental structures to the improved imaging of teeth, dental implants, and supporting soft tissues as well as other vital structures so critical for oral diagnostic procedures.

The opening chapter of the book, "Ultrasonic Imaging: Physics and Mechanism", provides the reader the fundamentals on the physics of ultrasonic imaging that includes the "what," "how," and "why" of this technology to help the learner better understand the unique aspects of this imaging technology to noninvasively identify soft and hard tissues in the oral cavity. The next chapter on Ultrasonic Imaging in Comparison to Other Imaging Modalities highlights how ultrasonic approaches compare to other traditional imaging techniques such as 2D intraoral radiography and 3D cone-beam computed tomography. Dr. Aps shows how the use of ultrasonic imaging can complement and/or in some cases potentially replace the use of other more invasive approaches to identify oral structures. Chapter 3, System Requirements for Intraoral Ultrasonic Scanning, gives a nice highlight of the platforms, system requirements, and new units coming onto the medical and dental marketplace for the application of these technologies to the oral cavity. This aspect is changing rapidly in the decision-making challenges with the changing landscape of manufacturers of imaging devices. In Chap. 4, Current Digital Workflow for Implant Therapy: Advantages and Limitations, Drs. Siqueira, Soki, and Chan assemble very well the role of ultrasonography to interface with the digital workflow so important in dental implant treatment planning. There are many opportunities to combine existing 2D and 3D radiography with ultrasound for preoperative, but also intraoperative diagnosis of structures for optimal dental implant positioning to enhance function and esthetics. The team goes on to demonstrate how these imaging approaches can be coupled with chairside 3D printing or CAD/CAM for the fabrication of implant guides to improve the workflow for more ideal implant placements. Chapter 5 focuses on the use of Ultrasound for Periodontal Imaging and while an emerging area with accumulating research activity, this approach to identify tooth-supporting structures offers good potential for the better assessment of periodontal diseases and the status of soft and hard tissues adjacent to teeth.

Implant dentistry using tooth replacement oral implants has revolutionized reconstructive dentistry. This therapy has allowed patients to be rehabilitated with endosseous titanium prostheses that can replace missing teeth in partially or fully edentulous individuals to improve their function and esthetics. The next five major chapters of the book (Ultrasonic Imaging for Estimating the Risk of Peri-Implant Esthetic Complications, Ultrasound Indications in Implant-Related and Other Oral Surgery, Ultrasonic Imaging for Evaluating Peri-Implant Diseases, Ultrasonography for Wound Healing Evaluation of Implant Related Surgeries, and Ultrasonic Evaluation of Dental Implant Stability) provide in-depth and useful material related to dental implant position and status. Given the tremendous health care costs, time involved, and increasing prevalence of peri-implant diseases, the use of a technology such as dental ultrasonography provides a unique approach to noninvasively identify the position, bone, and soft tissue support of dental implants. The beneficial evidence provided in these chapters will aid the clinician to better consider ultrasound in progressive disease states or during oral wound healing situations where traditional methods result in more invasive assessments that may be unjustified.

The final chapters in the book focus on Photoacoustic Ultrasound for Enhanced Contrast in Dental and Periodontal Imaging and Volumetric Ultrasound and Related Dental Applications. These sections of the book highlight the use of these dynamic imaging approaches that have implications in other dental presentations such as in the diagnosis of dental caries, tooth pulpal pathology, and other hard–soft tissue pathologies including traumas that can cause fractures or cracks on the teeth that often are challenging for the clinician to diagnose. The final chapter on volumetric and quantitative aspects has tremendous potential for use in the longitudinal assessment of bony and soft tissue changes following augmentation procedures or disease progression scenarios.

Motivated by this comprehensive approach in noninvasive dental imaging of ultrasonography, this might be an "enlightenment period" in biomedical imaging in dentistry. This state-of-the-art technology now allows us to firmly consider the many options available to us as clinicians to better prepare and treatment plan our cases to optimize the delivery of oral healthcare. This textbook by Drs. Chan and Kripfgans lays out a contemporary and exciting look for us as clinicians, researchers, and students alike to better understand the many exciting possibilities for the use of dental ultrasonography for innovative research and clinical care.

Boston, MA, USA   William V. Giannobile
July 2020

Preface

Healthcare is an ever-evolving field that navigates through many expectations. It should be set to be conservative with a negligible chance of error to maintain the promise of the hippocratic oath of *do no harm*. *Harm* does not have to be physical harm but can manifest itself in a variety of ways. Investment of resources into new developments obviously takes those resources away from patients and could be seen as *harm* to them. Healthcare providers come with a range of objectives besides their dedication to care and support. Universities serve the public with teaching and research. University (dental and medical) hospitals and clinics provide healthcare to patients today and contribute to advancing knowledge to provide better healthcare tomorrow.

This book is the first attempt to advance ultrasound imaging in the field of *Dentistry*. Current diagnostic methodologies in dental care consist of radiographic and optical methods. X-rays and cone-beam CT are established imaging methodologies for providing a high level of dental care. Optical methods are also available and contribute diagnostic information. Ultrasound is a well-established imaging modality in medicine. It has propagated into many specialty areas and shows high levels of acceptance from patients. However, there is little or no use of ultrasound in dental care, except for the intersection of medicine and dental, i.e. oral and maxillofacial surgery. This is surprising for two reasons: First, ultrasound has excellent soft tissue contrast and provides real-time cross-sectional images without any ionizing radiation. Second, many oral diseases start from inflammation in soft tissues. Thus, ultrasound would be an excellent diagnostic modality. However, for a long time, several limitations hindered its practical use in the dental clinic. Image resolution was low due to the absence of high-frequency ultrasound probes. In addition, such probes were too large for use in the oral cavity.

Advances in electronics, signal processing, integration, and miniaturization have allowed medical ultrasound to enter new areas. These include imaging in preclinical rodent studies as well as the use of ultrasound in settings that require very little tissue penetration, such as dermatology. Dental soft tissues also require very little penetration. Gingiva and mucosa tissues are thin compared to those imaged in the traditional use of ultrasound. Thus, the current state of the art of ultrasound may be a strong addition to contemporary dentistry and it may help caregivers to offer precise diagnosis and prognosis to their patients. Precision oral care is largely dependent on quantitative subclinical and clinical data for dentists to make clinical decisions and evaluate treatment outcomes. Many established and yet to-be-studied quantitative ultrasound parameters may be found applicable to diagnose periodontal and peri-implant diseases, among other oral lesions. One of the objectives of this book is to provide first-hand information regarding our research results, the advantages and limitations of dental ultrasound, and practical implementations to the readers.

It should be noted that dental and medical nomenclature are used in parallel in this book. While they share a substantial fraction of their extent, they also differ in some aspects. This is where the readers can find themselves between the two worlds. For example, the definition of *lateral*. Picture a 2D cross-sectional sagittal mid-facial scan of the right maxillary central incisor. Dental nomenclature defines the "lateral" position with respect to such a scan to be either toward the mesial or distal side of the scan plane. Medical ultrasound nomenclature would define the same direction to be the elevational plane toward either the mesial or distal direction, whereas the lateral (ultrasound) direction is defined to be in-plane in the scan, perpendicular to the axial (depth) extent of the scan.

Ann Arbor, MI, USA   Hsun-Liang (Albert) Chan
Ann Arbor, MI, USA   Oliver D. Kripfgans
February 2020

Disclaimer

Any commercial products shown are not meant to be endorsed by the authors but rather are examples of available products. The authors do not receive any financial or other in-kind contributions from any of the manufacturers of the products shown.

Acknowledgements

We would like to thank our coworkers and colleagues for numerous discussions and valuable input for this book. We also thank the reviewers for their time and constructive feedback.

We thank Dr. Aps for contributing his chapter "Ultrasonic Imaging in Comparison to other Imaging Modalities" to guide the readers through the landscape of the current dental imaging technologies. Drs. Siqueira and Soki graciously co-wrote the chapter "Current Digital Workflow for Implant Therapy: Advantages and Limitations" with us, thereby contributing their radiological and clinical expertise regarding the current digital workflow for implant therapy. We thank Drs. Le, Nguyen, Kaipatur, and Major for contributing their chapter "Ultrasound for Periodontal Imaging," a cornerstone of dental ultrasound as periodontal (gum) disease is a prevalent oral disease, affecting approximately 40% of the US adults. We thank Drs. Hériveaux, Nguyen, Vayron, and Haïat for contributing their chapter "Ultrasonic Evaluation of Dental Implant Stability." Their extensive studies demonstrate ultrasound could provide quantitative implant stability evaluation. We thank Drs. Moore and Jokerst for their chapter on "Photoacoustic Ultrasound for Enhanced Contrast in Dental and Periodontal Imaging." Dental soft tissue structures are especially attractive for photoacoustics due to their superficial nature and thus the ability to potentially deliver sufficient light in situ. In addition to dermatology and ophthalmology, dentistry might be the third promising healthcare application for photoacoustics.

We would like to take this opportunity to appreciate our research group members, including Dr. Shayan Barootchi, Dr. Ali Bushahri, Dr. Nikhila Goli, Mr. Luis Hernandez, Dr. Xiangbo Kong, Mr. Eric Larson, Dr. Jad Majzoub, Mr. Preston Pan, Dr. Khaled Sinjab, Dr. Fabiana Soki, Dr. Mustafa Tattan, Dr. Lorenzo Tavelli, and Mr. James Wishart, for their efforts toward dental ultrasound research. The leadership, faculty, and staff at the University of Michigan School of Dentistry and Medical School have provided a rich environment and resources, allowing us to generate fundamental research results that made the production of this in-depth book possible. Dr. Jonathan Rubin deserves our gratitude for his clinical and scientific insight in ultrasonic imaging in general and blood flow and elasticity imaging in particular. Dr. J. Brian Fowlkes has been a great mentor and an endless supporter of our research endeavor. From the dental side, special thanks are given to Dean McCauley, the University of Michigan School of Dentistry, Dr. William

Giannobile, former Chair of the Department of Periodontics and Oral Medicine (POM), now Dean at Harvard School of Dental Medicine, Dr. Hom-Lay Wang, the Graduate Periodontal Program Director, Dr. Tae-Ju Oh, Dr. Robert Eber, and Dr. Jeffery Johnston for their mentorship and guidance. Mrs. Alicia Baker, Graduate Periodontal Clinics Coordinator, Mrs. Cynthia Miller, Dental Assistant Senior, Mrs. Veronica Slayton, and all staff have meticulously ensured a seamless clinical workflow. Mrs. Alice Ou, our clinical research coordinator, diligently contacted and scheduled patients and volunteers for human subject studies and always gracefully managed complicated work schedules of the participating investigators. Dr. Kimberly Ives deserves our gratitude for supporting our preclinical studies with her veterinary skills and decades of preclinical experience. From grant writing, to study approvals, to manuscript writing, Kim has always been *the* go-to colleague due to not only her wealth of knowledge but also her positive spirit. Mr. Patrick Lagua and Mrs. Jeanni Goormastic, our grant managers, have been of tremendous help in managing our grants.

We would like to thank Dr. Mitra Aliabouzar and Dr. Donald MacQueen for help with editing. It is impossible to write a book and read it as an independent. We appreciate both Mitra's content review as well as Donald's professional language editing.

Grants and funding that financially support our research have been graciously provided by the following organizations: the National Institutes of Health (NIH), the Michigan Institute for Clinical and Health Research (MICHR), the Delta Dental Foundation, the Osteology Foundation, the School of Dentistry Research Collaborative Sciences Award, the POM Clinical Research Supplementary Grant, the Kuwait Foundation for Advancement of Sciences, the American Academy of Periodontology Sunstar Research Grant, and BRS Award for Interim Support and New Initiative Proposals.

Last but not least, we would like to thank our families, Naki Kripfgans, Sophie Kripfgans, Alexander Kripfgans, Chu-Chun (June) Hsiao, and Claire Chan, for the time away from them for the writing and the editing of the chapters and assembling the final book.

Ann Arbor, MI, USA   Hsun-Liang (Albert) Chan
Ann Arbor, MI, USA   Oliver D. Kripfgans
March 2020

Contents

Acronyms and Definitions

1D, 2D, ...	One-dimensional, two-dimensional, and so on
AAOMR	American Academy of Oral and Maxillofacial Radiology
AAP	American Academy of Periodontology
ABC	Alveolar bone crest
ABS	Acrylonitrile butadiene styrene
AC	Angle correction
AGD	Auxiliary geometric device
AIUM	American Institute of Ultrasound in Medicine
ALARA	As low as reasonably achievable
ANOVA	Analysis of variance
AR-PAM	Acoustic-resolution photoacoustic microscopy
B-mode	Ultrasound scanner imaging mode showing anatomical structure encoded in 2D grayscale images. The brightness of each pixel represents the amount of ultrasound reflected or scattered from the corresponding anatomical location
BIC	Bone–implant contact
BII	Bone–implant interface
BL	Bone level, sometimes also bone loss
BOP	Bleeding on probing
bpm	Beats per minute
BT	Bone thickness
C-scan	Cross plane scan, i.e. both dimensions of the image plane are parallel to the aperture
CAD	Computer-aided design
CAL	Computer-assisted localization
CAM	Computer-aided manufacturing
CB	CEREC Bluecam
CBCT	Cone-beam computed tomography
CBT	Crestal bone thickness
CBW	Crestal bone width
CEJ	Cemento-enamel junction
CGIP	Computer-guided implant placement
CGS	Computer-guided surgery
CI	Confidence interval

CNV2	Maxillary nerve, i.e. the second branch of the trigeminal nerve
Color flow	Ultrasound scanner imaging mode showing blood flow as color pixels overlaid to the B-mode image. The color pixels represent mean blood velocity within each pixel and its flow direction
CS	Carestream
CST	Crestal soft tissue
CT	Computed tomography
dB	Decibel, logarithmic unit to measure amplitudes and intensities of sound for example
DICOM	Digital imaging and communications in medicine data
DLP	Digital light processing
DPT	Panoramic radiograph
EFP	European Federation of Periodontology
f#	f-number
FM	Facial mucosa
FST	Facial soft tissue
FDA	Food and Drug Administration of the United States of America
FDM	Fused deposition modeling
FDP	Fixed dental prosthesis
FDTD	Finite-difference time-domain
FOV	Field of view
GBR	Guided bone regeneration
GM	Gingival margin
GPC	Greater palatine canal
GPF	Greater palatine foramen
HU	Hounds field units
IA	Implant abutment angle
IAC	Inferior alveolar canal
IAN	Inferior alveolar nerve
IOS	Intraoral scanning devices
ISQ	Implant stability quotient
kHz	Unit of frequency, 1 thousand oscillations per second
M-mode	Ultrasound scanner imaging mode showing moving anatomical structure
MAR	Metal artifact reduction
MB	Mature bone
MBL	Mesial bone level
MHz	Unit of frequency, 1 million oscillations per second
MM	Mylohyoid muscle
MRI	Magnetic resonance imaging
MSK	Musculoskeletal [medicine]
MSCT	Multi-slice computed tomography

MT	Mucosal thickness
MU	Muscle
NB	Newly formed bone
NIR	Near-infrared
NMR	Nuclear magnetic resonance
OB/GYN	Obstetrics/gynecology
OPG	Panoramic radiograph
OPT	Panoramic radiograph
OR-PAM	Optical-resolution photoacoustic microscopy
PCF	pounds per cubic foot, lb/ft^3
PD	Probing depth
Pulsed wave Doppler	Ultrasound scanner imaging mode showing blood flow within a region of interest of the B-mode image. Pulsed wave Doppler information is displayed in a secondary part of the screen and shows spectral flow information as a function of time
PL	Periodontal ligament
PLA	Polylactic acid
PLY	Polygon file format or the Stanford triangle format
PM	Palatal mucosa
PRF	Pulse repetition frequency
PST	Palatal soft tissue
QUS	Quantitative ultrasound, i.e. ultrasonic imaging with derived quantitative measures
RFA	Resonance frequency analysis
ROI	Region of interest
S-mode	Tomographic imaging mode, where contrast is determined by the spectral slope
SLA	Stereolithography
SLS	Selective laser sintering
Sound	Mechanical wave traveling in a medium such as water or biological tissues
STH	Soft tissue height
STL	Stereolithography, it also includes backronyms such as *Standard Triangle Language* and *Standard Tessellation Language*
STT	Soft tissue thickness
TSBC	Tricalcium silicate-based cement
UI	Ultrasonic indicator
Ultrasound	Sound wave beyond 20 kHz
UTV	Ultrasound transmission velocity, a methodology for determining the speed of sound in a material
VAS	Visual analogue scale
WF	Wall filter, used to suppress soft tissue motion in Doppler imaging
X-ray	Radiograph

Ultrasonic Imaging: Physics and Mechanism

1

Oliver D. Kripfgans and Hsun-Liang (Albert) Chan

1.1 Introduction

Ultrasound is a physical phenomenon with widespread use, including non-destructive testing and evaluation [1–3], cleaning [4], imaging [6–9], and therapy [10–18]. Medical ultrasound ranges from audio feedback only [19, 20] to 4D image sequences [21, 22] and comprises a multitude of specializations depending on the individual objectives. This section presents a brief overview of the mechanism of ultrasound. It explains how ultrasound is generated and what governs the propagation of ultrasound. The chapter also discusses ultrasonic exposure, i.e. the quantification of ultrasound with respect to safety and FDA regulations [21, 22]. Section 1.3 addresses ultrasonic imaging. This is the controlled transmission and reception of ultrasound in order to create diagnostic images. The concept of transducer arrays is introduced. Beamforming is explained with examples of steering and focusing of ultrasound beams. Spatial resolution is introduced and set in relation to physical quantities such as frequency, image depth, and aperture size. Penetration depth is explained and also placed in relation to user-controlled parameters such as transmit frequency. A number of basic and advanced imaging modes are introduced, and examples are provided. These include imaging anatomy and function. The latter is concerned with blood flow imaging in soft tissues. Advanced examples include harmonic imaging. While this mode was introduced for cardiac and liver imaging, it proves to be quite useful in dental imaging as

O. D. Kripfgans (✉)
Department of Radiology, Medical School, University of Michigan, Ann Arbor, MI, USA
e-mail: greentom@umich.edu

H.-L. (Albert) Chan
Department of Periodontics and Oral Medicine, School of Dentistry, University of Michigan, Ann Arbor, MI, USA
e-mail: hlchan@umich.edu

© Springer Nature Switzerland AG 2021
H.-L. (Albert) Chan, O. D. Kripfgans (eds.), *Dental Ultrasound in Periodontology and Implantology*, https://doi.org/10.1007/978-3-030-51288-0_1

beam clutter is also seen when imaging the interdental papilla. The reader will also become acquainted with ultrasound scanner displays and ultrasound phantoms used to assess the performance of ultrasound systems and transducers. Section 1.4 closes this chapter with a discussion of imaging artifacts. These are important to know and recognize as ultrasound images frequently evince them. Real-time imaging allows the user to modify machine settings or transducer placement to avoid or minimize these artifacts.

1.2   Physics of Ultrasound

1.2.1   Generation of Ultrasound

A series of excellent textbooks positioned along a spectrum between solely physics and solely clinical are available [6, 9, 23–29].

This chapter is therefore meant as an abbreviated introduction to prepare the reader for the subsequent chapters of this book. The reader seeking an in-depth textbook on diagnostic ultrasound is referred to listed textbooks.

Sound is a mechanical wave and relies on the interaction of mechanical forces. In a loudspeaker, the speaker cone is pulsing in and out of the basket, mechanically driven by a coil. This coil in turn is driven by a magnet and the magnet by an electrical current. The entire system is thus converting electrical power into mechanical power and therefore electrical information into mechanical information. Again, in terms of audible sound, such as music from a radio, the electrical information of the music is converted into mechanical information, i.e. the sound. Ultrasound is exactly the same concept but at a frequency that is beyond the range audible to the human ear. This threshold is at 20 kHz. While some animals can hear and produce sound beyond 20 kHz, humans cannot. Current medical ultrasound for imaging is typically at even higher frequency, ranging approximately from 1 to 100 MHz. Figure 1.1 illustrates the concept of sound and ultrasound generation. Piezo crystals or similar materials are used to produce ultrasound. When a disc made from a piezo material is exposed to an electric potential, i.e. voltage, then the disc will either contract or expand in the direction of the voltage potential. In Fig. 1.1 this is illustrated on the right side by three scenarios. For negative voltage the crystal expands, for positive voltage the crystal contracts. In both cases, sound and ultrasound, loudspeaker and piezo crystal, an accelerated motion is required to produce (ultra-)sound. Were the loudspeaker cone or piezo-crystal to move linearly, no sound would be emitted. Figure 1.2 illustrates whether a moving surface can produce sound or not. In particular, four motion types are shown, i.e. two linear motions and two accelerated motions. Linear motion (panels a and c) does not produce a sound wave; accelerated motion (panels e and g), here a sinusoidal motion, does produce a sound wave. In medical ultrasound the displacement is typically a modulated sinusoidal function similar to rows four and five (panels e and f). Mathematically this can also be recognized by the wave equation. It describes how temporal changes in sound pressure p (left side of Eq. (1.1)) travel in space

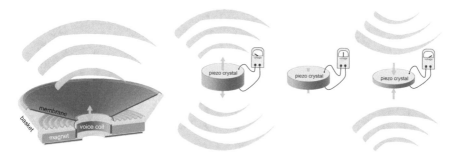

Fig. 1.1 Mechanics of generating sound and ultrasound. Left: Schematic of a loudspeaker illustrating how an electrical signal excites the magnet which then moves the cone to produce a (mechanical) sound wave. Right: Ultrasound can be generated by using a piezo crystal, whose thickness expands and contracts when exposed to negative or positive voltage, respectively (as indicated by the voltmeter)

(x) with sound speed c. A linear change has a zero second derivative and there is therefore no traveling pressure wave. Note that Eq. (1.1) is the most simplistic description of an ultrasound wave, it does not account for attenuation (absorption and scattering) nor diffraction or nonlinear effects.

$$\frac{\partial^2 p}{\partial t^2} = c^2 \frac{\partial^2 p}{\partial x^2} \tag{1.1}$$

The most common material to convert an electric signal into an acoustic wave is a piezoelectric crystal. Specialized piezoelectric composite materials have been developed from piezoelectric crystals to accommodate the unique needs of medical imaging, including efficiency and sensitivity of electrical-to-acoustic conversion. Figure 1.3 shows the composition of a typical ultrasound transducer. The expression *transducer* emphasizes the conversion of energy from one mode to another, i.e. here from electrical to mechanical. An incoming electrical signal causes the piezoelectric element to change its thickness and thus generate an acoustic wave, which then emerges on the front and back sides of the element. To eliminate the unwanted backside wave, an acoustic absorber is included in the housing. In addition, a backing block is placed on the rear side of the element. It is used to dampen the temporal extent of the piezo oscillation and dampen waves emerging from the back side of the crystal. Without this block, the piezo would continue to vibrate even after the electrical signal ceased and waves emerging from the rear of the crystal could ultimately interfere with the forward-traveling wave as well as received waves.

Piezoelectric materials differ significantly from human tissue in their mechanical/elastic composition. This difference causes acoustic waves to be reflected from human skin unless a *matching layer* is used. The matching layer is engineered to maximize the amount of acoustic energy that enters the human body when placed onto skin. Similarly audible waves traveling in air are reflected from rigid walls. In addition to the matching layer, there is a fixed-focus mechanical lens to focus

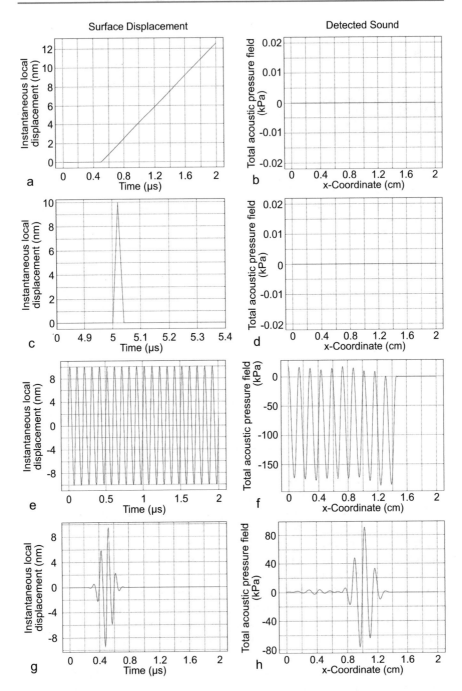

Fig. 1.2 Generation of sound and ultrasound. Left: Displacement of the sound-producing surface. Ordinate (x-axis) time in seconds, abscissa (y-axis) displacement in meters. Right: Resulting sound pressure. Ordinate space in centimeters, abscissa sound pressure in Pascals. First row: Linear

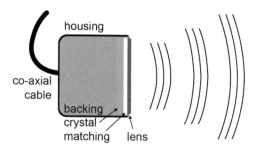

Fig. 1.3 Schematic overview of an ultrasound transducer. The piezoelectric crystal (element) generates a sound wave when driven by an alternating electric signal. It is encased by a matching layer in the front and a backing layer in the back. When placed in contact with human skin, sound travels through the matching layer into the soft tissue. Sound also travels through the backing block but is removed by the adjacent acoustic absorber

the generated sound at a specific distance from the transducer. Depending on the clinical use, a smaller or larger focal distance is desired. Vascular imaging typically demands a shallower focus than abdominal imaging, for example.

1.2.2 Propagation of Ultrasound

Ultrasound requires a medium to travel in. Medical ultrasound typically requires a medium similar to water. Human soft tissue has mechanical properties that are similar to water. Table 1.1 shows mechanical parameters significant for the propagation of an ultrasonic wave.

1.2.2.1 Speed of Sound
Speed of sound, as the name suggests, is the speed at which sound travels in the respective medium. Human soft tissue has a sound speed of approximately 1540 m/s; thus sound travels approximately 1.54 millimeters per microsecond. Ultrasonic imaging relies on timing. First the transducer emits an ultrasound wave (see Fig. 1.4) at which time a stopwatch is started. Any returning sound waves, i.e. those scattered by tissue structures or reflected from tissue boundaries, are recorded as a signal pair consisting of time and amplitude. The amplitude is a measure of how strong the scattering or reflecting structure is, and is depicted in the ultrasound

←

Fig. 1.2 (continued) displacement (monodirectional) of the surface after 0.5 μs, without resulting sound wave, since the displacement is linear. Second row: Also linear displacement (bidirectional), also without resulting sound wave. Third row, sinusoidal displacement with resulting sinusoidal pressure in the field. The field snapshot was taken after 10 μs, by which time the pressure wave had not yet arrived at the 1.5 cm x-coordinate. More about this effect is in Sect. 1.3.1. Fourth row, truncated sinusoidal pulse, also results in a truncated sinusoidal pressure wave. All data were produced by a one-dimensional finite element analysis using COMSOL Multiphysics™

Table 1.1 Acoustic properties relevant to the propagation of ultrasonic waves

Material	Speed of sound c [m/s]	Mass density ρ [kg/m^3]	Characteristic impedance Z [MRayl]	Attenuation coefficient a [dB/MHz^b/cm]	b
Water	1489	1000	1.489	0.0021	2
Air	340	1	0.00034	40.5	2
Skin	1720	1093–1190	1.88–2.05	3.5 ± 1.2	–
Fat (subcutaneous)	1476	916	1.35	0.6	–
Muscle cardiac	1589–1603	1038–1056	1.65–1.69	0.24	1.04
Bone (cortical)	3850–4040	1990	7.66–8.04	4.34	–
Blood (whole)	1560	1060	1.65	0.12–0.16	1.19–1.23
Liver	1587	1050–1070	1.67–1.70	0.4	–
Gum	1540	1071	1.65	–	–
Tooth, cementum	3200	2090–2240	6.69–7.17	11.1	–
Tooth, dentine	4000	2030–2350	8.12–9.40	4.44	–

Note: Characteristic impedance is computed from c and ρ here [6, 30–36]

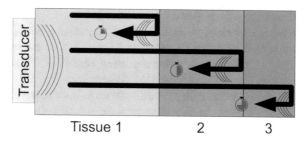

Fig. 1.4 Ultrasonic imaging relies on knowing the sound speed in the tissues imaged. Spatial information is derived from timing data. Received ultrasound signals are recorded as pairs of time and amplitude. By combining time and sound speed, the distance to the scattering or reflecting structure is computed and the recorded amplitude is displayed at that distance as a shade of gray. This is a simplified method by which an ultrasound image is generated

image by a gray scale. Light gray is a strong signal and dark gray is a weak signal. Time is used to determine where the reflection or scattering originated from and is computed as

$$s = c \cdot t \tag{1.2}$$

where s is the distance to the reflection or scattering structure, c is the speed of sound, and t is the elapsed time between the original transmission and when the signal was recorded. A structure at 1 cm depth is recorded at 20 mm divided by 1.54 mm/µs, i.e. 13 µs. Since the sound has to travel to a depth of 1 cm, i.e. 10 mm, and return as well, the distance has to be doubled. Forgetting to double the travel path is a common mistake.

1.2.2.2 Acoustic Impedance

The product of speed of sound c and mass density ρ defines the characteristic acoustic impedance Z of a medium (Eq. 1.3). When ultrasound travels from medium 1 into medium 2 a certain fraction of sound pressure is reflected at the interface. This sound pressure fraction R is directly proportional to the difference in acoustic impedance between the two media and is defined in Eq. (1.3). The transmitted sound pressure fraction T is defined in relation to impedances Z_1 and Z_2 as well as R.

$$Z = c \cdot \rho$$

$$R = \frac{Z_2 - Z_1}{Z_2 + Z_1}$$

$$T = \frac{2Z_2}{Z_2 + Z_1} \tag{1.3}$$

$$T = 1 + R$$

Given Eq. (1.3) and acoustic properties from Table 1.1, sound propagating through soft tissue is reflected by bone at 60%. In addition, sound entering the bone will also be reflected at 60% when propagating back into soft tissue. Bone is therefore difficult to image in the frequency range discussed here (1–100 MHz). Dentine is comparable to cortical bone and reflects 66%. Sound propagation is inhibited when traveling between media with significant differences in their characteristic acoustic impedances. Small changes in the characteristic acoustic impedance between soft tissues, such as skin, fat, muscle, liver, and gum, result in small reflection coefficients and thus allow for excellent propagation.

1.2.2.3 Acoustic Attenuation

Acoustic waves are also diminished when traveling within a single medium. Acoustic absorption and scattering contribute to the acoustic amplitude attenuation coefficient α which is shown in Eq. (1.4). An acoustic wave with initial intensity I_0 is attenuated by $e^{-\alpha x}$ after traveling x centimeters within a medium with attenuation coefficient α. This is known as the Lambert–Beer Law. As the intensity diminishes exponentially, the attenuation coefficient is often provided in logarithmic units of decibel (dB).

$$I(x) = I_0 e^{-\alpha x} \tag{1.4}$$

The attenuation coefficient α is measured by comparing sound pressures or intensities before and after traveling inside the investigated medium. The natural computation of the attenuation coefficient is done by solving Eq. (1.4) for α. This leads to

$$\alpha_{Np} = \ln\left(\frac{I_0}{I(x)}\right) \tag{1.5}$$

The units of α_{Np} are called Neper, hence the subscript of Np. The relation of Neper to the above-mentioned unit of decibels, i.e. dB, is $8.686 = 20 \times \log_{10}(e^1)$. The definition of α in units of decibels and the relation of acoustic pressure amplitudes p to acoustic intensities $I \propto p_{rms}^2$ lead to therefore:

$$\alpha_{dB} = 10 \; \log_{10}\left(\frac{I_0}{I(x)}\right)$$
$$\tag{1.6}$$
$$\alpha_{dB} = 20 \; \log_{10}\left(\frac{A_0}{A(x)}\right)$$

Acoustic waves with higher frequencies are more attenuated than those with lower frequencies. A general description of the relationship between acoustic attenuation and frequency is given by Eq. (1.7). For a linear dependence of α to f, $b = 1$ and a

equals the constant acoustic attenuation defined above. In biological tissues b varies between 1 and 1.3 [30].

$$\alpha(f) = a \times f^b \qquad (1.7)$$

As imaging frequencies range from 1 to 100 MHz, resulting attenuation can therefore vary significantly. A 10 MHz ultrasound wave traveling 1 cm through muscle loses 99.6% of its amplitude due to attenuation. Approximately 1/5 of the attenuation is due to scattering, which is the signal used for imaging. Ultrasound scanners have a wide dynamic range to accommodate the reception of weak signals. Current electronics and signal processing allows for a 120 dB dynamic range and corresponds to 1:1,000,000, i.e. received signals can range from 1 V to 1 μV.

1.2.3 Ultrasonic Exposure

Currently the FDA regulates two bioeffects of medical ultrasound [23, 24], namely cavitation effects and thermal effects. Those unfamiliar with cavitation may have seen pictures or video clips of ship propellers in water as they rapidly increase their rotating speed. Clouds of gas bubbles emerge around the propeller blades. They are produced by the blade surfaces that move away from the water. When the propeller turns, one side of each blade turns into the water, i.e. pushes the water in front of it away and the opposite side of the blade moves away from the water. That side is where the gas bubbles are created. When this side of the blade moves away from the water facing it, it creates a significant underpressure, as water tries to rush into the space that the blade leaves from. Figure 1.5 shows the generation of gas bubbles by a moving propeller as well as the resulting effects on the steel surface of the blades. While the forces in this example are much greater than those expected from diagnostic ultrasound, the underlying mechanism and the resulting effects are the same. The FDA regulates the mechanical and the thermal indices, i.e. the MI and TI, respectively. The MI is a measure for the likelihood of cavitation and is defined as the ratio of the acoustic wave peak negative pressure measured in MPa, divided by the square root of the center frequency of the acoustic wave (Eq. 1.8). An acoustic wave produces positive and negative pressures relative to the ambient static pressure. Figure 1.2, panel h, shows a pressure waveform similar to those from an ultrasound scanner. Its peak negative pressure is almost −80 kPa, whereas its peak positive pressure is 90 kPa. High-intensity waves show a larger amplitude discrepancy between the positive and negative pressures and the negative pressure causes cavitation, not the positive pressure. Per the FDA, the maximum safe MI in the absence of gas bodies in the field of view is 1.9. Examples of in situ gas bodies are gas pockets in the lung and in the intestine as well as any administered ultrasound contrast agent, which consists of microscopic gas bubbles. Ultrasound can also cause thermal effects, hence the TI. As mentioned above, acoustic attenuation is divided into scattering and absorption. The latter converts acoustic energy into heat. When same body part is scanned for a long time at highly repetitive acoustic

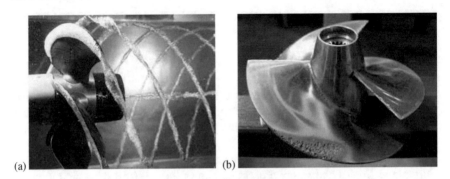

(a)   (b)

Fig. 1.5 Ship propellers are a classic example for cavitation. An example is shown in panel (**a**). The consequences of this effect are severe damage to the propeller blade as shown in panel (**b**). When cavitation bubbles collapse on the surface of the blade, they pinch the metal, and over time a substantial amount of the material is removed. In vivo, cavitation can destroy cells and can generate free radicals. That is why the FDA regulates acoustic output of ultrasound scanners to avoid unwanted cavitation in vivo. Copyright Wikimedia Commons (web pages: https://images. app.goo.gl/wRsXxYRKS3N7aLok8; https://images.app.goo.gl/iqxV5aJrzhmEtxup6)

pulses, the temperature of that region will rise. A TI of 1 corresponds to the amount of energy W_p that raises the local temperature by $1\,°C$ (web page, 2019: https://webstore.ansi.org/standards/nema/nemaud2004r20091358693).

$$MI = \frac{p^- \,[\text{MPa}]}{\sqrt{f}\,[\text{MHz}]}$$

$$TI = \frac{W_p\,[\text{Nm/s}]}{W_{1\,°C}\,[\text{Nm/s}]}$$

(1.8)

Safe use of ultrasound follows the ALARA (As Low As Reasonably Achievable) principle (web page, 2019: https://www.aium.org/officialStatements/39), which states that [ultrasound scanner] controls for acoustic output should be adjusted and transducer dwell times are minimized to reduce the risk of biological effects.

1.3 Imaging

1.3.1 The Concept of Beamforming

Ultrasonic images are generated by a technique called beamforming. As the name suggests, acoustic beams are generated, and images are created from these beams. This is not done by single piezoelectric elements but rather an array of these elements. The goal is to create images with large fields of view and sufficient spatial resolution depending on their ultimate clinical use. Beamforming is typically done for transmitting and for receiving a wave. Exceptions are discussed below.

1.3.1.1 Transducer Arrays

Imaging a two-dimensional region requires a one-dimensional ultrasound array of piezoelectric elements. A single piezoelectric element would only be able to determine the axial distance to the imaged object. By using a one-dimensional ultrasound array (1D array) geometric triangulation allows for differentiating objects in the lateral direction. This is achieved by steering and focusing the ultrasound beam in a desired direction and recording reflected and scattered signals. Transmitting and receiving ultrasonic signals is a symmetric process, i.e. the beamforming is equal, at least conceptually.

Transmit Beamforming Figure 1.6 shows simulations of transmitted ultrasound from an array of 16 elements. Four cases are shown. In the first case all elements are delayed by the same amount (panel (a)). The blue-colored sinusoidal signal symbolizes the electrical excitation of each piezoelectric array element (termed channel on the ordinate). The result is a planar wave front as seen in panel (b). Each array element emits a spherical wave (blue circles). The superposition of these spherical waves results in the planar wave front at 2 mm axial depth. In fact panel (a) shows the travel time needed for the wave front to reach the axial depth of 2 mm, i.e. 1.3 μs, since ultrasound travels 1.54 millimeters per microsecond. For steering the planar wave front off-axis, a linear increasing delay must be added when exciting the array elements (panel (c)). An approximately 1 μs difference between the first and last element causes a 15° steered wave front. Focusing of the wave requires a complex delay that is approximately parabolic (panel (e)). The case shown focuses the wave at 2 mm axially, 0 mm laterally. When steering the beam also laterally, here to approximately 4.5 mm, an additional linear delay must be added (panel (g)).

Receive Beamforming When in receive mode, the ultrasound array records time-amplitude signal pairs for each element and stores this information for receive beamforming. If a strong reflection or scattered signal were to originate from an axial depth of 2 mm and lateral position of approximately 4.5 mm, then the recorded time-amplitude signal pairs would show strong amplitudes at specific times for each array element. These times are exactly the same as when focusing a transmit beam to the same location, which means that the specific times are the same as those shown in the bottom left graph of Fig. 1.6. Ultrasonic receive beamforming is therefore also called delay-and-sum beamforming.

1.3.1.2 Array Types

Ultrasound arrays are the acoustics analog to radio antennas. They transmit and receive (acoustic) waves and have specific design features. There are four common basic array types used in ultrasonic beamforming (see Fig. 1.7). A linear array is an assembly of typically 128 elements in one row spaced at the wavelength λ in the target medium, i.e. soft tissue. For a 10 MHz array and an average soft tissue speed of sound of 1540 m/s, the wavelength is 154 μm and thus a 128-element array is approximately 2 cm wide. To prevent mechanical cross-talk

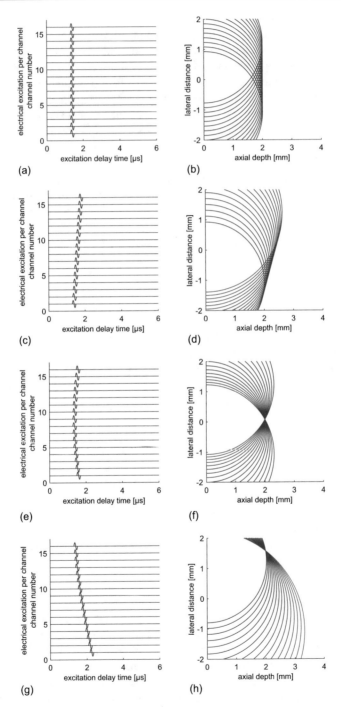

Fig. 1.6 Simulation of delayed transmission from a linear array of 16 elements. The left side graphs show the delay time in microseconds for each element. Simultaneous excitation of all

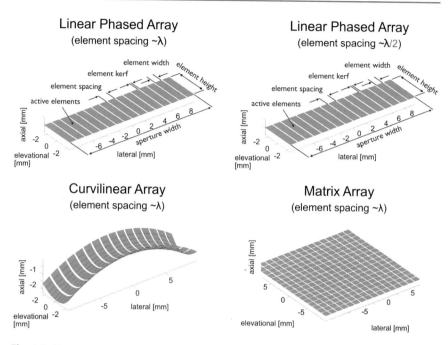

Fig. 1.7 From a beamforming point of view, there are four types of imaging arrays. The most common is the linear array (top left), whose elements are spaced at the wavelength λ. Element width equals the element spacing minus a trench between adjacent elements, termed kerf. Element height is multiples of the element width. Apertures are typically 128 or 192 elements wide and have a lens mounted in front of them to focus the beam in the elevational direction. This lens effect is illustrated in the bottom left panel (exaggerated curvature). For a larger field of view the array elements can be mounted in an arc shape in the lateral direction (bottom left panel). A phased array (top right) has all the features of a linear array, except that its elements are spaced by λ/2 ("2" intentionally in red). This feature allows for ±90° beam steering in lateral direction, whereas linear arrays can only steer ±20°. Vector arrays (2D array, matrix array, bottom right) can steer beams in the axial and lateral directions and thus image a 3D volume. These arrays are expensive and require significantly more resources due to the large number of elements (2000–15,000). All graphics produced using Field II [5]

between adjacent elements a gap is placed between them, termed kerf. Element kerf may be approximately 10% of the element spacing. The emitted acoustic power is proportional to the radiating surface area. To achieve sufficient acoustic power the element height is therefore typically a multiple of the element width and a 10 MHz element may be several millimeters tall. While lateral focusing is achieved

---

Fig. 1.6 (continued) elements results in a planar wave front (panels (**a**) and (**b**)). Adding a linear delay between elements (panels (**c**) and (**d**)) results in a planar wave front that is steered. Focusing is achieved by delaying the excitation in an approximately parabolic fashion (panels (**e**) and (**f**)). To focus off-axis, a linear delay is added to the focus delays (panels (**g**) and (**h**))

by phase or excitation delays of the array elements, elevational focusing for a one-dimensional array relies on a fixed focus placed on top of the array elements. The focus of this lens depends on the intended application of the ultrasound probe. A small parts or peripheral vascular application benefits from a shallow focus (~2–3 cm) and an abdominal or OB/Gyn application from a more distal focus (~10–15 cm).

Curvilinear arrays are used in applications that require a large lateral field of view and provide a large acoustic window, i.e. allow for using a large aperture. The radius of curvature in the lateral direction depends on the lateral width of the aperture and is generally of the same order. For example, a 3 MHz abdominal probe (510 µm wavelength) would be 65 mm wide and thus have a 65 mm radius of curvature. The above 10 MHz could have a much tighter 20 mm radius of curvature. Both arrays, linear and curvilinear, use variable fractions of the aperture, i.e. not all elements are always in use. Which elements are used depends on the imaging depth.

Phased arrays have all the features of linear arrays, except that the element spacing is only half the wavelength, i.e. $\lambda/2$. While a linear array can only steer $\pm 20°$ in the lateral direction, a phased array can steer $\pm 90°$, i.e. in the entire 2D image plane. This feature makes the phase array attractive for applications with small acoustic windows. Examples include liver and cardiac imaging, where the acoustic access is limited by the rib cage. Phased arrays always use the entire aperture, i.e. all elements.

Vector arrays have independent elements in the lateral and elevational directions, which requires up to 128×128, i.e. 16,384 elements. Economically and technically this was a major barrier, if not prohibitive. While achieving a true two-dimensional array has the said barriers, arrays of various dimensions (D) have been developed. Table 1.2 lists fractional dimension arrays with their features and characteristics. A 1.25D array is essentially an array with an electronically adjustable aperture, which changes the elevational beam shape. Instead of one row of elements, there are 3, 5, or 7 rows. For a given application, these rows can be enabled or disabled. Typically more rows are enabled when imaging deeper and are symmetric to the main (middle) row. A 1.5D array consists of a limited number of elevational elements that can be individually amplitude-controlled but not delayed; thus elevational focusing can

Table 1.2 Features and characteristics of multidimensional ultrasonic arrays

Dimension (D)	Feature	Characteristics
1D	One row of elements	Classic linear or phased array
1.25D	Additional rows of elements (symmetric to main row)	Change elevational aperture size. No electronic elevational focusing or steering
1.5D	Limited 2D set of elements	Elevational electronic focusing, not steering
1.75D	No. of elevational elements ≪ no. of lateral elements	Elevational electronic focusing, limited steering
2D	No. of elevational elements ~ no. of lateral elements	Full elevational electronic focusing and steering

be controlled, but there is no elevational steering. A 1.75D array possesses fully independent array elements with full amplitude and delay control in the lateral and elevational directions. However, there are fewer elements in the elevational direction than in the lateral direction. It is therefore possible to freely focus the beam in the lateral and elevational directions, allowing full steering in the lateral direction and limited steering in the elevational direction. A 2D array has none of these limitations.

1.3.2 1D, 2D, 3D Imaging

Conceptually, imaging is based on recording an electrical signal with timestamps and associating spatial locations to it using the speed of sound. A zero-dimensional imaging array, i.e. 1 element only, can resolve axial positions only. Figure 1.8a illustrates this scenario. A one-dimensional imaging array (b), i.e. a row of transmit/receive elements, can in addition provide lateral information and therefore create a two-dimensional image (Fig. 1.8b). The most sophisticated is a two-dimensional imaging array (c). It can provide triangulation in all three dimensions and thus deliver image volumes. The current standard is one-dimensional arrays for

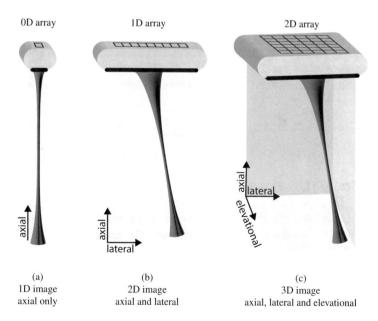

Fig. 1.8 Illustration of imaging in one or more dimensions. (**a**) A single ultrasound element can only image in 1 dimension. It can only resolve the axial (or radial) distance from the element if the speed of sound is known. (**b**) A one-dimensional array can use axial-lateral triangulation to image features in a single image plane. (**c**) A two-dimensional array can steer the ultrasound beam in lateral and elevational directions and thus image a 3D volume

two-dimensional imaging. Established, albeit very specialized, are single-element Doppler imaging devices for fetal heart rate, to be introduced and discussed later. Two-dimensional arrays exist as well and are mostly found in cardiology, though they are currently also entering the realm of abdominal imaging and other applications.

1.3.3   Resolution (Axial, Lateral, and Elevational)

Resolution is the measurement that determines what feature size can be imaged, i.e. resolved. Ultrasound beams have significant differences in their axial, lateral, and elevational resolution. The best resolution is achieved in the axial direction (Δx) and equals the product of the number of cycles in the transmit pulse (N) and the wavelength λ. Lateral resolution is proportional to the product of λ and the f-number ($f\#$). The latter is defined as the ratio of distance to the focus (F) divided by the lateral extend of the emitting aperture D_{lat}, i.e. F/D_{lat}. The elevational beam width is defined in the same way, except that the elevational aperture size must be used. A one-dimensional array has a fixed elevational aperture but a variable (electronic) lateral aperture. When imaging shallow features, only a small fraction of the aperture is active. When imaging a larger depth feature, the full aperture is active. Which part of the aperture is active is controlled by a constant $f\#$ approach. Typically an $f\#$ of 3 or 4 is used. For a focus at 2 cm depth, an aperture width of 5 mm ($f\# = 4$) is used. For a 10 MHz array ($\lambda = 154\,\mu m$), this corresponds to approximately 32 elements. Assuming a transmit wave with one cycle ($N = 1$), the axial resolution is 154 μm (Eq. 1.9). For an $f\#$ of 4, the lateral resolution is 616 μm. Assuming an elevational aperture of 2 mm yields a 1.54 mm elevational resolution.

$$\Delta x = N \cdot \lambda \qquad \Delta y = \lambda \cdot \frac{F}{D_{lat}} \qquad \Delta z = \lambda \cdot \frac{F}{D_{ele}} \qquad (1.9)$$

1.3.4   Grating Lobes and Side Lobes

Beamforming using finite arrays creates grating and side lobes. These overlap with the main beam and produce clutter. Side lobes are generated due to the finite length of the used array. The elements at the ends, i.e. the first and last array element, have only one neighbor, whereas elements 2 to second-to-last have neighbors on both sides. This creates an imbalance in the transmitted wave, termed *side lobes*. *Grating lobes* originate from spacing array elements too far apart from each other. The relationship between the direction of existing side (θ_s) and grating lobes (θ_g) is given as

$$\Theta_s = \arcsin \frac{\lambda n}{a}$$

$$(1.10)$$

$$\Theta_g = \arcsin \frac{\lambda n}{p}$$

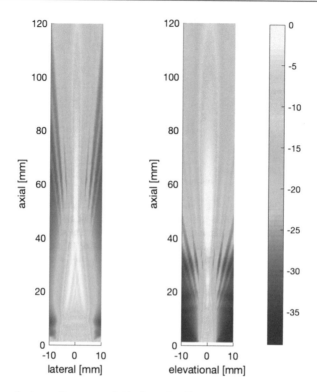

Fig. 1.9 Acoustic transmit pressure field plots of a linear array transducer (3.75 MHz center frequency). Left: Lateral-axial plane. Right: Elevational-axial plane (right). The lateral focus was set at 50 mm, whereas the elevational focus, given by the lens of the transducer, was 20 mm. The color bar shows the transmit pressure in dB relative to the maximum at 50 mm axially. Side lobes can be seen in symmetry to the main lobe. Note: The color bar is showing pressure in dB. Pressure fields computed using Field II [5]

where λ is the wavelength, n is the order of the side or grating lobe, a is the size of the aperture, and p is the pitch. Side lobes can be suppressed by driving edge elements at lower electric power. This is termed apodization. Here the aperture is driven non-uniformly using a tapering function, such as a Hamming window or other functions. Grating lobes are avoided by spacing array elements sufficiently close to each other. Linear arrays are spaced at λ and must not be steered more than approximately 20° to avoid grating lobes. Phased arrays are spaced at $\lambda/2$ and do not have a steering limitation.

An example of side lobes is shown in Figs. 1.9 and 1.10. The field of an array spaced at λ is shown, i.e. a linear array. As the beam is not steered, only side lobes are visible and no grating lobes. These could be suppressed using apodization. Techniques for such are presented in the textbook literature [6, 25, 26, 37].

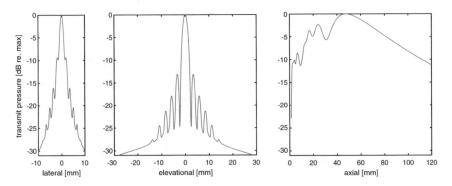

Fig. 1.10 Cross-sectional plots of the linear array transducer transmit pressure fields shown in Fig. 1.9. Left: Lateral beam profile through the axial focus. Middle: Elevational beam profile through the axial focus. Right: Axial beam profile. Maximum pressure at focus, i.e. at 47.1 mm. Pressure amplitudes are in logarithmic units, i.e. in dB, relative to the maximum in the field. Therefore all resulting pressures are negative and the maximum is zero. Acoustic pressures computed using Field II [5]

1.3.5 Penetration

Ultrasound waves attenuate as they travel. Frequency and medium dictate to what maximum depth one can image. Theoretically, a 10 MHz probe on a clinical ultrasound scanner with 120 dB dynamic range can image to a depth of 120 dB $=$ 2×0.5 dB/MHz/cm × 10 MHz × d cm, therefore $d = 12$ cm. However, many ultrasound scanners display an effective dynamic range for a given imaging application. A more realistic value would be a 70 dB dynamic range, for which the resulting image depth would be 7 cm. Even that may be too generous, but on the correct order of magnitude.

1.3.6 Ultrasonic Imaging Modes

1.3.6.1 B-Mode

Ultrasound images are commonly known as grayscale images. Formally they are called B-mode images. The letter "B" stands for brightness, which encodes the strength of the scattered or reflected wave. The example image in Fig. 1.11 was acquired using a linear array and a so-called *phantom* (CIRS Inc., model 040GSE). This is typically a container filled with a base material, either agar, some other type of gel, or rubber, and it is meant to mimic structures of the human body and concurrently allow for quality control of the ultrasound probe and system. The base material contains sub-wavelength scatterers to mimic such structures in human tissue. These produce the speckle pattern that is seen throughout the image. It is not noise, as can be easily observed, as the pattern does not change unless the probe moves. In fact, if the probe moves but returns to the same exact position, then the exact same, seemingly random, speckle pattern returns as well. The grayscale to

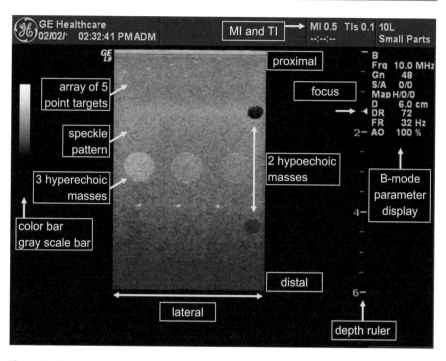

Fig. 1.11 Example of a B-mode ultrasound image, acquired using a linear array. B-mode is the most common imaging mode in ultrasound. It encodes scattering or reflecting structures in grayscale or brightness, hence B-mode. The annotations are elaborated on in the main text and in Table 1.3

physical intensity mapping is shown as the grayscale bar, commonly called a *color bar* on the left side of the image. It consists of 255 steps and can be a linear mapping or follow some kind of gamma correction or curve. Quantitative image analysis uses this information as it linearizes intensity. Several B-mode parameters are displayed on the screen. They are typically displayed in a section. Here the section starts with "B" indicating that the information relates to the B-mode. Other modes could be shown simultaneously, hence the label. Please refer to Table 1.3 for a discussion of these parameters. Most ultrasound images are shown with the probe located on the top of the image (proximal label). The field of view is 6 cm (distal label) as indicated by the depth ruler on the right. Zero centimeters is at the probe location. There is commonly no ruler for the lateral image extend. The authors know of only one exception to the probe being located on the top of the image, namely fetal echo, i.e. fetal cardiac ultrasound, where the image convention is upside down from the format shown here. It is possible that in the future manufacturers will allow for additional flexibility in image orientation. In dentistry it may be helpful, since intuitive, to position the probe on the left side of the image when obtaining a sagittal view of a tooth.

Table 1.3 Example listing of user controlled B-mode parameters on a diagnostic ultrasound scanner

Parameter	Definition
Frq	Center frequency of the transmitted beam, here 10 MHz
Gn	Receive gain the scanner applies to the acoustic echoes
S/A	Image filtering specific to this brand/model
Map	Mapping of physical wave intensities to display grayscale
D	Image depth
DR	Dynamic range, here 72 dB
FR	Frame rate, here 32 frames per second, 32 Hz
AO	Acoustic output, here 100%
MI	Mechanical index
TI	Thermal index, here for soft tissue (TIs), TIc stands for cranial bone and TIb for bone

User controllable parameters differ across scanner models and brands

While the overall ultrasound image is of lateral uniform brightness it can be observed that its axial brightness tapers off after approximately 4 cm depth. In fact there is a local enhancement across the lateral range at 1.5 cm depth. This is due to a user setting, the imaging focus. A yellow triangle can be found near the depth ruler. It indicates where the beamformer focuses the transmit beam. As can be seen in the image, the focused beam results in a brighter scatter from that depth. This is not because of the phantom but because of a stronger acoustic illumination at that depth. Not all ultrasound scanners allow the user to specify a focus location, but set it automatically. The system shown here is a GE Logiq 9 as branded on the top left side of the ultrasound image. This logo shows if the user swapped the ultrasound image left to right. Since most ultrasound probes can be held in reverse (with respect to left-right), scanners allow the user to flip the image left to right. If the image below was flipped, the logo would appear on the right.

Five types of phantom features can be observed in the ultrasound image. First the uniform background. Any broken piezoelectric elements in the ultrasound probe or broken signal channels in the ultrasound scanner could potentially produce a non-uniformity in the *lateral* direction of the image. On the very top of the image, within the first millimeter of the image is a bright line across the entire lateral width. This brightness is caused by the piezoelectric elements ringing down after their electric excitation, plus any reverberation of the launched acoustic waves within the matching layer and the elevational focus lens. The second feature is an array of five-point targets (100 μm diameter, actual nylon monofilaments oriented elevationally) at 1–5 mm away from the top end of the gel. Note that the imaging array reads approximately 2.2 mm to the first target. The difference of 1 mm may be the surface cover of the phantom. While 100 μm is not much smaller than the wavelength (here 154 μm), it is possible to measure the apparent axial and lateral extent of these filaments to obtain performance information of the ultrasound probe and scanner. While the filaments are 100 μm across, if the lateral resolution of the ultrasound beam is 600 μm (example from above), then the filaments diameter would image as 600 μm. In other words, for a known transmit frequency and focal distance, one can measure the lateral aperture size. The same holds for the axial measurement: for a known transmit frequency one can compute the number of transmit cycles in the acoustic wave.

Two hypoechoic cylinders (labeled as mass) are shown on the right side of the image. These are to evaluate clutter. Actual ultrasound beams are very complex. They not only point in the direction of the beamformer but also have side and grating lobes (discussed on Sect. 1.3.4). These extra lobes contribute to the received acoustic signal and cause hypoechoic areas to be filled to a certain degree. The top mass shows a stronger contrast to the background, i.e. is darker on the interior compared to the surrounding base material, than the lower mass that is filled with lighter gray pixels. This demonstrates that a sonographer might miss a mass or a lesion if it is filled with too much clutter signal. Three large cylinders are positioned across the image. Two of them have defined contrast compared to the background. The right two are +6 and +3 dB above background. The left cylinder is not specified. When performing quantitative image analysis these numbers can be tested for quality control. The bottom three-point targets can serve two purposes. First they are meant to calibrate the scanner for horizontal distance measurements. They are separated by 20 mm. Second, they demonstrate beam widening. While they are also 100 μm in diameter, they appear significantly wider than those closer to the aperture, indicating a larger f# since the distance to the aperture increases and the aperture size may have reached its maximum size. In addition, the center frequency of the beam may have decreased at this depth due to frequency dependent attenuation, thus increasing λ and therefore the lateral resolution.

1.3.6.2 M-Mode

A major area of use for ultrasound is cardiac imaging, as ultrasound is a real-time modality and naturally able to image moving structures. B-mode can image at frame rates of up to 100 Hz on a radiological ultrasound scanner and up to 800 Hz on some cardiac scanners. While human hearts move significantly more slowly, rodent hearts can reach 600 bpm, i.e. 10 Hz. Extra sampling speed is required to temporarily resolve valve motion. Left ventricular wall motion of a Sprague Dawley rat is shown in Fig. 1.12. The top image is a sector scan B-mode image from a phased array typically used in cardiac imaging. The yellow dotted line in the image reaches from the probe aperture to the distal end of the field of view. This line marks the spatial part of the B-mode image that feeds into the M-mode image, which is shown on the bottom part of Fig. 1.12. The vertical axis of the M-mode is space. Here this space is 2 cm, shown on the left-side depth ruler of the B-mode image and the right side depth ruler of the M-mode image. One can see that the focus is set at 1.25 cm. The horizontal axis is time. In real-time this image continuously rolls from the right to the left. Note that zero time, i.e. now, is on the right. The left end of the time axis is −1 s, i.e. there are approximately seven heart beats within one second, i.e. 420 bpm. In the M-mode image, the cardiac motion can be seen as contractions and dilations

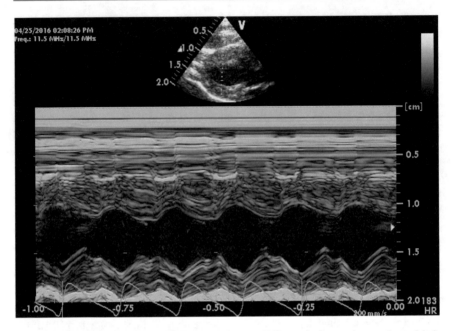

Fig. 1.12 Example of an M-mode ultrasound image. "M" stands for motion mode, and it is intended to display moving structures such as heart valves. As there are no inherent moving structures in dental imaging, its description is included as the reader may find a dental application of this mode

of the ventricle over time. The anterior and posterior walls move periodically in- and outwards.

1.3.6.3 Extended View

Linear arrays have the smallest field of view (FOV), but the highest image quality. To extend the view, it is possible to enable a virtual convex view, which adds approximately 20° to each lateral side. Above it was mentioned that a linear array can steer the beam by up to 20° without compromise due to grating lobes. Another way to extend the FOV is to modify the ultrasonic probe, i.e. mount the elements on a curved housing, which is what a curvilinear array is. An alternative to that is the phased array, which also has a large FOV. However, both are still limited in the sense that they only capture the region in front of their aperture. To further extend the FOV, the ultrasound scanner allows the user to slide the probe laterally and track the changing image with real-time image correlation. This mode is essentially analogous to the panoramic image mode for digital photography. An MSK ultrasound, i.e. musculoskeletal ultrasound, example is given in Fig. 1.13.

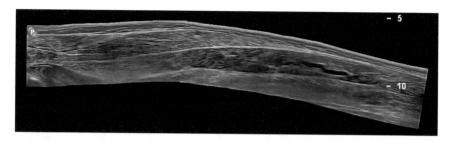

Fig. 1.13 Example of extended view of ultrasound image. This mode is analogous to the panoramic mode for digital photography. The ultrasound probe is moved laterally along the calf muscle. Following a significant curvature requires in-plane image correlation and image stitching. The scale can be derived from the depth indication on the right marking a 5 cm step

1.3.7 Blood Flow Imaging Modes

Ultrasonic blood flow imaging is based on methodologies that require the blood to be in motion. It is literally blood *flow* imaging, not imaging blood per se, but the movement of blood. In B-mode, blood appears hypoechoic, i.e. darker than the surrounding tissue. Blood consists of blood plasma and blood cells. The former does not contribute to ultrasound backscatter; the latter does.

1.3.7.1 Pulsed-Wave Doppler

Pulsed-Wave Doppler is the traditional blood flow imaging mode which is commonly known and produces real-time images as well as an audio signal. Though not conveyable in a book, the audio consists of the positive and negative velocity information of the pulsed-wave spectrum, transmitted through the left and right stereo audio speaker of the ultrasound system. Figure 1.14 shows the annotated screen interface of pulsed-wave Doppler, also known as PW Doppler, pulsed-wave, or as spectral Doppler. A B-mode image forms the central part of the display, where an additional line indicates where the spectral Doppler is obtained from. The line extends axially through the entire field of view and contains a gate with a short perpendicular line at the beginning and end of the gate. Within that gate the line is interrupted. Here is where the Doppler information is obtained. As shown in the example image, this part of the line should be positioned over the artery, vein, or as here, the lumen of the flow phantom. The length of the gate can be adjusted. Its current length is 8 mm and is shown as "SV" in the PW parameters section (see Fig. 1.14 and Table 1.4) towards the right of the PW section of the screen.

The PW display is similar to the M-mode display as it contains a horizontal time axis with zero on the right-hand side. Velocity is shown on the vertical axis, which is, in this example, shifted and inverted. The maximum is approximately −30 cm/s and the minimum +10 cm/s. Flow away from the transducer is shown as a positive velocity. A user control allows the axis to be flipped and negative velocities to be on the top. In addition, only negative velocities are present; for such, the baseline on the display can be shifted to use a larger range for negative velocities and a shorter

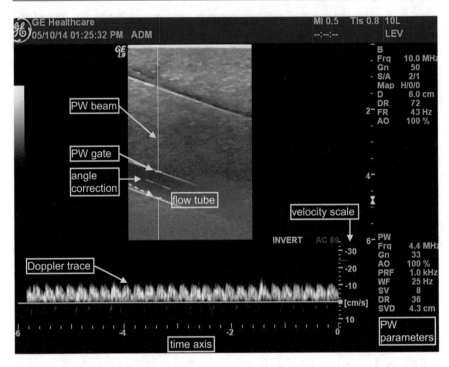

Fig. 1.14 Example of pulsed-wave (PW) Doppler imaging. PW-mode is used to display blood flow within a range gate as a function of time. The range gate is positioned within the accompanying live B-mode image. Annotations are elaborated on in the main text and in Table 1.4

Table 1.4 Example listing of user controlled PW-mode parameters on a diagnostic ultrasound scanner

Parameter	Definition
Frq	Center frequency of the transmitted beam, here 4.4 MHz
Gn	Receive gain the scanner applies to the acoustic echoes
AO	Acoustic output, here 100%
PRF	Pulse repetition frequency, here 1 kHz
WF	Wall filter, 25 Hz
SV	Sample volume, i.e. the length of the Doppler gate
DR	Dynamic range, here 36 dB
SVD	Sample volume depth, here 4.3 cm

User controllable parameters differ across scanner models and brands

range for positive ones. The Doppler equation governing the obtained velocities is

$$\Delta f = 2 \cdot f_0 \cdot \frac{v}{c} \cdot \cos(\alpha) \tag{1.11}$$

where Δf is the Doppler frequency shift for a transmitted wave with center frequency f_0 in a medium of speed of sound c, imaging an object moving with velocity v along a path with angle α with respect to the Doppler beam. The factor 2 is due to the fact that the scatterer is moving; hence it sees a Doppler shifted incoming wave and also becomes a moving source as it scatters the ultrasound. The angle α is shown as the dashed line on the center of the Doppler gate and its numerical value is shown as "AC" (angle correction) on the top right of the Doppler spectrum. In the example a 69° angle correction was dialed in. Angles that are too large (>60°) produce beam artifacts that yield unreliable velocity information. For such angles the AC is displayed in red color, as in this example. For those cases the user should reposition the ultrasound probe to find a better acoustic path with a shallower angle. Changes in the AC will directly change the labels on the velocity axis. The Doppler spectrum itself will not change.

1.3.7.2 Color Flow/Power Mode

Color flow (CF) is a blood flow imaging mode in which flow is shown as color overlaid on the B-mode image. Red and blue pixels indicate flow towards and away from the transducer, respectively. Unlike PW Doppler, no temporary (past) information is shown, only real-time. A two-dimensional region of interest, called *color ROI*, is chosen in which color flow is acquired and displayed. Figure 1.15 shows an example with an angled (steered) color ROI, framed by a yellow beige line. A color bar replaces the B-mode gray scale bar and depicts the association between color and velocity. In the example, light blue indicates a velocity of +10 cm/s, whereas −10 cm/s corresponds to yellow. Both colors transition to 0 cm/s from the extremes. In the middle around 0 cm/s is a black-colored range, which represents the wall filter (WF), i.e. its velocity range spans from $-v_{WF}$ to $+v_{WF}$. In the example in Fig. 1.15 the WF is set to 103 Hz. Given a PRF and maximum velocity of 1.3 kHz and 10 cm/s, $v_{WF} = 10\,[\text{cm/s}] \times 103\,[\text{Hz}]/1.3\,[\text{kHz}] = 0.8\,[\text{cm/s}]$.

The purpose of the wall filter is to literally remove signal originating from the lumen wall. A pulsatile lumen may contribute Doppler signals not only from the flowing blood but also from a pulsatile wall. As the lumen pressure changes throughout the cardiac cycle, the wall will displace. Two factors enhance the contribution of this motion to the Doppler processor. First the orientation: While blood most often moves at an angle with respect to the Doppler beam, the expanding or contracting wall moves directly to or from the transducer aperture, i.e. in-line with the Doppler beam. Hence its contribution to the Doppler signal is undiminished (angle α is zero, i.e. $\cos(\alpha) = 1$). Second, the wall is a very strong reflector. Compared to the blood cells, its signal is orders of magnitude larger, and it would dominate the Doppler processing chain. The wall filter removes velocities, i.e. frequencies, slower/smaller than the WF setting. There is a range of displays for the

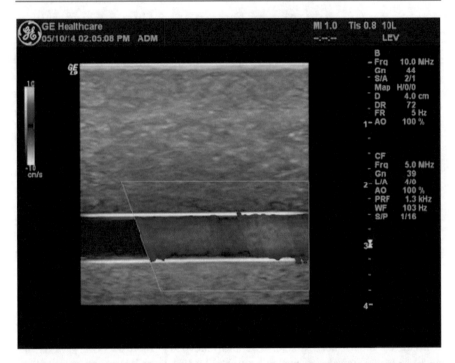

Fig. 1.15 Example of color flow imaging, which is used to display blood flow within the 2D B-mode image. For such, a color box is placed in the region of interest, i.e. across the lumen of interest. Within this box the ultrasound scanner detects temporal changes in the echoes and displays them as color pixel. In this example blue indicates blood moving towards the ultrasound probe and red moving away, as indicated by the color bar on the left. Since the lumen is parallel to the ultrasound probe, the color box is slanted to create an artificial angle and display blood flow parallel to the probe

WF, including straight frequency in Hz, or as a fraction of the maximum velocity or PRF, or qualitatively as low, medium, or high.

There are several parameters associated with color flow imaging. Some of them are listed in Table 1.5. *Packet size* is one of them: and it controls how many firings are averaged before they are displayed. In other words it controls quality but also responsiveness. A packet size of 8 will be able to update velocities twice as fast as a packet size of 16. As indicated in Fig. 1.15 the frame rate dropped to 5 Hz, as opposed to 43 Hz in the PW Doppler example in Fig. 1.14. Where PW Doppler only images one line, color flow images close to 50.

1.3.7.3 Aliasing

One of the most important parameters of flow imaging is the *pulse repetition frequency* (PRF). It controls how often the scanner transmits a beam to track the flow. A PRF that is too large will essentially transmit too often and waste resources, or even produce heating in the field of view. On the screen this is reflected as

Table 1.5 Example listing of user controlled color flow-mode parameters on a diagnostic ultrasound scanner

Parameter	Definition
Frq	Center frequency of the transmitted beam, here 5 MHz
Gn	Receive gain the scanner applies to the acoustic echoes
L/A	(Lateral) line density (4) and frame averaging (off)
AO	Acoustic output, here 100%
PRF	Pulse repetition frequency, here 1.3 kHz
WF	Wall filter, 103 Hz
S/P	Spatial filtering (1) and packet size (16)

User controllable parameters differ between scanner models and brands

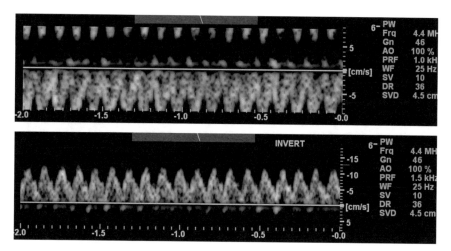

Fig. 1.16 Example of pulsed-wave Doppler aliasing. Aliasing occurs when a recording device is slower than the action being recorded. The reader may recall movies in which wheels of forward moving cars appear to be reversing. This is due to the frame rate of the camera being slower than the rotation of the wheels. If blood moves at a rate faster than the PW Doppler firings, i.e. the pulse repetition frequency (PRF), then flow aliases. This manifests itself as flow going to opposite direction. In the top panel, reverse flow at a maximum speed of 10 cm/s exceeds the display limit of 9 cm/s. This limit results from the PRF of 1 kHz. Flow beyond 9 cm/s is depicted as forward flow reaching from 9 to 8 cm/s, i.e. the flow waveform tops are clipping and display upside down from the top of the display. After increasing the PRF to 1.5 kHz and reversing the display, the waveform is no longer clipped

a mismatch between displayed velocity range and measured velocity range. In Fig. 1.14 the maximum flow velocity is approximately 10 cm/s, yet, the scale reaches up to 30+ cm/s. This range is too large; the PRF, here 1 kHz, could be reduced by a factor of 3 or more. A PRF that is too small will result in aliasing. Two scenarios are shown in Fig. 1.16. For a PRF of 1 kHz the imaged flow in the top panel aliases, i.e. its fastest velocities exceed the display range and wrap around to the opposite end of the range, here from maximum negative to maximum positive flow. There are three steps to change the scanner configuration. First, increase the PRF to capture the flow more often, here to 1.5 kHz. Second, change the baseline to show a velocity range suitable for the observed flow, here approximately −5 to +15 cm/s. Third, invert the display to show systole on the top side of the PW display.

1.3.8 Advanced Image Modes

Ultrasonic imaging has evolved from simple delay-and-sum beamforming as described above to overcome economic and physical limitations to produce greater image detail and increase contrast.

1.3.8.1 Harmonic Imaging

Harmonic imaging is a method by which a wave with frequency f_0 (e.g., 5 MHz) is transmitted into the body and a wave with twice the frequency, i.e. $2 \times f_0$ (10 MHz), is expected back [38]. Two times f_0 is the first harmonic of f_0, hence the name *harmonic imaging*.

Equation (1.1) introduced the linear wave equation. Sound at f_0 entering the body will be reflected and scattered at the same frequency. A nonlinear wave equation is needed to theoretically describe the creation of harmonics. Several solutions have been offered in the literature, including the Westervelt equation [39], the Burgerséquation [40], and the KZK equation [41, 42]:

$$\frac{\partial^2 p}{\partial z \partial t} = \frac{c_0}{2} \nabla^2_\perp p + \frac{\delta}{2c_0^3} \frac{\partial^3 p}{\partial t^3} + \frac{\beta}{2\rho_0 c_0^3} \frac{\partial^2 p^2}{\partial t^2}$$

(1.12)

$$\beta = 1 + \frac{B}{2A}$$

While these theoretical descriptions exceed the scope of this book chapter, they can illustrate the complexity of the underlying formalism as well as the dependence on the biological medium (Table 1.6). Generally speaking, driving human tissue with sound pressures above 0.5 MPa results in harmonics [38]. Insonification at less than 0.5 MPa only returns the original frequency. While ultrasound scanners do not display information on the current sound pressure, they do display the mechanical index (MI). By use of Eq. (1.8) one can compute the rarefactional sound pressure from the MI and the transmit frequency.

Figure 1.17 shows the transmit receive beam profile of an ultrasound beam with $f_0 = 24$ MHz at f#4. The left panel shows the beam profile with a dynamic range of 36 dB, starting at 0 dB. In the focus at 10 mm, the beam's full width at half maximum is approximately 250 μm. This size is suitable to image the interdental papilla (also termed interdental gingiva) soft tissue without interference from the adjacent teeth. However, the ultrasound beam is wider than 250 μm (as shown in the right-hand panel of Fig. 1.17) and even though the beam intensity drops significantly, the

Table 1.6 Listing of tissue parameters B/A for nonlinear sound propagation [30, 43]

Tissue	B/A
Blood	6.1
Brain	6.5
Fat	10
Liver	6.8
Muscle	7.4
Skin	7.8
Water	5.2

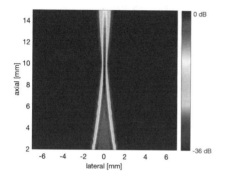 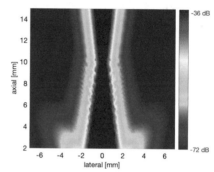

Fig. 1.17 Objective for harmonic imaging. Imaging is based on beamforming to locate the scattering structures that contribute to the receive signal. Left: The first 36 dB (i.e., -36 to 0 dB) of the imaging beam simulated here are fairly confined to a tight beam for good lateral spatial resolution in the focus at 10 mm axially. Right: The next 36 dB, i.e. -72 to -36 dB, are contributing lateral components, spreading the beam considerably. At the 10 mm focus the -36 dB beam is 4 to $5\times$ wider than the full width at half maximum ($\sim 250\,\mu$m). Any strongly reflecting structures would contribute clutter signal to the ROI in the center of the beam. Driving the transmit beam at high sound pressure generates nonlinear tissue scattering. This nonlinearity transforms an incoming wave at f_0 to a scattered wave at $2 \times f_0$. Using frequency filtering can remove the linear scattering clutter signals

scattering or reflecting objects, i.e. the adjacent teeth, have a much larger reflection coefficient than soft tissue. This causes what is known as clutter, i.e. off-beam contributions to the receive signal that shadow on-beam structures. By driving the ultrasound transducer at higher sound pressure the central part of the beam causes the illuminated soft tissue to scatter $2 \times f_0$, which can be filtered out from the receive signal. Therefore, off-beam clutter contributions at f_0 can be removed by frequency filtering. Figure 1.18 shows example images for two traditional cases where the same frequency is used for transmit and receive and one case where harmonic imaging is used, i.e. the transmit is a $f_0 = 12$ MHz and the receive signal is filtered to remove f_0 and only allow $2 \times f_0 = 24$ MHz. The harmonic imaging case shows less fill-in of hypoechoic structures than the straight f_0 cases.

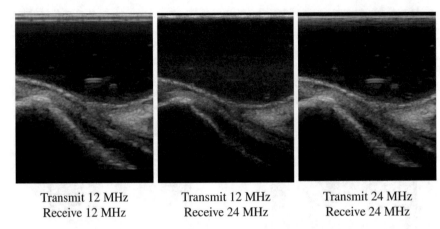

Transmit 12 MHz   Transmit 12 MHz   Transmit 24 MHz
Receive 12 MHz   Receive 24 MHz   Receive 24 MHz

Fig. 1.18 Three examples of harmonic imaging. The same oral structure was imaged three times, with varying transmit (TX) and receive (RX) frequencies. In general higher frequencies produce better spatial resolution and better contrast unless penetration is limited. Left and right sides show the cases where TX and RX are at the same frequency, 12 and 24 MHz, respectively. The latter shows better delineation than the former. However, the middle case with TX at 12 MHz and RX at 24 MHz shows less clutter than the right side. Hypoechoic regions are more pronounced and less filled with clutter

1.3.8.2 Image Compounding

Ultrasound images of specular reflectors suffer from lack of signal at essentially non-perpendicular insonification angles. In other words, when an ultrasound beam impinges on a reflecting surface at an angle other than 90°, then the beam is reflected away from the receiving transducer and is thus not recorded. The result is no signal, a hypoechoic region. This is the case for blood vessels, bones, roots, implants, abutments, etc. A possible solution is to vary the image angle and combine images from a range of angles. This method is called *spatial compounding* and is illustrated in Fig. 1.19.

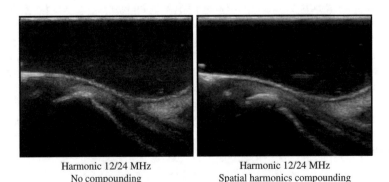

Harmonic 12/24 MHz   Harmonic 12/24 MHz
No compounding   Spatial harmonics compounding

Fig. 1.19 Examples of spatial image compounding. Underlying imaging is harmonic imaging with a 12/24 MHz pair. Right side is (spatial harmonics) compounded, left side is not. Compounding enhances spatial delineation

1.4   Artifacts

Ultrasonic imaging artifacts can be multifactorial and their manifestations in diagnostic imaging are well documented in the literature. General artifacts discussion and classifications are given by Prabhu et al. [44], Hindi et al. [45], Scanlan [46], Kirberger [47], Park et al. [48], and Feldman et al. [49], as well as Kremkau and Taylor [50]. Reverberations and comet tail artifacts, as are visible in dental ultrasound, are discussed in particular by Lichtenstein et al. [51]. Slice-thickness artifacts are discussed by Goldstein and Madrazo [52]. Three-dimensional ultrasound artifacts are addressed by Nelson et al. [53]. Color flow and spectral Doppler artifacts are discussed by Jenssen et al. [54]. Improving images that suffer from artifacts is the topic of a review by Ortiz et al. [55]. Examples of image artifacts are presented in the following subchapters.

1.4.1   Coupling, Shadowing, and Enhancement

Sound propagation relies on the ambient acoustic impedance Z and speed of sound c to be in a range typical for medical imaging, i.e. $Z = 1.54$ MRayl, $c = 1540$ m/s. Placing an ultrasound transducer on the skin without using ultrasound coupling gel or similar will prevent the sound from penetrating the skin, as the majority of the sound energy is reflected on the air gap between the transducer aperture and the skin. The speed of sound in air is 340 m/s and its acoustic impedance is $Z = 0.0034$ MRayl. Figure 1.20, left panel, illustrates the effect of poor coupling. Part of the left side aperture is not correctly coupled to the imaged phantom. Shadowing is an artifact where a strong reflector causes a significant reduction of the forward-propagating acoustic wave, which manifests itself as an artifactually hypoechoic tissue region (middle panel). Enhancement is the opposite effect. Here a lower background reflector or scatterer yields a forward-propagating acoustic wave that then manifests itself as an artifactually hyperechoic tissue region (right panel).

1.4.2   Refraction

Analogous to optics, ultrasound beams are refracted when they transverse from medium 1 with speed of sound c_1 to medium 2 with speed of sound c_2 [56]. This is known as Snell's Law, where the ratio of c_1/c_2 equals the ratio of $\sin(\alpha_1)/\sin(\alpha_2)$, where α_1 is the incident beam angle with respect to the interfacial surface and α_2 is the refracted beam angle. Ultrasound imaging systems assume a constant speed of sound of $c = 1540$ m/s. Using that speed c, the system maps temporal information t from receiving beam information to spatial coordinates ($s = c \times t$). Figure 1.21 shows simulation and imaging examples of beam refraction [57]. In the simulation (left panel) a sound beam travels upwards through ultrasound gel (medium ①) towards a human skin interface (double parallel curved lines, medium ②). Due to

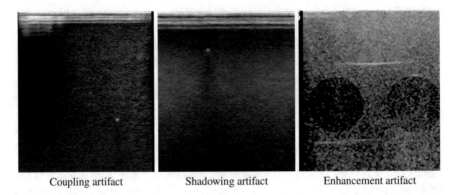

Coupling artifact   Shadowing artifact   Enhancement artifact

Fig. 1.20 Examples of image artifacts. Left panel: Effect of poor coupling. Ultrasound coupling gel is applied to the center and the right side of the aperture. The sound emitted on the left side of the aperture is reflected by the air gap between the aperture and the surface of the imaged ultrasound phantom. Middle panel: A point target comprised of a 100 μm, nylon monofilament is imaged in cross-section. Its acoustic impedance differs from the surrounding host material and causes a strong specular reflection. The reflected acoustic energy diminishes the forward going wave and thus casts a shadow distal to the point target. Right panel: Hypoechoic regions can produce enhancement on their distal side as the penetrating sound wave does not *lose* as much energy, i.e. the backscattered energy from the hypoechoic region is less from than the surrounding tissue. The image shows two hypoechoic cylinders in cross-section. Their distal region is enhanced, whereas the background tissue in-between the cylinders appears darker

the shallow incidence angle between the beam and the skin surface, the incident beam is split into two beams, one refracted and one reflected. The refracted beam leaves a shadow region behind the skin in medium ③. Without the speed of sound changes between the three media, the incident beam would travel straight, whereas here the beam is split. A clinical example is shown in Fig. 1.21 (right panel), i.e. an ultrasound scan of breast tissue. The incident beam also enters the field of view from the bottom. The bright curved 45°-oriented line is the skin surface. This setting is analogous to the simulation in the left panel. There is a shadow region due to beam refraction, which is circled in blue. Clinically this shadow is covering a region which is prone to cancers. Health-care providers need to recognize this artifact and find ways to circumvent the image degradation to adequately support their medical assessment.

1.4.3 Noise

Noise is always a part of any signal. Every ultrasound image contains noise. However, in most meaningful diagnostic images, the noise has a much smaller amplitude than the remaining signal, i.e. the signal to noise ratio, as known as SNR, is high. Figure 1.22a shows a case with poor system choices. A high frequency probe with a shallow elevational, i.e. fixed focus, lens is set up to image relatively deep in an attenuating phantom, here 2.5 cm and 0.5 dB/MHz/cm, which is deep for this combination of lens, frequency, and phantom. The result is image noise. A still image cannot convey how image noise appears on the screen. Speckle "noise" is the typical ultrasound image granularity. It does not change over time, only when the ultrasound probe moves. Non-speckle, electronic, traditional noise changes over time. For an ultrasound probe remaining at exactly the same spatial position over time, the image portion that contains noise will fluctuate. This fluctuation is the best indicator for image noise. Typically noise appears in the image beginning from the distal side, progressing to the proximal side, since the ultrasound wave diminishes over space.

1.4.4 Mirroring

Mirror artifacts are not uncommon in the human body. They occur when the ultrasound beam or the scattered signal is reflected by a finite surface (see Fig. 1.22b). This can include bones, implants, and gas interfaces, such as the lung (diaphragm), stomach, intestine, etc. The user can challenge mirror image appearances by changing the probe position and reevaluating the image.

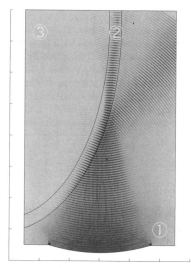
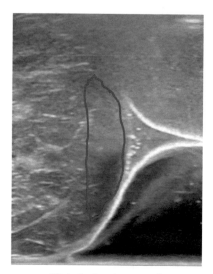
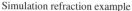

Simulation refraction example   Clinical refraction example

Fig. 1.21 Examples of refraction image artifacts. Left panel: Simulation of an acoustic beam emerging from the bottom, traveling through ultrasound coupling gel (medium ①) and being refracted to the right by the curved skin surface (medium ②) into breast tissue (medium ③) [57]. Right panel: Clinical refraction example of a hypoechoic region below the skin surface [57]

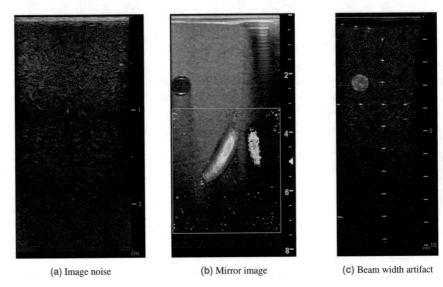

(a) Image noise   (b) Mirror image   (c) Beam width artifact

Fig. 1.22 Examples of image artifacts. (**a**) Example of image noise. The displayed image is from a 24 MHz transmit with a 7 mm elevational focus, yet the image depth is 2.5 cm. At this high frequency and shallow elevational focus, it is not possible to obtain an image at this great depth. The result is noise. (**b**) Example of mirror image. The displayed image shows color flow visualizing a flow tube in a phantom. The right-hand side of the image is not fully coupled as can be seen from the right-side aperture. However, there are two flow tubes in the images, whereas the phantom contains only one. Moreover, the two lumens appear to be in part symmetric to each other. The right-hand lumen is truncated compared to its left side counterpart. It is produced by ultrasound beams being reflected from the right-hand housing wall of the phantom, thus producing a mirror image. (**c**) Example of beam width artifacts. The displayed image demonstrates how lateral resolution decreases with depth. The shown axial wire targets are all of the same physical size yet appear larger as depth increases. This is due to the decreasing lateral resolution of the ultrasound beam as it penetrates deeper tissues

1.4.5 Beam Width

Ultrasonic beams are shaped with electronic and mechanical lenses. The beam-former uses electronic delays to focus the beam and a certain aperture size to create an intended beam width. For 1D arrays the fixed-focus elevational lens on the transducer shapes the beam depending on the application of the probe. It can be for superficial imaging of teeth or peripheral blood vessels or for deep imaging, such as abdominal imaging. The beam width is minimal in the focal region and widens as it progresses beyond that spatial point. Figure 1.22c shows a 10 cm field of view in a phantom for spatial calibrations. The beam width can be estimated and measured by examining the apparent width of the (axial) wire targets. This width increases with depth and can be explained with Eq. (1.9), where the lateral beam width is related to the frequency and the $f\#$. Since $f\#$ is defined as focal length F divided by the aperture width D, i.e. $f\# = F/D$, it is obvious that at the point where the aperture cannot widen more yet the focal length increases, the beam width has to increase as well. This is the case in Fig. 1.22c. It is also possible that the actual frequency of the acoustic wave decreases and thus the wavelength increases, but that is beyond the scope of this chapter.

1.4.6   Reverberation and Comet Tail Artifacts

Ultrasonic imaging assumes a continuously forward-propagating wave and speckle scattering from the penetrated tissue. However, some tissue structures or foreign body inclusions may change the acoustic path. Figure 1.23 left shows reverberation artifacts within a crown. The speed of sound and mass density of teeth are greater than those of soft tissue. In addition, the distal side of the crown is exposed to air, whose speed of sound and mass density are significantly lower than soft tissue. Therefore, the proximal and distal interface of the crown trap a certain amount of the incident sound wave and cause it to reflect within the crown multiple times, each time with diminishing energy. The ultrasound scanner associates the time of any received acoustic wave relative to the time when the original beam was transmitted and computes the distance of an associated structure based on the assumed speed of sound of 1540 m/s. As a result, the reverberating sound within the crown is interpreted as a structure that is equally spaced and distal to the front surface of the crown. Distinct parallel lines are visible when the front and back side of the underlying structure are parallel as well (left panel in Fig. 1.23). Any appreciable

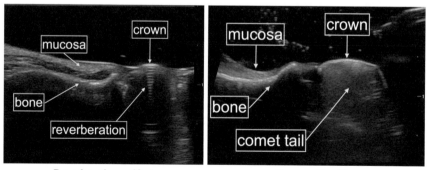

Reverberation artifact   Comet tail artifact

Fig. 1.23 Example of reverberation and comet tail artifacts. Sound, much like any wave, is reflected when it encounters an impedance change. In dental ultrasound the wave is reflected on bones, crowns, roots, implants, and others. For structures with parallel boundaries, crowns, and implants, for example, the sound can reverberate (left image) within them and slowly "leak" out towards both parallel boundaries. The sound "leaking" towards the ultrasound probe is received and displayed as a structure in the axial direction. Reverberating waves where individual reflections blend into a continuous wave, right image, are called *comet tail* or *vail* artifact

curvature, with respect to the acoustic wavelength in the structure, causes a diffuse reverberation, which is termed a *comet tail* or *vail artifact* (right panel in Fig. 1.23).

References

1. Gholizadeh S. A review of non-destructive testing methods of composite materials. Proc Struct Integr. 2016;1:50–7. ISSN: 2452-3216.
2. Drinkwater BW, Wilcox PD. Ultrasonic arrays for non-destructive evaluation: a review. NDT E Int. 2006;39(7):525–41. ISSN:0963–8695.
3. Hunter AJ, Drinkwater BW, Wilcox PD. Autofocusing ultrasonic imagery for non-destructive testing and evaluation of specimens with complicated geometries. NDT E Int. 2010;43(2):78–85. ISSN: 0963-8695.
4. Jenderka K-V, Koch C. Investigation of spatial distribution of sound field parameters in ultrasound cleaning baths under the influence of cavitation. Ultrasonics. 2006;44:e401–6. ISSN: 0041-624X.
5. Jensen JA. Field: a program for simulating ultrasound systems. In: 10th Nordic-Baltic conference on biomedical imaging published in medical & biological engineering & computing. Vol. 34, Issue: 1; 1996. p. 351–53.
6. Szabo TL. Diagnostic ultrasound imaging: inside out. London: Academic Press; 2004. ISBN: 0126801452.
7. Saini K, Dewal ML, Rohit M. Ultrasound imaging and image segmentation in the area of ultrasound: a review. Int J Adv Sci Technol. 2010;24.
8. Fenster A, Downey DB. 3-D ultrasound imaging: a review. IEEE Eng Med Biol Mag. 1996;15(6):41–51. ISSN: 0739-5175.
9. McGahan JP, Goldberg BB. Diagnostic ultrasound. Vol. 1. London: Informa Health Care; 2008. ISBN: 1420069780.
10. Caskey CF, Hu XW, Ferrara KW. Leveraging the power of ultrasound for therapeutic design and optimization. J Control Release. 2011;156(3):297–306. ISSN: 0168-3659. https://doi.org/10.1016/jjconrel2011.07032. %3CGo%20to%20ISI%3E://WOS:000298555000004.
11. Hynynen K. Focused ultrasound for blood-brain disruption and delivery of therapeutic molecules into the brain. In: Expert Opin Drug Deliv. 2007;4(1):27–35. ISSN: 1742-5247. https://doi.org/1.1517/1742524741.27. %3CGo%20to%20ISI%3E://WOS:000252825100004.
12. Bailey MR, et al. Physical mechanisms of the therapeutic effect of ultrasound (a review). Acoust Phys. 2003;49(4):369–88. ISSN: 1063-7710. https://doi.org/10.1134/1.1591291. %3CGo%20to%20ISI%3E://WOS:000184769300001.
13. Baker KG, Robertson VJ, Duck FA. A review of therapeutic ultrasound: biophysical effects. Phys Ther. 2001;81(7):1351–8. ISSN: 0031-9023. https://doi.org/10.1093/ptj/81.7.1351. %3CGo%20to%20ISI%3E://WOS:000169684600007.
14. Jiang XX, et al. A review of low-intensity pulsed ultrasound for therapeutic applications. IEEE Trans Biomed Eng. 2019;66(10):2704–18. ISSN: 0018-9294. https://doi.org/10.1109/tbme.2018.2889669 %3CGo%20to%20ISI%3E://WOS:000487192000001.
15. Gorick, CM, Chappell, JC, Price, RJ. Applications of ultrasound to stimulate therapeutic revascularization. Int. J. Mol. Sci. 2019;20(12):3081. ISSN: 1422-0067. https://doi.org/10.3390/ijms20123081. %3CGo%20to%20ISI%3E://WOS:000473756000231.
16. O'Reilly MA, Hynynen, K. Emerging non-cancer applications of therapeutic ultrasound. Int J Hyperthermia. 2015;31(3):310–8. ISSN: 0265-6736. https://doi.org/10.3109/02656736.2015.1004375. %3CGo%20to%20ISI%3E://WOS:000355926300012.
17. Ebbini ES, Ter Haar, G. Ultrasound-guided therapeutic focused ultrasound: current status and future directions. Int J Hyperthermia. 2015;31(2):77–89. ISSN: 0265-6736. https://doi.org/10.3109/02656736.2014.995238. %3CGo%20to%20ISI%3E://WOS:000353167300002.
18. Miller DL, et al. Overview of therapeutic ultrasound applications and safety considerations. J Ultrasound Med. 2012;31(4):623–34. ISSN: 0278-4297. https://doi.org/10.7863/jum.2012.31.

4.623. %3CGo%20to%20ISI%3E://WOS:000302446100014.

19. Wells PNT. A range-gated ultrasonic Doppler system. Med Biol Eng. 1969;7(6):641–52. ISSN: 0025-696X.
20. Lawson G, Dawes GS, Redman CWG. A comparison of two fetal heart rate ultrasound detector systems. Am J Obstet Gynecol. 1982;143(7):840–2. ISSN: 0002-9378.
21. Kurjak A, et al. How useful is 3D and 4D ultrasound in perinatal medicine? J Perinatal Med. 2007;35(1):10–27. ISSN: 1619-3997.
22. Yagel S, et al. 3D and 4D ultrasound in fetal cardiac scanning: a new look at the fetal heart. Ultrasound Obstet Gynecol. 2007;29(1):81–95. ISSN: 0960-7692.
23. Barnett SB, Maulik, D. Guidelines and recommendations for safe use of Doppler ultrasound in perinatal applications. J Matern Fetal Med. 2001;10(2):75–84. ISSN: 1057-0802.
24. Barnett SB, et al. International recommendations and guidelines for the safe use of diagnostic ultrasound in medicine. Ultrasound Med Biol. 2000;26(3):355–66. ISSN: 0301-5629.
25. Morse PM, Ingard KU. Theoretical acoustics. Princeton: Princeton University Press; 1986. ISBN: 0691024014.
26. Cobbold RSC. Foundations of biomedical ultrasound. Oxford: Oxford University Press; 2006. ISBN: 0199775125.
27. Kinsler LE, et al. Fundamentals of acoustics. In: Kinsler LE, Frey AR, Coppens AB, Sanders JV, editors. Fundamentals of acoustics. 4th ed. Weinheim: Wiley-VCH; 1999, p. 560. ISBN 0-471-84789-5.
28. Azhari, H. Basics of biomedical ultrasound for engineers. London: Wiley; 2010. ISBN: 0470561467.
29. Hoskins PR, Martin K, Thrush, A. Diagnostic ultrasound: physics and equipment. Cambridge: Cambridge University Press; 2010. ISBN: 1139488902.
30. Duck, FA. Physical properties of tissues: a comprehensive reference book. London: Academic Press; 2013. ISBN: 1483288420.
31. Herring N, Paterson DJ. Levick's introduction to cardiovascular physiology. Boca Raton: CRC Press; 2018.
32. Chivers RC, Hill, CR. Ultrasonic attenuation in human tissue. Ultrasound Med Biol. 1975;2(1):25–9.
33. Barootchi S, et al. Ultrasonographic characterization of lingual structures pertinent to oral, periodontal and implant surgery. Clin Oral Implants Res. 2020;31(4):352–9.
34. Branham ML, et al. Effect of ultrasound-facilitated fixation on oral mucosa density and morphology. Biotech Histochem. 2012;87(5):331–9.
35. Hosokawa A, Otani T. Ultrasonic wave propagation in bovine cancellous bone. J Acoust Soc Am. 1997;101(1):558–62.
36. Bond LJ, Chiang C-H, Fortunko CM. Absorption of ultrasonic waves in air at high frequencies (10–20 MHz). J Acoust Soc Am. 1992;92(4):2006–15.
37. Schmerr LW Jr. Fundamentals of ultrasonic phased arrays. Vol. 215. Berlin: Springer; 2014.
38. Anvari A, Forsberg F, Samir AE. A primer on the physical principles of tissue harmonic imaging. RadioGraphics. 2015;35(7):1955–64.
39. Shevchenko I, Kaltenbacher, B. Absorbing boundary conditions for nonlinear acoustics: the Westervelt equation. J Comput Phys. 2015;302:200–21.
40. Hamilton MF, Blackstock DT, et al. Nonlinear acoustics. Vol. 237. San Diego: Academic Press; 1998.
41. Rozanova, A. The Khokhlov–Zabolotskaya–Kuznetsov equation. C R Math. 2007;344(5):337–42.
42. Pinton GF, et al. A heterogeneous nonlinear attenuating full-wave model of ultrasound. IEEE Trans Ultrason Ferroelectr Freq Control. 2009;56(3):474–88.
43. Wells PNT. Ultrasonic imaging of the human body. Rep Prog Phys. 1999;62(5):671.
44. Prabhu SJ, et al. Ultrasound artifacts: classification, applied physics with illustrations, and imaging appearances. Ultrasound Q. 2014;30(2):145–57.
45. Hindi A, Peterson C, Barr, RG. Artifacts in diagnostic ultrasound. Rep Med Imaging. 2013;6:29–48.

46. Scanlan KA. Sonographic artifacts and their origins. Am J Roentgenol. 1991;156(6):1267–72. ISSN: 0361-803X.
47. Kirberger RM. Imaging artifacts in diagnostic ultrasound—a review. Vet Radiol Ultrasound. 1995;36(4):297–306. ISSN: 1058-8183.
48. Park RD, et al. B-mode gray-scale ultrasound: imaging artifacts and interpretation principles. Vet Radiol. 1981;22(5):204–10. ISSN: 0196-3627.
49. Feldman MK, Katyal S, Blackwood MS. US artifacts. RadioGraphics. 2009; 29(4):1179–89. ISSN: 0271-5333.
50. Kremkau FW, Taylor KJ. Artifacts in ultrasound imaging. J Ultrasound Med. 1986;5(4):227–37. ISSN: 1550-9613.
51. Lichtenstein D, et al. The comet-tail artifact: an ultrasound sign ruling out pneumothorax. Intensive Care Med. 1999;25(4):383–8. ISSN: 0342-4642.
52. Goldstein A, Madrazo BL. Slice-thickness artifacts in gray-scale ultrasound. J Clin Ultrasound. 1981;9(7):365–75. ISSN: 0091-2751.
53. Nelson TR, et al. Sources and impact of artifacts on clinical three dimensional ultrasound imaging. Ultrasound Obstet Gynecol. 2000;16(4):374–83. ISSN: 0960-7692.
54. Jenssen C, et al. Ultrasound artifacts and their diagnostic significance in internal medicine and gastroenterology—part 2: color and spectral Doppler artifacts. Z Gastroenterol. 2016;54(6):569–78. ISSN: 0044-2771.
55. Ortiz SHC, Chiu T, Fox, MD. Ultrasound image enhancement: a review. Biomed Signal Process Control. 2012;7(5):419–28. ISSN: 1746-8094.
56. Sommer FG, Filly RA, Minton, MJ. Acoustic shadowing due to refractive and reflective effects. Am J Roentgenol. 1979;132(6):973–9. ISSN: 0361-803X.
57. Jintamethasawat R, et al. Acoustic beam anomalies in automated breast imaging. J Med Imaging (Bellingham). 4(4):045001. ISSN: 2329-4302 (Print) 2329-4302 (Linking). https://doi.org/10.1117/1.JMI.4.4.045001. https://www.ncbi.nlm.nih.gov/pubmed/29057289.

Ultrasonic Imaging in Comparison to Other Imaging Modalities

2

Johan Aps

2.1 Introduction

The famous picture of the radiograph taken of Roentgen's wife's hand, was the start of a new era. On 12 January 1896, merely two weeks after Roentgen's discovery of X-rays was published, Dr. Otto Walkhoff probably took the first dental radiograph which initiated the birth of dental radiography. In Fig. 2.1, a timeline shows what the images looked like back then and how long the exposures had to be. It also shows important events and discoveries that changed the field of medicine and dentistry. The author is pretty sure that this is not the end of that timeline, as new technologies and improvements of current technologies will be explored and applied.

Since 1896, a new era was born and ever since, dental radiographs have proven their significant value in dental and maxillofacial diagnosis. For many years two-dimensional intraoral radiography and extraoral radiography was the only radiographic modality, but in recent years, three-dimensional imaging in dentistry (CBCT, i.e. Cone Beam Computed Tomography) has become common ground. Challenges regarding tomography of the skull were battled by the Finish Professor Paatero, who developed the first panoramic machine. Many of us refer to the panoramic radiograph as 'pan', 'pano', 'panorex', 'DPT', 'OPT' or 'OPG'. Other advanced imaging modalities such as Multi-Slice Computed Tomography (MSCT), Magnetic Resonance Imaging (MRI) and ultrasound imaging are also available to the clinician. Both MSCT and MRI are too expensive to be used in a dental environment, but they have their applications in dentistry. Ultrasonography is in some countries around the world better accepted than in others for diagnostic purposes in the dental and maxillofacial region. Without a doubt ultrasonography

J. Aps (✉)
Dentomaxillofacial Radiology, Discipline Lead Dental and Maxillofacial Radiology, Division Head Oral Diagnostic and Surgical Sciences, University of Western Australia–Dental School–OHCWA, Perth, WA, Australia

© Springer Nature Switzerland AG 2021
H.-L. (Albert) Chan, O. D. Kripfgans (eds.), *Dental Ultrasound in Periodontology and Implantology*, https://doi.org/10.1007/978-3-030-51288-0_2

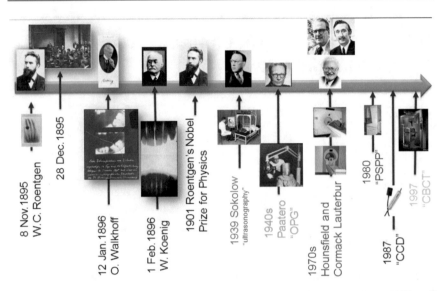

Fig. 2.1 Timeline showing introductions of innovation in diagnostic imaging from 1895 until 2019

or echography, as it is also called, has definitely a place in our armamentarium. In contrast to MSCT and CBCT and plain radiography, MRI and ultrasonography do not use ionizing radiation, and can therefore be considered 'safer' than the other imaging modalities. Infrared thermography, near-infrared transillumination and laser fluorescence are gaining more ground in dentistry too. The first one is used for soft tissue pathology (e.g. cancer) and the two latter rather for caries diagnosis. Further research will show how reliable these two latter techniques are and if they can replace ionizing radiation (e.g. bitewing radiographs). Figure 2.1 also shows the introduction of ultrasonography in 1939 by Dr. Sokolow, who managed to image soft tissues when patients were submerged in water or when a bag of water was placed over the patient to allow ultrasound waves to penetrate the patient's tissues. The principle of and need for a watery medium will be discussed elsewhere in this book. As is clear from the timeline in Fig. 2.1, the introduction of magnetic resonance imaging (MRI) took place around the same time as the introduction of multi-slice computed tomography (MSCT). Drs. Hounsfield and Cormack, the inventors of MSCT, stuck to the use of ionizing radiation, while Dr. Lauterbur suggested the future lie in magnetic resonance imaging, or nuclear magnetic resonance imaging (NMR), as it was first called. In the last decade of the twentieth century, cone beam computed tomography (CBCT) was introduced into dentistry in particular. This technology has rushed like a tsunami over dental imaging and it seems, assessing the literature published about dental imaging in the last 20 years, that there is more than plenty written and researched about CBCT. However, CBCT uses ionizing radiation and therefore carries a potential risk to patients, which is something, especially in paediatric dentistry, of great concern, as this technique is proposed to be used in orthodontic planning and follow-up. Though it is not the scope of this book to address this issue, the author wishes, nevertheless, to draw the reader's attention to this issue, as the main technique this book is emphasizing on is not using ionizing radiation at all. This chapter will further focus on the different imaging modalities that are available within the dental field. Table 2.1 shows an overview of intraoral and extraoral techniques, two- and three-dimensional imaging and ionizing versus non-ionizing diagnostic imaging. Table 2.1 is further explained in the following paragraphs, each describing the particular diagnostic imaging techniques. The reader who is interested in more detailed information is kindly referred to the textbooks mentioned in the reference list of this chapter.

2.2 Ionizing Radiation or X-rays

All X-ray machines consist, generally speaking, of the same components [1–4]. A vacuum glass tube contains the negatively charged cathode, which looks like an incandescent light bulb's filament, and the anode, which is a flat surface allowing for electron collisions, which will subsequently cause production of X-rays if the energy of the incoming colliding electrons from the cathode is high enough. The number of electrons is determined by the Amperage (usually milli-Ampere or mA) and is proportionate to the number of X-rays and hence to the X-ray dose. Both anode and cathode are usually made of Tungsten (W) or Molybdenum (Mo). The electrons are attracted to the anode due to a high voltage across both. That (kilo-)voltage determines the penetration power (energy) of the X-rays that are produced. Most medical X-ray machines have a rotating anode to dissipate the heat better, as they use longer exposure times, higher kV and mA settings. Approximately 99% of all electron collisions are after all only causing heat and no X-rays. The vacuum glass tube is therefore surrounded by oil, in order to cool down the machine. Lead lining around the machine is essential, as X-rays should only be exiting the machine through the collimator, which is aimed at the patient and the image detector. Before the X-rays exit the machine, they pass through an aluminium filter, which ensures only high enough X-rays will exit the machine. Lower energy X-rays would only add to the patient's absorbed dose and not benefit the image. Therefore filtering out the low energy X-rays is essential. The latter will benefit image quality (less scattered radiation) and will also decrease the patient's absorbed radiation dose. In medical diagnostic X-ray machines, the collimation can easily be changed and the machines are manufactured with a diaphragm light bundle to visualize the surface that will be irradiated. This is not the case in dental radiography equipment.

Table 2.1 Overview of dental imaging techniques, their implementation, advantages and disadvantages

Imaging technique	Imaging modality [two- or three-dimensional (2D or 3D)]	Place of image detector [intraoral (IO) or extraoral (EO)]	Place of X-ray source [intraoral (IO) or extraoral (EO)]	Dental applications	Advantages	Disadvantages
Bitewing radiography	2D	IO	EO and stationary	• Caries diagnosis • Periodontal bone height assessment • Dental development assessment	• Easy technique • Quick acquisition • Commonly available in dental office	• 2D only • Limited field of view • Not accurate soft tissue information • Challenging geometry • Some patients do not tolerate procedure
Periapical radiography	2D	IO	EO and stationary	• Caries diagnosis • Periodontal bone height assessment • Periapical assessment • Dental development assessment	• Easy technique • Quick acquisition • Commonly available in dental office	• 2D only • Limited field of view • Not accurate soft tissue information • Challenging geometry • Some patients do not tolerate procedure
Occlusal/oblique occlusal radiography	2D	IO	EO and stationary	• Alternative to periapical radiography • Dental development assessment • Extended periapical view and assessment	• Easy technique • Quick acquisition • Image detector not against palate or in floor of mouth	• 2D only • Not accurate soft tissue information • Prone to distortion (challenging geometry)

Modality						
Oblique lateral radiography	2D	EO	EO (opposite side) and stationary	• Alternative to periapical and bitewing radiography • Dental development assessment • Extended periapical view and assessment	Image detector not against palate or in floor of mouth	• 2D only • Not accurate soft tissue information • Prone to distortion (challenging geometry) • Equipment not commonly available in dental office
Cephalometric radiography	2D	EO	EO (opposite side) and stationary in case of one shot technology—otherwise mobile (translational movement)	• Lateral skull radiograph for orthognathic surgery/treatment	• Reproducible in time due to cephalostat, which enables standard patient positioning	• 2D only • Not accurate soft tissue information • Special equipment required
Dental panoramic tomography (DPT/OPG/Pan)	2D	EO and mobile	EO and mobile in synchronicity with image detector (rotational movement)	• Panoramic overview of the jaws and immediate adjacent anatomical tissues • Extended periapical view • Lateral view of the mandibular condyles	• Broader overview of the jaws than intraoral radiograph series	• 2D only • Not accurate soft tissue information • Distortion in the image • Ghost images inherent to technique • Equipment not always available in dental offices

(continued)

Table 2.1 (continued)

Imaging technique	Imaging modality [two- or three-dimensional (2D or 3D)]	Place of Image detector [intraoral (IO) or extraoral (EO)]	Place of X-ray source [intraoral (IO) or extraoral (EO)]	Dental applications	Advantages	Disadvantages
Cone beam computed tomography (CBCT)	3D	EO and mobile	EO and mobile in synchronicity with image detector (rotational movement)	• Adjunct to 2D imaging when 2D has inadequate or incomplete diagnostic yield	• 3D • Bone and teeth can be visualised very well	• Not accurate soft tissue information • Streaking artefacts with radiodense materials • Relative high radiation dose compared to all techniques mentioned above in this table • Equipment is expensive and not commonly available in dental offices
Multi-slice computed tomography (MSCT)	3D	EO and mobile	EO and mobile in synchronicity with image detector (rotational movement)	• Adjunct to 2D imaging in cases where soft tissue and hard tissue diagnostic information is required (e.g. tumour) • Acute head trauma imaging	• 3D • Hard and soft tissue information	• High radiation dose compared to all techniques above in this table • Streaking artefacts with radiodense materials • Not available in dental office as equipment requires

Magnetic resonance imaging/nuclear magnetic resonance imaging (MRI/NMR)	3D	Not applicable	Not applicable as is using non-ionizing radiation	Adjunct to 2D imaging where soft tissue information is required for diagnosis	• 3D Non-ionizing radiation • Ideal for soft tissue imaging	special maintenance and imaging technicians to operate • Expensive equipment • Impossible with claustrophobic patients • Machine makes a lot of noise • Cannot be used with ferro-magnetic objects in or on the patient's body (artefacts when ferro-magnetic objects are inside the patient's body—severe accidents can happen with ferro-magnetic objects in the MRI room) • Very expensive equipment that requires a special room and technical support to run the machine • Not available in dental offices

(continued)

Table 2.1 (continued)

Imaging technique	Imaging modality (two-2D- or three dimensional - 3D)	Place of Image detector [intraoral (IO) or extraoral (EO)]	Place of X-ray source [intraoral (IO) or extraoral (EO)]	Dental applications	Advantages	Disadvantages
Ultrasound imaging/ultrasonography/ echography (US/Echo)	2D and 3D	IO and EO possible	Not applicable as is using non-ionizing radiation—though, transducer can be IO or EO (manual operation—transducer is both emitter and receiver)	• Adjunct to 2D imaging when soft tissue information is required for diagnosis • Soft tissue imaging in head and neck (e.g. salivary glands)	• 3D and 2D possible • immediate acquisition of images • Live imaging • Can be performed as often as one wants • Equipment ranges from a couple of 100 to 100k US Dollars (hand-held or tablet connected to stand alone 3D machines)	• Operator dependent image quality (pressure on tissue differs per operator) • Special equipment not commonly available in dental offices
Thermography	2D	Not applicable	Not applicable as is using non-ionizing radiation	Soft tissue facial diagnosis	• No ionizing radiation • Can be repeated as often as one wants	• 2D only • Only soft tissues • Superficial layers only • Not commonly available in dental offices • Experimental at this moment

Near-infrared light (NIR)	2D	Not applicable	Not applicable as is not using ionizing radiation	• Dental caries diagnosis • Alternative and/or adjunct to bitewing radiography	• No ionizing radiation • Can be repeated as often as one wants • Recordable • Educational towards patients	• 2D only • Not commonly available in dental offices • Accuracy still under investigation
Laser fluorescence imaging	2D	Not applicable	Not applicable as is not using ionizing radiation	• Dental caries diagnosis • Alternative and/or adjunct to bitewing radiography	• No ionizing radiation • Can be repeated as often as one wants • Recordable • Educational towards patients	• 2D only • Not commonly available in dental offices • Accuracy still under investigation

2.3   Intraoral Imaging

2.3.1   Bitewing and Periapical Radiography

In intraoral radiography the image detector is placed inside the patient's mouth and the X-ray machine is positioned extraorally, and stationary, aiming at the image detector. There are three ways of obtaining intraoral radiographs: parallel technique, bisecting angle technique and occlusal technique. The latter two techniques are somewhat different, as the X-rays are not aimed perpendicular at the image detector, but perpendicular at the imaginary bisecting angle between the long axis of the tooth and the long axis of the image detector [1–4]. Under ideal circumstances, a periapical and bitewing radiograph requires the image detector to be as parallel and close as possible to the teeth, with the X-ray beam aligned perpendicular to the image detector. This is the so-called parallel technique. This creates geometrically accurate images of teeth and alveolar bone levels. To obtain proper alignment one should use image detector holders (e.g. Rinn® and Hawe Neos®) with extraorally placed guidance rods and rings, which definitely help properly aligning the X-ray machine with the image detector. Unfortunately the image detector cannot always be placed ideally inside the patient's mouth due to anatomical restrictions (e.g. shape of the palate, the level of the floor of the mouth or a mandibular torus), or due to the patient not tolerating the intraoral placement of the image detector. In some cases, the parallel technique cannot be performed as the patient does not tolerate the image detector placement parallel to the teeth. In that case, one can attempt the bisecting angle technique. This technique requires one to aim the X-ray beam perpendicular at an imaginary bisecting line between the long axis of the tooth and the long axis of the image detector as mentioned above. This is a more difficult technique as there is usually no image detector holder involved with an extraoral guide to aid with the X-ray machine alignment. There is, however, an image detector holder on the market that allows for proper alignment using the bisecting angle technique: the Rinn® BAI (bisecting angle instrument). Unfortunately it is usually the image detector holder that causes issues for patients and as a consequence this holder is less frequently used.

2.3.2   Occlusal Radiography

If neither the parallel nor the bisecting angle technique is possible, then one more alternative is still possible: the occlusal radiograph. For this technique, one uses best a photo stimulable phosphor storage plate, as these come in different sizes and allow for proper placement in the patient's mouth. For primary teeth, a size 2 will suffice, while for permanent teeth, a more useful size would be size 4. These images will not always produce the perfect geometrically aligned images as is the case with the parallel technique, but can still provide sufficient diagnostic yield. Intraoral radiography is the standard diagnostic imaging technique to assess interproximal caries, and also interproximal periodontal bone levels. Bitewing radiographs are good examples of the latter, whereas periapical radiography and occlusal radiography are better for evaluation and assessment of the periapical regions of the jaws. The major limitation of intraoral radiography is that it is only a two-dimensional imaging modality which is not very good at differentiating between soft tissues (see Table 2.1). That being said, it should be emphasized that occlusal radiographs can be useful in identifying radiopaque sialoliths in the floor of the mouth, despite the fact that the musculature and glandular tissue cannot be differentiated.

2.4 Extraoral Imaging with Stationary X-ray Tube

2.4.1 Cephalometric Radiography

The cephalometric radiograph [4] is very often used in orthodontic and orthognathic surgery planning. The technique requires a specialized X-ray machine which provides a reproducible lateral skull view. That reproducibility is important as certain structures in the skull, and especially the sella turcica, have to be used as reference to verify growth or the impact of disease or surgery. A dental cephalometric radiograph is therefore unique and that is exactly why the machine is equipped with a so-called cephalostat. This device helps position the patient with the midsagittal plane of the skull perpendicular to the floor, by putting an ear rod in each external acoustic meatus, while a support on the bridge of the nose reassures the patient's head is in a natural position. The patient should have the teeth in occlusion during the exposure. Some manufacturers use a one-shot approach, which implies a 1 s X-ray exposure and hence very little chance for motion artifacts. Other manufacturers use an anterior to posterior or vice versa scan of the skull, which takes several seconds, hence a higher chance for motion artifacts during the exposure. Technically the latter machines are therefore not stationary X-ray tube machines. Cephalometric images should always show the soft tissues overlying the face and neck, as these outlines are also used for planning purposes in several orthodontic and orthognathic analyses. By convention, the image is supposed to be viewed with the patient facing to the right-hand side. It needs to be emphasized that one cannot distinguish between the different soft tissues (e.g. salivary glands from muscular tissue) on a cephalometric radiograph. The medical lateral skull radiograph differs significantly from a dental cephalometric image, as the first one does not use a cephalostat, and therefore reproducibility is impossible. Medical lateral skull radiographs are rarely used in dentistry. Many clinicians do not realize that the cephalostat can also be rotated and allows one to take other skull radiographic projections, which are more common in medicine: anterior-posterior skull, posterior-anterior-skull, submento-vertex skull and any deviation or variation of the former positions. Since the use and availability of cone beam computed tomography (CBCT) have increased, most of these techniques have become obsolete, as these views of the skull can be easily regenerated from a CBCT scan, while providing more information as the latter technique offers three-dimensional images.

2.4.2 Oblique Lateral Radiography

A technique which is often forgotten is the oblique lateral radiograph [1, 4]. This technique is overlooked by many, but definitely has a place in paediatric dentistry imaging and imaging in patients with special needs. In the hands of an experienced clinician/radiographer this technique can provide very good diagnostic information. This being said, it needs to be emphasized that there is a learning curve to produce good oblique lateral radiographs. This technique requires a stiff cassette with a phosphor storage plate inside and an X-ray machine that is used for intraoral radiography. The exposure time is only 0.16 s at 65 or 70 kV. The image detector should not bend as that would cause significant distortion in the image. The cassette should be held against the side one wishes to image, and should be in contact with the tip of the nose and the cheek. Part of the cassette should be inferior to the inferior border of the mandible. Subsequently the patient has to turn the head towards the side the cassette is leaning against. This creates a radiographic key-hole on the opposite side between the cervical spine and the posterior border of the ramus of the mandible. The X-ray machine, with circular collimator, is now aimed perpendicular at the cassette, with the central X-ray beam following the occlusal plane. For the latter one can use the lips as a guide. If the geometry was correct, the image should be a perfect circle. If one sees an oval, it means the X-rays were not aimed perpendicular at the cassette. It is obvious that this technique is only to be considered an alternative for a panoramic radiograph or a periapical or bitewing radiograph in cases where patients are not able to cope with the procedure. Oblique lateral radiographs have the same limitations as intraoral radiographs and cephalometric radiographs regarding soft tissue diagnosis.

2.5 Extraoral Imaging with Revolving X-ray Tube

2.5.1 Panoramic Radiography

Dental panoramic tomography is often called, depending on the region in the world, a panorex, a pan, an OPG, an OPT, a DPT, just to name a few. They all refer to the same technique and the same image that is generated [1–4]. This technique implies that the X-ray source and the image detector, placed opposite of each other, rotate synchronous around the patient's head, with the image detector passing as close as possible to the patient's face. By doing so, one creates a focal trough, or a slice with a particular thickness. The shape of the focal through is a three-dimensional horse shoe, which, ideally, follows the shape of the dental arches as good as possible. The thickness of the slice depends on the width of the X-ray beam. The narrower the beam, the thinner the slice. The latter means a more sharp image, but there is a threshold of course, below which one should not go, as the image would become non-diagnostic. Some machines allow for adjustments to the shape and size of the focal trough, while others do not. The latter are usually cheaper and assume one size fits all. It is evident that this is incorrect and that if the shape of the jaw can be followed more accurately, the image will be better as well. The most recent machines use technology that collects information from different image layers, without radiation dose increase, but with image quality improvement. The X-ray beam used in panoramic radiography is collimated as a vertical narrow slit beam, which can be adjusted in height to accommodate for adult or paediatric settings. This collimation is essential when imaging children as it will reduce the radiation burden and avoid unnecessary parts of the head to be exposed. The X-ray beam is also angled slightly upwards (8–12°), which explains why structures in the neck, like, for instance, a forgotten necklace or a lead (equivalent) apron over the shoulders and neck, will be projected on the patient's chin in the final image. It also deserves to be emphasized that the upward angulation of the X-ray beam causes distortion and magnification in a panoramic image, which is about 1.3 in magnitude. Therefore measuring tooth length or bone height, for instance, on a panoramic radiograph is not accurate at all, as differences in patient positioning may cause additional distortion in the final image. Due to the technique there are always ghost or phantom images in panoramic radiography, which makes interpretation of the image sometimes challenging. Just like the previous techniques, also this radiographic imaging technique is not good at differentiating between soft tissues.

2.5.2 Cone Beam Computed Tomography

Cone beam computed tomography (CBCT), as the name of the technique implies, uses a conical (actually pyramidal) shaped X-ray beam, which revolves in a single rotation arc around the patient's head, while the image detector (flat panel) moves in synchronicity on the opposite side of the skull [1–4]. The image that is obtained is therefore a cylinder, providing three-dimensional images, and is captured as a whole and not in segments as is the case in multi-slice computed tomography. The latter technique, also called medical CT, uses a fan shaped beam which revolves multiple times around the patient (see further), hence causing a higher radiation dose. In CBCT, one can decide where the pivoting point or rotation axis has to be positioned, in order to get the region of interest in the centre of the scan volume. Some CBCT manufacturers allow for the field of view, or the size of the volume that is scanned, to be changed. Ideally the field of view should be as close as possible to the area of interest, in order to keep the radiation dose as low as possible to the patient. The latter implies that some machines, due to their design, do not allow the field of view to be altered, and therefore might be covering much more volume than they should. Besides the field of view, CBCT manufacturers have autonomy regarding the design of the machine. There are machines that have a chair fixed to the machine (e.g. Morita® Accuitomo 170) and there are machines that have no chair (e.g. Planmeca® 3D Max). The latter usually allows for patients to either stand, or sit on a stool, or sit in a wheelchair for the exposure. It is obvious that the wheelchair should not interfere with the machine. In machines with a chair, the patient will be moved to the correct position for the axis of rotation to fall through the centre of the region of interest. In machines that have no chair attached to their frame, the C-arm manoeuvres around the patient's head to ensure the correct position of the rotation axis. The resulting images from both machines are similar though. The image resolution has to be decided before the patient is exposed and has to be justified for the purpose. One has to bear in mind that the higher the resolution, the higher the radiation dose will be, as the exposure time will increase. This has to be balanced with the goal of the study. A high resolution (e.g. 76 µm) is indicated for endodontic purposes, while a lower resolution (e.g. 200 µm) would suffice for root resorptions or eruption issue cases. With regard to the rotation arc, it deserves to be mentioned that some manufacturers allow it to be altered, for instance from 360° to 180° rotation. This reduces the radiation dose with approximately 50%, without affecting the image quality significantly [5, 6]. The latter should definitely be considered when imaging children. Unfortunately the soft tissue resolution of CBCT is low, and as such for soft tissue imaging this technique is not really suited, if one is interested in differentiating between soft tissue layers.

2.5.3 Multi-Slice Computed Tomography

Sir Godfrey Hounsfield invented computed tomography in 1973 and together with Dr. Cormack worked on the development of the first scanner [1, 4, 7–11]. Since then many improvements have been realized to increase image quality of these three-dimensional images, as well as patient comfort. Professor Willi Kalender is credited for his significant contributions to develop helical computed tomography. Commonly this technique is called 'CT'. It is, however, very different from the cone beam computed tomography (CBCT) that was discussed above. Multi-slice CT uses a collimated narrow fan shaped beam, which revolves several times around the patient, while on the opposite side of the patient, image detectors capture the image. The patient is simultaneously moved slow or fast through that revolving X-ray field. If done fast, the resolution will be low, as the slices will be thicker (large pitch), whereas if done slowly, the slice thickness is thinner (smaller pitch) and hence the resolution is higher (maximum 350 µm, compared to CBCT where the highest resolution today is 70 µm). However, one has to keep in mind that the higher the resolution, the higher the radiation dose will be. As these machines require the patient to lie on a table, while the table is moved into the machine's gantry, their footprint is considerable and therefore they will not be found in a dental setting. Because of the radiation dose and the need for a radiographer to obtain the images, these machines belong in hospital environments. At the writing of this chapter, the fourth generation CT scanners have been developed and are referred to as stationary-rotate geometry scanners as the X-ray tube rotates within a stationary circle of detectors. Technology allows the detectors to be arranged in a continuous circular array containing as many as forty thousand individual detectors. Whereas in the past scanning time could be substantially long (minutes), today that scanning time is merely a few seconds anymore. The latter causes less movement artefacts to be present in the image, which is a great advantage. However, the resolution of the image can be affected negatively by this fast scanning, as the patient is moved faster through the gantry. Reducing the speed would increase the resolution, but also the radiation dose. It is obvious that this is a trade-off that needs to be made for the pathology one is investigating. That decision lies with the radiologist/radiographer team and the purpose of the diagnostic investigation. MSCT is ideal for hard and soft tissue imaging and as its exposure settings and algorithms are standardized, one can obtain information about the type of tissue one is assessing. The soft tissue resolution is much better than that of CBCT and one can distinguish several tissues from one another (e.g. salivary gland versus muscle), as for the use of the so-called Hounsfield units, which allow for finer diagnosis in assessing the nature of a lesion or a tissue (e.g. haemorrhage in the brain). It is obvious that MSCT, because of its high radiation dose associated, is not an imaging modality one would order for common dental pathology, such as dentigerous cyst or radicular cyst. However, patients who suffered a severe trauma with risk of intracranial haemorrhage would benefit from being submitted for MSCT immediately after the accident, as it could save their lives. This technique is also indicated for pathology involving the jaws which invades the surrounding soft tissues (e.g. squamous cell carcinoma, osteosarcoma).

2.6 Non-ionizing Radiation Techniques

2.6.1 Magnetic Resonance Imaging

Magnetic resonance imaging (MRI) was initially called nuclear magnetic resonance (NMR), but because the public's erroneous perception that there was a connotation with nuclear energy made the medical profession change the name to MRI [1–4, 8, 9, 11]. This technique does not use ionizing radiation, but magnetism and the fact that hydrogen atoms, hence the original name nuclear imaging, can be influenced in their precession when a high magnetic field is applied. The principle is to place the patient in a very strong magnetic field (1.5 or 3.0 T), several times higher than the Earth's magnetic field (approximately $0.5\,\mu T$). This will have an effect on the hydrogen atoms (protons) in the human body, which can be considered as positively charged randomly spinning tops. These hydrogen atoms will respond to the high magnetic field and will start spinning in a particular direction and at a specific speed and with a particular magnitude. Since the hydrogen content is different per type of tissue in the body, every type of tissue will emit a different signal when the magnetic field is switched on and off. When the magnetic field is turned off, the hydrogen atoms return to their resting state. The speed of this, as just mentioned, depends on the tissue (amount of hydrogen atoms and their chemical bonds). The software translates these returns into an image of grey values, which allows for differentiation between soft tissues very well. Therefore MRI is the preferred technology to image soft tissue and soft tissue pathology. Tissues with a lot of hydrogen atoms will give a strong signal (e.g. salivary glands are bright white) and tissues with a low amount of hydrogen will result in a low signal (e.g. cortical bone is black). Both hard and soft tissue diagnosis is possible, however, the technique gets more credit for imaging soft tissues. In order to obtain the best image, several so-called sequences can be used, which result in images with differences in appearance of the tissues. In a T1 sequence, fat will give a high signal (white), while water will give a low signal (dark), whereas in a T2 sequence, water will give a high signal (white) as will fat. Some other examples of particular sequences that are used are: spin echo, fluid attenuated inversion recovery or FLAIR, short time inversion recovery or STIR and turbo spin echo or TSE. In its physical appearance the MRI machine shows some resemblance with the MSCT machine, but as explained, the technology is completely different. Caution is required when entering the MRI area in the hospital. All ferro-magnetic materials need to be banned from the room and its immediate surroundings as it would cause harm to the patients and damage the machine. Since the magnetic field in the MRI is several hundred times stronger than the earth's magnetic field ($30\,\mu T$ near the equator and $70\,\mu T$ at the poles), objects like scissors, oxygen tanks, metal carts, for instance, would be attracted into the magnet with great force. Accidents have happened and as such precaution is key when entering the zone around an MRI machine. Audible and visual warning signs are always in place to announce visitors of potential risks entering the zone. MRI in dentistry is indicated if the patient has soft tissue pathology that requires imaging (e.g. ranula, salivary gland tumour) or a temporomandibular joint disorder that affects the muscles and/or condylar disc. In the latter case MRI will enable one to visualize the disc clearly (low signal as the disc does not contain as much hydrogen atoms as muscle, for instance) in the joint space. One also has to keep in mind that MRI machines produce a banging sound (sometimes more than 95 dB, which requires ear plugs or head phones to be worn by the patient), which might be frightening and which may require some patients to be sedated. Claustrophobia is another issue as often a mask (magnetic coils) is placed over the patient's face, which again may be another reason for patients to be sedated. The high cost of the machine, the large footprint, the specialized technical support and the special requirements for the room make this piece of equipment unique and therefore highly unsuited for a dental office environment.

2.6.2   Ultrasonography

Ultrasonography or echography is another imaging modality that does not use ionizing radiation [1–4, 8, 9, 11]. However, compared to MRI, this machine is very cheap (thousands of dollars versus millions). This technique is probably best known for its application in OB/GYN medicine to visualize the unborn child in the womb. The technique uses ultrasonic waves which are generated in a piezoelectric crystal inside the so-called transducer, which not only emits but also receives the ultrasonic waves. An example of a linear and hockey stick type transducer is shown

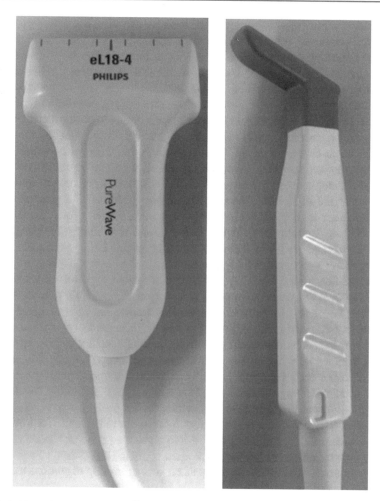

Fig. 2.2 Example of linear Philips® transducers (left-hand side is a traditional linear transducer and right-hand side is a hockey stick type transducer, which can be used intraorally on the cheek or tongue, for instance)

in Fig. 2.2. The speed of sound is affected by the compressibility of the medium (acoustic impedance), therefore it travels faster in rigid materials which are more resistant to compression and it travels slower in fluids and gases as these are more susceptible to compression. Reflection of the sound is paramount in this technique as the sound will be reflected at boundaries of tissues. Tissues or pathology that reflect little to no sound waves will produce no 'echo', hence the typical jargon hypoechoic or anechoic, respectively, whereas tissues or pathology that do reflect the sound waves will return an echo and will be identified as echoic or hyperechoic (high signal or white shadow). The particular characteristics of each of the soft tissues will enable one to distinguish between them (e.g. healthy salivary gland tissue shows a homogenously grey echo, whereas muscular tissue is hypoechoic). When the ultrasound beam hits a boundary between two materials with different acoustic impedance, some of the beam will be reflected and the remainder will be transmitted. For diagnostic imaging, an ultrasound frequency between 2 and 20 MHz (mega Hertz) is required. This is initiated inside the transducer, which is held in contact with the soft tissues. However, since air is a bad medium for sound, a so-called coupling agent (a gel or a gel pad) is required to ensure a good contact. If ultrasound is used intraorally, saliva or a gel pad will be the coupling agent. This is the principle earlier described by Sokolow in 1939, who used a water bath as coupling agent or medium. The frequency affects the travel depth or penetration of the ultrasound waves. The lower the frequency, the deeper the ultrasound will travel, while the higher the frequency, the more superficial the penetration will be. The images from the latter will, however, have a higher resolution than the former. Colour Doppler is a feature in ultrasound that allows for visualization of vascularization. That is a feature that will be useful in live image identifying pathology (e.g. hypervascularisation in a tumour) or to assess healing tissue (e.g. check blood flow after a flap or major orthognathic surgery). Variation in operators, in terms of application of amount of pressure on the patient's tissues with the transducer, will result in different images. But then again, ultrasonography does not pose any danger for the patients and can be repeated as often as needed, if one requires to check the patient again. In the field of dentistry, ultrasonography is useful in patients with, for instance, salivary gland problems (e.g. sialolith, mumps), muscular issues and hypertrophy of lymph nodes (lymphadenopathy). Since it requires special training and is not yet often used in the dental setting, this imaging modality will usually be available in specific hospital settings or private specialty clinics. The harmless character of ultrasonography and the small footprint of the modern machines (some can be plugged into a mobile phone or a tablet) and the fact that this technique allows for quick and live image assessment of soft tissues inside and outside the oral cavity make this a very promising diagnostic technique in modern oro-dental medicine.

2.7 Conclusion

The majority of imaging in dentistry is mostly covered by intraoral radiography, as this technique often provides sufficient diagnostic yield. However, in other cases where there is substantial involvement of pathology spreading within the jaws, additional imaging modalities should be used. Panoramic radiography provides a large overview of the maxillofacial complex and can provide adequate diagnostic information in several cases, though this two-dimensional imaging modality with its distortions is sometimes simply not good enough. For the latter, cone beam computed tomography, which provides three-dimensional images, may be the solution, especially if the information one is after is to be found in hard tissues, such as teeth and bone. However, if one suspects the pathology involves hard and soft tissues, a multi slice computed tomography scan is the best choice. After all, one has to balance which technique is beneficial in each individual clinical case: two-dimensional versus three-dimensional and ionizing radiation versus non-ionizing radiation. These latter techniques all use ionizing radiation, which hold potential risk for the patient to develop a fatal cancer over time (stochastic effects of ionizing radiation). At the other end of the diagnostic imaging spectrum, there are magnetic resonance imaging and ultrasonography, both techniques which are not using ionizing radiation and which also can provide three-dimensional images. However, the applicability of these techniques is quite different. While magnetic resonance imaging can also provide important information about hard tissue (e.g. bone) involvement in the pathology that is mainly occupying soft tissue, ultrasonography is a more affordable imaging modality, compared to magnetic resonance imaging, and can be used in a chairside setting in a dental office to investigate soft tissues in the head and neck region (e.g. salivary glands, tongue). Even intraoral use of ultrasonography is possible (e.g. gingiva measurements, apical bone lesions). Other imaging modalities, such as thermography and near-infrared light, certainly deserve our attention, as they may be playing a role in the future, once their accuracy has been proven for diagnosis in the head and neck region. This chapter has not addressed the cost of the equipment in detail, but it is obvious that multi slice computed tomography and magnetic resonance imaging are too expensive to be used in a dental setting, let alone their foot print which would not suite a dental office anyway.

References

1. Whaites E, Drage N. Essentials of dental radiography and radiology. Amsterdam: Elsevier; 2013. ISBN: 0702045993.
2. White SC, Pharoah MJ: Oral radiology-E-Book: principles and interpretation. Amsterdam: Elsevier; 2014. ISBN: 0323096344.
3. Haring JI, Jansen L. Dental radiography: principles and techniques London: WB Saunders; 2000. ISBN: 0721685455.
4. Aps J. Imaging in pediatric dental practice. Berlin: Springer; 2019.
5. Hoff MN, et al. Can cephalometric parameters be measured reproducibly using reduced-dose cone-beam computed tomography? J World Fed Orthod. 2019;8(2):43–50. ISSN: 2212-4438.
6. Yeung AWK, Jacobs R, Bornstein MM. Novel low-dose protocols using cone beam computed tomography in dental medicine: a review focusing on indications, limitations, and future possibilities. Clin Oral Investig. 2019;23(6):2573–81. ISSN: 1432-6981.
7. Mahesh M. MDCT physics: the basics-technology. In: Image quality and radiation dose, vol. 62. Philadelphia: Lippincott Williams & Wilkins; 2009.
8. Graham D, Cloke P, Vosper, M. Principles and applications of radiological physics. London: Churchill Livingstone; 2011. ISBN: 0702043095.
9. Armstrong P, Wastie M, Rockall AG. Diagnostic imaging. London: Wiley; 2010. ISBN: 1444391232.
10. Upton AC, Mettler FA Jr. Medical effects of ionizing radiation. Philadelphia: WB Saunders; 1995.
11. Hendee WR, Ritenour ER. MyiLibrary medical imaging physics. London: Wiley; 2002.

System Requirements for Intraoral Ultrasonic Scanning

3

Oliver D. Kripfgans and Hsun-Liang (Albert) Chan

3.1 Introduction

System requirements for any medical device are specific to the intended applications. Ultrasound comes in four or more specific applications: radiology, cardiology, OB/Gyn, and point of care. There are very specific needs to each of them, even though it is (now) possible to create a hybrid ultrasound scanner which encompasses all of the combined needs. Dental ultrasound is in its infancy and the system requirements stated here are likely to change as the field progresses and the benefits of ultrasound in dental diagnostics are better understood. Manufacturers will most likely respond first with software changes as they are cheaper and have a faster turn-around time than hardware changes. However, the spatial restrictions in the oral cavity will require ultrasound transducers with smaller scan heads, i.e. hardware changes. While buccal side scans of the frontal incisors and canine teeth are accessible when using larger transducers, lingual scans of any teeth as well as scans of posterior teeth do require a smaller transducer housing. An active dialogue will be necessary between manufacturers, researchers, and clinicians. Existing technology needs to be adapted to the specific requirements of dental ultrasound.

O. D. Kripfgans (✉)
Department of Radiology, Medical School, University of Michigan, Ann Arbor, MI, USA
e-mail: greentom@umich.edu

H.-L. (Albert) Chan
Department of Periodontics and Oral Medicine, School of Dentistry, University of Michigan, Ann Arbor, MI, USA
e-mail: hlchan@umich.edu

© Springer Nature Switzerland AG 2021
H.-L. (Albert) Chan, O. D. Kripfgans (eds.), *Dental Ultrasound in Periodontology and Implantology*, https://doi.org/10.1007/978-3-030-51288-0_3

3.2 Review of Commercial Scanning Systems

Commercial ultrasound has entered many clinical areas and has opened niches previously unknown to ultrasound, such as clinical dental imaging. Ultrasound as an imaging modality is highly dependent on electronics and real-time signal processing. The evolution of electronics has lead to greater availability of specialized real-time hardware required for ultrasound systems. Moreover, where previously many stages of complex hardware were required for transmit and receive electronics, suitable for clinical ultrasound, now minimal hardware is sufficient and software takes the place of the remaining processing steps. In part this is due to the development of faster clock-cycle CPUs and parallel processing of GPUs. Other important developments are cheaper and greater performance off-the-shelf digital to analog (DA) and analog to digital (AD) converters with low noise and large dynamic range. This allowed more companies to enter the market of commercial ultrasound and drive the development of specialized systems for diverse clinical areas and also provide more opportunities for entering niches. There are at least 21 different companies providing scanners for clinical imaging, they include (in alphabetical order): Alpinion, BK, Biosound Esaote, Butterfly Network, Canon, Chison, Edan, GE, Hitachi Aloka, Konica Minolta, Mindray, Philips, Samsung (Samsung Medison), Siemens Acuson, SIUI, SonoScape, Sonosite, SuperSonic Imagine, Terason, FUJIFILM VisualSonics, and Whale Imaging. Table 3.1 lists these companies along with the maximum frequency imaging probes that are currently available according to their official websites. Specific probe names are also listed as well as imaging applications associated with each probe.

In the following subchapters we are reviewing existing clinical scanners suitable for 2D real-time imaging at high resolution, hence we selected products from this review that reached at least a 20 MHz imaging frequency.

3.2.1 BK Medical

BK Medical offers a variety of transducers. The highest frequency found is the 20R3 (Fig. 3.1), a 3D capable probe for endocavitary (i.e., transvaginal or transrectal) and urological applications. Its frequency range extends from 3 to 20 MHz and supports B-mode scanning. Resulting 3D data can be used for distance, area, angle and volume measurements. The probe does not support pulsed-wave Doppler or color flow imaging.

3.2.2 Esaote

Esaote offers a high frequency linear array, the L8-24 (Fig. 3.2). It supports B-mode and blood flow imaging, as it is designed for small parts and vascular imaging. Its frequency range extends from 8 to 24 MHz.

Table 3.1 Review of commercial clinical ultrasound scanners

Company	Maximum frequency	Probes	Applications
Alpinion	17 MHz	L8-17X L8-17H L8-17 IO8-17 IO8-17T	Carotid, peripheral vascular, thyroid, testicle, MSK, superficial, breast, small parts
BK	20 MHz	3D 20R3	Transrectal, transvaginal, urology
Biosound Esaote	24 MHz	L8-24	Small parts, vascular
Butterfly Network	–	CMUT 2D array	General imaging
Canon	33 MHz	i33LX9	Subcutaneous imaging, superficial MSK
Chison	18 MHz	L18V	Small parts
Edan	15 MHz	L17-7HQ L17-7SQ	Small parts, MSK, nerve, and vascular
GE	22 MHz	L10-22-RS	Small parts, peripheral vascular, nerve block, musculoskeletal, and intraoperative
Hitachi Aloka	18 MHz	L64	Breast, small parts, thyroid
Konica Minolta	14 MHz	L14-6Ns	MSK, small parts
Mindray	20 MHz	L20-5	Breast, CEUS, interventional, MSK, nerve, ocular, pediatric, superficial, testicular, vascular
Philips	22 MHz	eL18-4	Small parts, micro flow imaging, elastography, and precision biopsy
Samsung	18 MHz	LA4-18B	Small parts, vascular, musculoskeletal
Siemens Acuson	17.8 MHz	18L6	Pediatric, small parts, MSK, strain elastography, contrast imaging
SIUI	–	–	General imaging
SonoScape	–	–	General imaging
Sonosite	15 MHz	HFL50x, HFL50xp	Breast, musculoskeletal, nerve
SuperSonic Imagine	18 MHz	SL18-5	Abdominal, breast, genitourinary, MSK, pediatrics, thyroid, vascular, general
SuperSonic Imagine	18 MHz	SL18-5	Abdominal, breast, genitourinary, MSK, pediatrics, thyroid, vascular, general
Terason	16 MHz	16HL7	MSK, venous
FUJIFILM VisualSonics	71 MHz	MX700	Vascular, embryology, superficial tissue, ophthalmology
Whale Imaging	–	–	General imaging

Listed are the company name, the maximum frequency if provided in their product description, the associated probe label as well as clinical target applications. All transducers are either linear or curvilinear arrays. Reviewed from companies official websites on August 20th, 2019. Dashes ('–') indicate information missing from the websites. Highlighted companies offer products with a maximum imaging frequency of 20 MHz or more

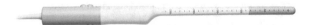

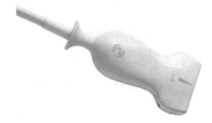

Fig. 3.1 Commercially available ultrasound probe from BK Medical with a scanning frequency of 20 MHz. The probe is designed for endocavitary and urological applications. The scanning aperture is on the far right side, pointing towards the right. Source: Corporate website [1]

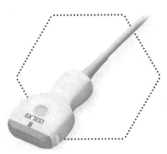

Fig. 3.2 Commercially available ultrasound probe from Esaote with a scanning frequency of 24 MHz. The probe is designed for small parts and vascular imaging. The scanning aperture is on the right side, pointing towards the bottom right. Source: Corporate website [2]

Fig. 3.3 Commercially available ultrasound probe from Canon Medical with a scanning frequency of 33 MHz. The probe is designed for subcutaneous imaging and superficial MSK applications. The scanning aperture is in the front. Source: Corporate website [3]

3.2.3   Canon

Canon Medical offers a 33 MHz ultra-high frequency linear array (i33LX9, Fig. 3.3). The probe is designed for 2D imaging and supports B-mode and blood flow imaging. The latter facilitates Canon's *superb micro-vascular imaging* (SMI) to visualize microvasculature. Subcutaneous imaging and superficial MSK are listed as clinical applications.

3.2.4   GE

GE Healthcare offers a linear array with a maximum frequency of 22 MHz (L10-22-RS, Fig. 3.4). Its range from 10 to 22 MHz is designed for use in peripheral

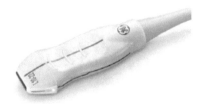

Fig. 3.4 Commercially available ultrasound probe from GE with a scanning frequency of up to 22 MHz. The probe is designed for peripheral vascular, small parts, nerve block, musculoskeletal and intraoperative applications. The scanning aperture is in the front left. Source: Website [4]

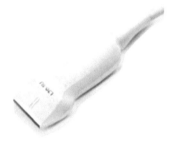

Fig. 3.5 Commercially available ultrasound probe (L20-5) from Mindray with a scanning frequency of 20 MHz. The probe is designed for MSK, nerve, small parts, and vascular imaging. The scanning aperture is in the front. Source: Corporate website [5]

vascular, small parts, nerve block, conventional/superficial musculoskeletal as well as intraoperative applications. Its footprint is 8.1×19.3 mm.

3.2.5   Mindray

Mindray offers a linear array probe (L20-5, Fig. 3.5) with up to 20 MHz imaging frequency and a field of view of 28.6 mm. Its clinical applications are MSK, nerve and small parts imaging as well as vascular imaging.

3.2.6   Philips

Philips offers a linear array probe (eL18-4, Fig. 3.6) with up to 22 MHz imaging frequency and is designed for vascular labs. It features a multi-row array which suggests good elevational slice thickness control. In addition to being capable of imaging blood flow, it is designed to image slow and weak blood flow, i.e. small phase shifts and small fractional blood volume.

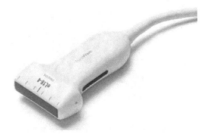

Fig. 3.6 Commercially available ultrasound probe (eL18-4) from Philips with a scanning frequency of 22 MHz. The probe is designed for vascular imaging. The scanning aperture is in the front. Source: Corporate website [6]

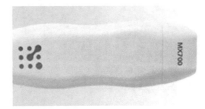

Fig. 3.7 Commercially available ultrasound probe (MX700) from FUJIFILM VisualSonics with a scanning frequency of 71 MHz. The probe is designed for vascular imaging, embryology, superficial tissue, and ophthalmology. The scanning aperture is on the right. Source: Corporate website [7]

3.2.7 FUJIFILM VisualSonics

FUJIFILM VisualSonics is known for preclinical ultrasonic imaging and offers exceptionally high frequencies. Its MX700 transducer reaches up to 71 MHz for an axial resolution of 30 µm (Fig. 3.7). Its clinical applications include vascular imaging, embryology, superficial tissue, and ophthalmology.

3.3   Medical Applications

Ultrasound application modes are usually subdivided into their physical and technical requirements onto the ultrasound scanner. For example, superficial tissues can be imaged with high frequency to obtain great spatial detail. Abdominal tissues cannot be imaged with high frequency since the long path length would for a given attenuation diminish the acoustic wave to the noise floor. Therefore it is necessary to choose a lower frequency which is adequate for the required image depth. Another parameter is the field of view. Superficial tissues rely on a large lateral aperture to create a large lateral field of view. The axial size is limited due to the superficial nature of the application. Contrary, abdominal imaging can benefit from transducers that create a sector format image, i.e. that of an phased array or of a curvilinear array.

High frequency applications have varying needs depending on the specific use of the transducer. The following sections will address the high frequency applications listed for the transducers in Sects. 3.2.1–3.2.7.

3.3.1 Transducer Geometry Specific Applications

Transrectal and transvaginal ultrasound scans allow for high frequency but require specific transducer geometries due to the spatial location of the tissues of interest. This also includes some urological scans. As seen in Fig. 3.1 the geometry is that of a transducer with an extended handle to maneuver it for endocavitary applications where the tissues of interest are only reachable by entering a body cavity with the transducer. Some of these scans can also be performed with abdominal arrays, however, in these cases only with a lower frequency due to the long path length and therefore cumulative attenuation.

3.3.2 Low Attenuation Applications

Subcutaneous, superficial, and ocular imaging benefit from typically low overall acoustic attenuation. In most cases low attenuation equals shallow image depths, i.e. for a given ultrasound probe, low attenuation tissue can be imaged to a deeper depth and shallow regions can be imaged at higher attenuation. Ocular imaging is different as the acoustic attenuation in the eye is low. The largest structure, the vitreous body consists of 98% water and has an acoustic attenuation of 0.08 dB/MHz/cm [8], i.e. little attenuation. The lens has higher acoustic attenuation (1.19 dB/MHz/cm [9]), however the lens is much shorter than the vitreous body, therefore the accumulative attenuation is less.

3.3.3 Non-Specific Applications

Some of the applications listed above are non-specific to the technical or physical requirements on the ultrasound transducer. Interventional, elastography (also known as strain imaging), contrast enhanced ultrasound (also known as CEUS), nerve, vascular, and precision biopsy do not specifically state where or what the regions of interest are and thus it is difficult to associate technical or physical requirements. Typically CEUS benefits from low rather than high frequencies since contrast agents are acoustically resonant at frequencies between 1 and 5 MHz. Nerve and vascular imaging is also non-specific, as nerves and blood vessels can be superficial or deep seated. The same reasoning holds for precision biopsy.

3.3.4 Other Applications

The eL18-4 from Philips is listed with MicroFlow imaging as a clinical application. Since the scanning frequency is up to 22 MHz, it is likely that only superficial regions can be imaged. Blood has lower acoustic backscatter than soft tissue which decreases the achievable signal to noise ratio for imaging at this high frequency. However, the backscatter of blood exponentially increases with frequency until 87 MHz [10]. Thus, there is a trade-off between the increasing acoustic attenuation between the transducer and a given blood vessel and the increasing backscatter of the red blood cells in the lumen.

Musculoskeletal ultrasound (MSK) typically benefits from high or very high ultrasound frequencies. This is however only true for superficial structures. Deep seated muscles, bones, or joints cannot be imaged at high frequencies. Breast ultrasound is similar. A 10 MHz ultrasound wave may penetrate approximately 4 cm of breast tissue. This depth can be reduced when the ultrasound beam is aberrated which is often caused by the heterogeneous structures within the breast. Higher frequencies will penetrate even less. Testicular ultrasound can be considered as a *Small Parts* application and requires little penetration depth, in, for example, the evaluation for a possible testicular torsion. Some acoustic attenuation may occur when seeking the location of an undescended testicle. Pediatric imaging allows in general higher frequencies than adult scanning simply due to the shorter path lengths in children. Neonatal imaging even allows for imaging the brain as long as the fontanelle remains open.

3.4 Ultrasound Imaging Modes

3.4.1 Harmonic Imaging

Harmonic imaging, as described in Sect. 1.3.8.1, is a concept to receive ultrasound at a frequency different from the transmit frequency. Normally ultrasound waves transmitted at f_0 are also received at f_0. If, however, the receive signal contains clutter at f_0, then an alternative strategy can be pursued. Clutter is unwanted scattered or reflected contributions to the image. Soft tissue scatters ultrasound at twice the incoming frequency ($f_0 \rightarrow 2 \times f_0$) when insonified at high enough sound pressure (typically above 0.5 MPa [11]). In this case soft tissue scattering becomes nonlinear, that means that the tissue does not scatter a signal twice as large when the incoming sound pressure is twice as large. Instead it scatters also signals at harmonics of the incoming signal, i.e. $n \times f_0$ for $n = 2, 3, 4, \dots$. Figure 3.8 illustrates this imaging mode. In addition, Fig. 3.9 shows example images for two fundamental frequencies, i.e. 12 and 24 MHz, as well as three types of harmonic modes, H24, CH24, and SH24. Mode "H" uses a single harmonic frequency, whereas "CH" uses a combination of fundamental and harmonic frequencies. Mode "SH" uses spatial harmonics.

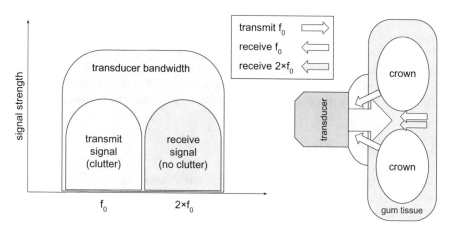

Fig. 3.8 Concept and use of harmonic imaging. Receiving ultrasound at twice the transmitted frequency is the underlying concept of harmonic imaging. It is useful when imaging structures that produce clutter signals, i.e. signals reflected from lateral structures that reflect more strongly than the intended region of interest (ROI). For example: When imaging the interdental papilla (also termed interdental gingiva) the ROI contains soft tissue

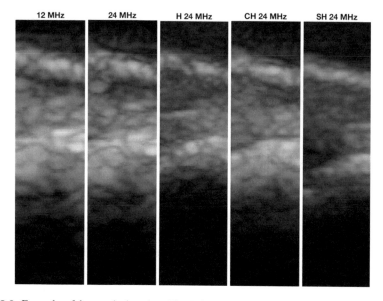

Fig. 3.9 Example of harmonic imaging. The Mindray ZS3 clinical scanner offers harmonic imaging for our L25-8 prototype transducer, namely: H—single harmonic frequency, CH—combination of fundamental and harmonic frequency, SH—spatial harmonics, otherwise one single frequency, one beam. These modes illustrate how spatial resolution and soft-tissue to hard-tissue contrast are enhanced by harmonic imaging

Typically only the second harmonic is used for imaging. This has at least two reasons. At first, the bandwidth of the transducer is limited, i.e. the range between the lowest to highest frequency that the transducer can operate at. Using the third harmonic requires a larger bandwidth than using the second harmonic. Second, the scattered signal at higher harmonics is weaker the higher the harmonics, i.e. the signal of the third harmonic is weaker than that of the second harmonic, etc.

3.4.2 Compounding

Compounding is a method by which ultrasonic imaging can minimize artifacts associated with specular reflections and speckle. Spatial compounding uses spatial features to remove artifacts. This includes scanning objects from a range of angles in the axial-lateral scan plane to include object surfaces that are non-parallel to the transducer aperture and would refract the transmit beam away from the receiving transducer aperture as illustrated in Fig. 3.10. Spatial compounding improves image quality for blood vessel and lesion delineation in medical imaging and can improve dental images where crowns, root, jaw bones, etc., are non-parallel to the transducer aperture. Frequency compounding utilizes beamforming at several center frequencies and combines the resultant images. The effect of this is the suppression of speckle related image features that then change with frequency (see examples in Fig. 3.11).

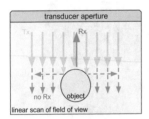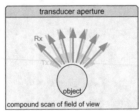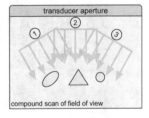

Fig. 3.10 Concept and use of spatial compound imaging. Left: In a non-compound scan, image beams are sent out parallel to each other. Those beams that impinge on a specular reflector and reflect away from the transducer are lost and leave the surface of that reflector as a hypoechoic region in the image. Middle: In a compound scan, image beams are ideally sent out at progressive angles to obtain reflections from specular reflector objects with surfaces non-parallel to the transducer aperture. Right: In reality, specular reflectors exist at various locations in the image and thus packets of parallel beams are sent out at progressive angles. Typically there are 3, 5, 7, etc., number of angles for which images are (beam-)formed and then compounded to obtain the final image. The example shows 3 angles with 5 parallel transmit beams each. In reality there are tens to hundreds of parallel transmit beams. Not necessarily transmitted concurrently but geometrically in parallel

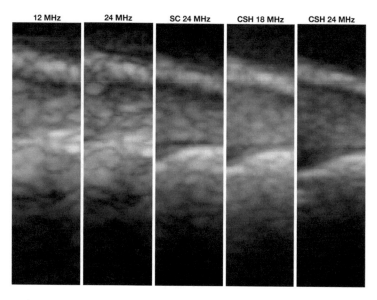

Fig. 3.11 Examples of image compounding. The Mindray ZS3 clinical scanner offers several imaging modes for our L25-8 prototype transducer, here: SC—spatial compounding, CSH—compound spatial harmonics, otherwise one single frequency, one beam. These modes illustrate how spatial resolution and soft-tissue to hard-tissue contrast are enhanced by compound imaging

3.4.3 Field of View

Image width and image depth determine the field of view. Image depth is easily changed by dialing in the desired depth on the user controls of the ultrasound scanner. However, the image depth is directly related to penetration (Sect. 1.3.5). Usually large increases in image depth require lowering the transmit frequency to warrant sufficient penetration. For a given transducer the lateral field of view is given by the size of the aperture of the array. The larger the aperture the larger the lateral field of view. Additional lateral view may be available by steering the transmit beam at the edges and thus creating a virtual convex field of view (see Fig. 3.12). Typically this yields an extra 20° on either side with more spatial gain on the distal side of the field of view as the additional space is triangular. Similar to cell phone cameras, the user may also extent the field of view by sliding the transducer array laterally across the region or object of interest and thus following a structure with a lateral size larger than the aperture.

3.4.4 Cine Loop

Ultrasound is a real-time image modality with image updates in the 10–100 Hz range, i.e. between 10 and 100 images per second. Cardiology scanners provide

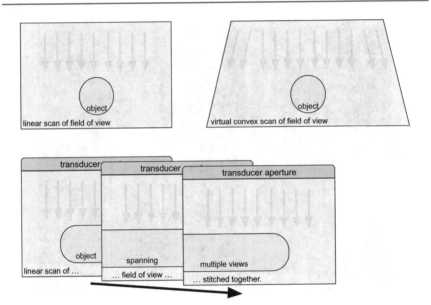

Fig. 3.12 The fundamental field of view constraints are aperture width and image depth (dictated by frequency, but user controllable). Some ultrasound scanners may allow the user to add additional lateral space by steering the left and right edge beams up to 20° and thus creating a virtual convex field of view (top-right). It may also be possible to laterally stitch images together by sliding the aperture sidewards and thereby recording an object which spans beyond the regular field of view (bottom)

the highest frame rate to follow fast moving heart valves. Radiology and OB/Gyn scanners show slower frame rates and better image quality, since slower frame rates allow for higher quality beamforming, i.e. more focal zones and higher line densities. As the name "cine loop" suggests, movie sequences can be acquired and reviewed retrospectively. Depending on the individual scanner a certain number of image frames is held in a temporary image buffer. This can be hundreds or thousands of images, which translates to several seconds or up to minutes of scanning. Upon freezing the scanning procedure, the user selects the displayed frame from the pool of available image frames from the cine loop buffer using the trackball of the keyboard. The cine loop buffer collects new images until the buffer is full. At that time the oldest image is discarded and the new current image stored. In other words, it is a first in, first out (FIFO) buffer. Some scanners flush their cine buffer, i.e. empty it, after the user unfreezes the scanning mode. Other scanners never flush the buffer even after repeated freeze–unfreeze maneuvers. For those scanners the user has to specifically trigger the flush using a dedicated key.

3.4.5 Other Imaging Features

Sonographers, cardiologists, radiologists, and other users of ultrasound scanners benefit from features that enhance workflow and aid in the diagnostic interpretation of the obtained image(s). This includes text and pictorial annotations as well as geometric measurement tools and others.

3.4.5.1 Annotations and Calipers

Annotations are used to identify lesions, masses, or other significant findings, etc. Text can be placed to describe these adjacent in the image (Fig. 3.13). Arrow can be used to point to them (Fig. 3.14). Quantitative measurement can be performed to obtain lengths, areas, volumes, angles, etc. Examples in Fig. 3.13 include an elliptical area measurement (#1) with a major axis of 0.77 cm and a minor axis of 0.70 cm. Its circumference is 2.31 cm and its area 0.42 cm^2. Distance measurements can be performed with concurrent depth information, as shown in example #2. Here the two point targets are 2.06 cm apart at a depth of 3.82 cm. A depth-only measurement is shown in example #3, showing a distance of 2.79 cm. Example #4 shows an angle measurement of 130°.

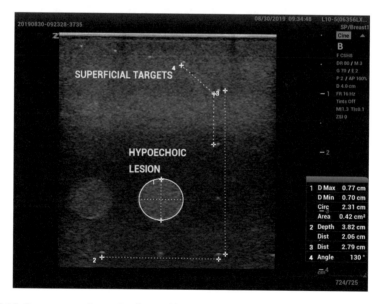

Fig. 3.13 Image annotation and calipers aid the reader when consulting images for diagnostic analysis. This image shows text annotations as well as linear, area, and angular caliper examples, that are available on this particular ultrasound scanner. These features may vary between manufacturers and models

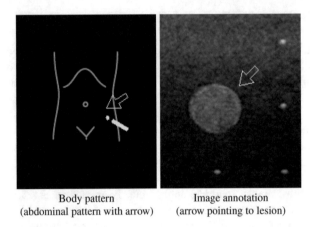

Body pattern   Image annotation
(abdominal pattern with arrow)   (arrow pointing to lesion)

Fig. 3.14 Body pattern example. Left: A selected body pattern with annotations to point to the region of interest, which was scanned and is displayed in the ultrasound image. Right: Actual ultrasound image with hyperechoic inclusion and arrow pointing to it

3.4.5.2 Body Patterns

Body patterns can be available to aid the annotation process. Depending on the selected scanner preset, here abdominal, a collection of abdominal pictograms are offered to the user. After selecting the most appropriate, additional pointers, arrows or markers can be placed on the pictogram as well as in the ultrasound image to illustrate the image site within the patient. Figure 3.14 shows an abdominal body pattern with an arrow as well as a marker on the patient's left side close to the left kidney. An arrow was also placed on the ultrasound image to point to the finding in the image (here a hyperechoic inclusion in the phantom).

3.5   Requirements for Dental Ultrasonic Imaging

Dental ultrasonic imaging is governed by the need for high spatial resolution at superficial regions of interest and a high constraints work environment. In the following sections specific requirements are reviewed and transformed into recommendations for creating an adequate imaging tool for use in dental diagnostics and follow-up.

3.5.1   B-mode Scan

Image quality is one of the most dominant features. As discussed above, frame rate is competing with image quality; however, there is no immediate need for high frame rate. High line density and possibly multiple focal zones would contribute to high spatial resolution and good signal to noise. Scan depths are typically less than 2 cm,

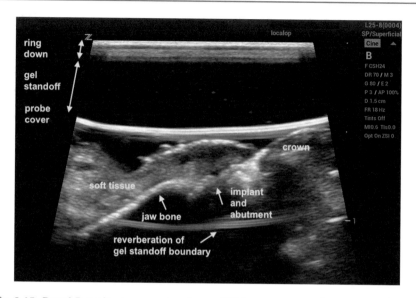

Fig. 3.15 Dental B-mode scan example using an L25-8 prototype transducer with an imaging frequency of 24 MHz. B-mode is operating in spatial harmonics compounding mode to image structures up to 1 cm depth. The hypoechoic first 5 mm are from a gel standoff pad to position the region of interest into the elevational focus of 7 mm. The strong reflection between gel pad and biological tissue is from the transducer probe cover. Ultrasound signal immediately adjacent to the aperture is called ringdown. It is caused by the finite time that the piezo crystal requires to stop vibration after it is electrically excited. At a depth of 4–5 mm one can see the strong reflection of the transducer probe cover. Beyond that is a layer of free ultrasound gel that couples to the soft- and hard-tissues in this image example. Those are gingiva and moucosa (soft-tissue) as well as jaw bone, implant/abutment, and crown (hard-tissue). A reverberation of the probe cover is seen as well and is naturally at a depth of 2 × 4–5 mm, i.e. 9 mm.

with most around 5 mm. Imaging structures at 5 mm or less is challenging as the transducer piezo crystal has a certain ringdown time that could interfere with image data and the elevational lens is set to a finite focal depth. Figure 3.15 shows the ringdown and a gel standoff that has been placed on top of the aperture to space the region of interest to the elevational focal zone of the transducer (7 mm). The strong reflection at 4–5 mm depth is from the boundaries between gel standoff pad, probe cover and ultrasound gel on the outside of the probe cover. Its duration is not insignificant (0.6 mm) for the total image depth of 1.5 cm and especially in regard to the effectively used 5 mm, i.e. from 5 to 10 mm depth.

3.5.2 Color Flow and Power Doppler Mode

Large dental blood vessels are typically on the order of 1 mm in diameter. Small blood volumes require good color flow sensitivity as the resulting power Doppler is small as well and bears low signal to noise ratio. Figure 3.16 shows an example

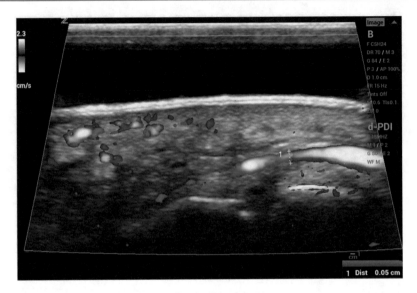

Fig. 3.16 Small lumen color flow example. Color flow is an imaging mode in which blood flow (physiology) is superimposed onto B-mode anatomy. Color flow usually indicates direction and velocity of blood flow. Direction is indicated by use of two distinct colors, such as red and blue. Velocity is indicated by the shade of the color. Note, the direction is *not* with respect to the blood lumen, but rather relative to the ultrasound probe, i.e. towards the ultrasound probe and away from it. In addition, velocity is not volumetric flow. The former is typically measured in centimeters per second and is biased by the angle between the ultrasound probe and the flow direction. This example does not encode velocity but power. Power is a measure for *how much* blood is flowing within each voxel. Bright white in this case means that the entire voxel is filled with moving blood. The wall filter will still exclude velocities too small, and aliasing occurs for velocities larger than v_{max}, here 2.3 cm/s. Note the measured lumen size of 500 μm

of directional power Doppler, i.e. traditional power Doppler, but also direction as in color flow. A minimum diameter of 500 μm is annotated on a lumen that is oriented laterally on the right image side. Several other power Doppler patches are showing. These may be noise or actual flow. A still image cannot convey this information reliably and it is the user's decision to properly exclude noise artifacts. A medium wall filter was chosen for this image. Dental imaging may show color flow or power Doppler noise when imaging molars or other difficult to reach teeth. In these cases it may be challenging to find proper support to hold the transducer still. Any motion due to lack of support will cause motion noise. This is also possible in abdominal scans and manufacturers have implemented the so-called flash artifact filters. Flash effects are moving tissue that is misinterpreted as blood flow. One way to distinguish tissue from blood is their level of echogenicity.

3.5.3   Ultrasound Transducer

Probably the most significant change towards dental ultrasound is rooted in the miniaturization of the transducer housing, as the oral cavity is challenging in terms of space and reach. The scaling may be proportional to the increase in frequency, i.e. the imaging frequency may triple and the housing may scale to ⅓ or similar. Above shown transducers reach up to 71 MHz, which is approximately 10× of that currently common. To scale transducer housings accordingly would be advantageous. However, heat dissipation of high frequency in small environments may be an issue.

3.5.3.1 Ergonomic Design and Size

A compact design transducer prototype is shown in Fig. 3.17. Its dimensions are comparable to that of a toothbrush and its cable runs perpendicular to the aperture allowing for sagittal scans even for second molars. The maximal transducer thickness is 15 mm. Its width is 17.2 mm and its length 30 mm. The latter is not a constraint as it provides space to actually hold the transducer with one's fingers. The aperture is approximately 13 mm wide, which allows for a sufficiently large lateral field of view (see Fig. 3.15) encompassing the gingiva, implant, abutment, and lower portion of the crown. The virtual convex image mode further increases the lateral width with axial depth.

3.5.3.2 Transducer Frequency

Oral tissues are commonly very shallow. As stated above, 5 mm image depths are often sufficient. However, in some situations, larger image depths are required. For those a lower frequency may be needed to allow for sufficient penetration. This includes imaging of the tongue, where a tissue path of up to 6 cm may be

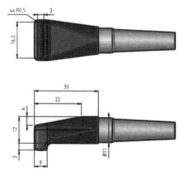
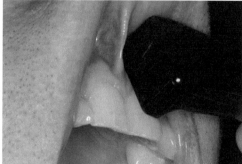

Fig. 3.17 Left: CAD drawings of prototype ultrasound probe for use on commercial clinical scanner (Mindray ZS3). Right: Photo of an in vivo scan. Note the probe geometry shown here. The transmitting and receiving surface of the probe, i.e. the aperture is transverse with respect to the probe cable. This allows the probe to enter into the oral cavity to reach the molars, where cable is required to run parallel to the tooth line to exit the mouth

encountered. The authors use a prototype imaging transducer at 24 MHz, which for a speed of sound of 1540 m/s, corresponds to 64 µm wavelength. Anatomically this is a competitive resolution when compared to CBCT, which is on the order of 100–200 µm. However, imaging at 71 MHz would yield 21.7 µm axial and lateral resolution which is becoming competitive with histology and more likely able to differentiate between soft tissue cell types. Overall, the transmit frequencies are likely going to continually increase with time as product development progresses, thus yielding better images. While penetration will diminish with increasing frequency, the trade-off is in favor for dental imaging with shallow image depths. Current systems already provide spatial resolution that is of immediate benefit for diagnostics.

3.5.3.3 Coupling System

Ultrasound requires gel for proper sound propagation. Any air pockets along the path will cause artifacts that may or may not hinder diagnostic use. Figure 3.18 demonstrates how an entrapped air pocket (or bubble) can cause an acoustic shadow in its distal region. To distinguish from actual hypoechoic tissue, the user would try to push the entrapped air bubble out. A gel standoff pad can be used to place regions of interest in the elevational focus of the transducer (see Fig. 3.19). While traditional contact scanning may handle sparse inclusion of air bubbles, dental ultrasound will most likely not. Traditional contact scanning makes a solid connection between the

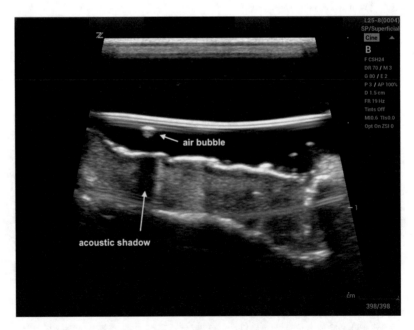

Fig. 3.18 Example for an air bubble inclusion in the acoustic path as well as the resulting acoustic shadow. The hypoechoic region past the air bubble could be hypoechoic tissue but is most likely a shadow artifact of the air bubble

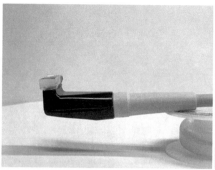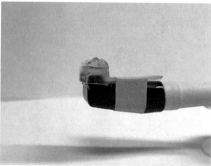

Fig. 3.19 Gel standoff for imaging superficial structures. Left: Transducer array from Fig. 3.17 with standoff pad as used in Fig. 3.15. Right: A 3D printed holder for securing the standoff pad to the aperture and preventing lateral or elevational slipping. The holder acts as a collar between the aperture of the transducer and the gel block (pad). For clinical scan an additional sheath is placed over the transducer as shown on the right to act as a barrier for infection transmission

transducer aperture and the skin. Any air inclusions will be removed by applying pressure from the transducer aperture to the skin. In dental ultrasound the aperture does not push against a flat surface. It is, therefore, possible that air inclusions will be trapped in the uneven surface morphology of the gum tissue, roots, or crowns, etc. Gel viscosity may also be important to prevent gel running from the transducer when angled in the oral cavity.

3.5.4 Imaging Features

3.5.4.1 Presets
Presets are essential for ultrasonic imaging as they lower the overhead of adjusting individual imaging parameters including frequency, image depth, gain setting, advanced imaging modes, color flow filter settings, etc. Besides being a time-saver, presets also prevent setup errors and set a safe imaging environment. Fetal or orbital ultrasound, for example, have presets with lowered acoustic output. Annotations also change with presets and are discussed next.

3.5.4.2 Annotations
Annotations need to be modified to include dental terminology. Such must encompass spatial terminology, landmarks, as well as diagnostic and pathologic keywords. Table 3.2 provides an overview of a minimal set of dental terminology.

3.5.4.3 Calipers
Calipers as available in the example shown in Fig. 3.13 set an adequate basis for dental imaging. Length, angle, and area measurements are essential for diagnostic annotations.

Table 3.2 Listing of desired labels for annotation of dental ultrasound images

Reference	Label
Spatial locations with respect to oral cavity	Midfacial, Mesial, Distal, Transverse, Epical, Buccal, Lingual, Mandibular, Maxillary
Oral cavity reference landmarks and soft and hard tissues	Crown, Root, Jaw, Mucosa, Implant, Abutment
Diagnostics and pathology	Baseline, Inflammation, Recession, Bone graft

Current labeling does not include a comprehensive set of annotations for dental applications

3.5.4.4 Registration

Multimodality image registration would be an excellent feature. Similar to existing ultrasound to CT or MRI registration would be ultrasound to cone beam CT (CBCT) and X-ray registration. CBCT and X-ray are the gold standard for dental imaging. Relating ultrasound findings spatially to existing or subsequent X-ray images would enhance the usability and acceptance of ultrasound into the field of dentistry.

References

1. Web page. https://www.bkmedical.com/transducers/?product=flex-focus
2. Web page (2020). https://us.medical.canon/products/ultrasound/aplio-i-series
3. Web page. https://pdfslide.net/documents/new-logiq-e-ultrasound-system-ge-mediadocumentscanadaproducts-gehealthcarecom.html
4. Web page (2020). https://www.esaote.com/en-US/ultrasound/probes/
5. Web page (2020). https://www2.mindraynorthamerica.com/Resona7-transducer-family-pdf
6. Web page (2020). https://www.usa.philips.com/healthcare/resources/feature-detail/ultrasound-el18-4-vascular
7. Web page (2020). https://www.visualsonics.com/product/transducers/mx-series-transducers
8. De Korte CL, Van Der Steen AFW, Thijssen JM. Acoustic velocity and attenuation of eye tissues at 20 MHz. Ultrasound Med Biol. 1994;20(5):471–80. ISSN: 0301-5629
9. Chivers RC, Round WH, Zieniuk JK. Investigation of ultrasound axially traversing the human eye. Ultrasound Med Biol. 1984;10(2):173–88. ISSN: 0301-5629
10. Save'ry D, Cloutier G. High-frequency ultrasound backscattering by blood: analytical and semianalytical models of the erythrocyte cross section. J Acoust Soc Am. 2007;121(6):3963–71. ISSN: 0001-4966
11. Anvari A, Forsberg F, Samir AE. A primer on the physical principles of tissue harmonic imaging. Radiographics 2015;35(7):1955–64

Current Digital Workflow for Implant Therapy: Advantages and Limitations

4

Rafael Siqueira, Fabiana Soki, and Hsun-Liang (Albert) Chan

4.1 Introduction

Digital technologies have been substantially incorporated into contemporary dentistry in the last decade to enhance the overall performance of dental treatment as it provides multiple advantages to aid in diagnosis, treatment planning, and procedure execution. The communication between clinicians, patients, and technicians has become more efficient with their introduction. The digital workflow is a sequential, predictable combination of data that permits the creation of three-dimensional (3D) structures and its final production with the desired material (Fig. 4.1). The initial stage is digital image acquisition, which can be from extra-oral, e.g., cone beam computed tomography (CBCT), a laboratory scanner, or intraoral means, e.g., an intraoral scanner (IOS). The introduction of IOS enables clinicians to obtain and store digital data of the surfaces of teeth and surrounding soft tissues in a reasonable time frame. Subsequent steps are usually referred as computer-aided design (CAD) and computer-aided manufacturing (CAM) (CAD-CAM) [1, 2]. This chapter is dedicated to discussing the concept of the digital workflow with emphasis on CBCT, IOS, and 3D-printing principles, accuracy, and their limitations.

4.2 CBCT in Implant Therapy

CBCT volumetric data provides three-dimensional (3D) radiographic imaging and became a valuable technology for the improvement of oral and maxillofacial diagnosis. Rapid technology development since the introduction of CBCT into the dental field resulted in the accessibility and spread of the 3D imaging to the

R. Siqueira (✉) · F. Soki · H.-L. (Albert) Chan
Department of Periodontics and Oral Medicine, School of Dentistry, University of Michigan, Ann Arbor, MI, USA
e-mail: rafasiq@umich.edu; fabisoki@umich.edu; hlchan@umich.edu

© Springer Nature Switzerland AG 2021
H.-L. (Albert) Chan, O. D. Kripfgans (eds.), *Dental Ultrasound in Periodontology and Implantology*, https://doi.org/10.1007/978-3-030-51288-0_4

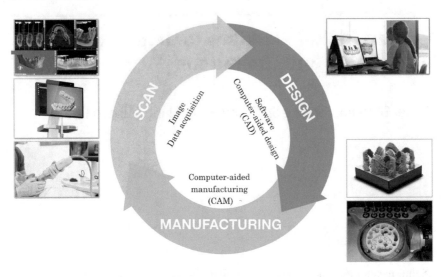

Fig. 4.1 The essential principle of digital workflow is based on three components: data acquisition, computer-aided design (CAD) software, and manufacturing of structures with the desired material through computer-aided manufacturing (CAM)

routine uses of dental practices. Currently, more than 85 different CBCT models are available with a variety of capabilities including multi-model systems with combined two dimensional (2D, panoramic and cephalometric) and 3D CBCT imaging, and less expensive panoramic units with limited 3D field of views. CBCT volumetric data is generated by a cone beam shaped X-ray that rotates with a reciprocating area detector around a fixed center which is the patient's region of interest (ROI). During the rotation, a series of sequential exposures are performed and multiple sequential planar projections are recorded into 2D individual planar images, constituting the raw primary data (basis, frame, or raw images). Software advanced algorithms transform the multiple raw data into a volumetric data set that can generate reconstructed images in the three orthogonal planes (axial, sagittal, and coronal). Generally, one rotational scan is sufficient to acquire enough data for volumetric reconstruction and the scan acquisition times are fast ranging from 5 to 30 s. Among many applications of CBCT imaging in oral and maxillofacial field, implant dentistry has been an area of great impact and the applications of CBCT has greatly expanded for not only the diagnostic, treatment planning, and post-surgical assessments but for advancement in areas where CBCT incorporates the digital workflow from the production of biomodels and surgical guides to surgical guidance assistance.

4.2.1 CBCT and Radiation Doses

Considerations in patient selection criteria and radiation effective doses are imperative for the correct prescription of CBCT imaging, given the higher radiation doses compared to other dental radiograph procedures. Based on the ALARA ("as low as reasonably achievable") principles, CBCT should be used as an adjunctive image modality when 2D radiographs are not sufficient to provide the information for the diagnosis and treatment of the patients and the potential benefits exceed and justify the individual detriment that radiation exposure may cause [3]. The American Academy of Oral and Maxillofacial Radiology (AAOMR), the American Dental Association ADA), and numerous consensus panels in implantology provide guidelines on the clinical applications, adequate prescription, radiation safety, and interpretation of CBCT imaging [4–6]. Given the great number and variety of commercially available CBCT units, a wide range of effective doses are present, based on the different FOV selections and CBCT units [7–10]. Approximately estimated values are provided in Table 4.1. Comparison with background radiation (approximately 8 μS/day) or with commonly used 2D radiographs: 4 posterior bitewings with effective doses of approximately 5 μS, Panoramic radiograph that ranges from 3 to 24 μS and a Full-Mouth series (~34 μS with rectangular collimator to ~170 μS with a round collimator) may be used as references to the different doses of CBCT units. Therefore, increased radiation doses in CBCT scan compared to some types of dental radiographs should be considered. However, the advantages of significantly lower radiation doses in CBCT imaging are greatly appreciated in comparison with a Multi-detector CT scan that has approximately 1000−2000 μS effective dose. It is important to understand that clinical parameters during image acquisition and machine parameters and protocol will affect both image quality and patient radiation dose. Optimal patient stabilization, use of coordinated pulsing X-ray generators and detectors, doses optimizations based on the patient size and diagnostic task, types of detectors, determination of the FOV or scan volume based on the patient's needs will reduce exposure, minimize scatter radiation, and increase the image quality.

Table 4.1 Effective dose range estimates in dental CBCT in adults and children at different field of views (FOV)

	Size of field of view (FOV)	Effective doses
Adult	Small FOV	5–652 μS
	Medium FOV	9–560 μS
	Large FOV	46–1073 μS
Child	Small FOV	7–521 μS
	Medium-large FOV	13–769

Adapted from Rios et al. [11]. μS—Microsievert

4.2.2   Advantages and Limitations of CBCT

Advanced technology in CBCT and software development not only improved the image quality with high-resolution scans but also optimized and facilitated the commercialization and availability of the CBCT units to the dental offices. In implant dentistry, it is well-established the benefits of multiplanar reformatting capacity in CBCT. Given the anatomic curvature present within the maxillary and mandibular arches, the basic orthogonal planes do not provide accurate visualization of the available buccolingual bone dimensions. Therefore, it is necessary that curved planar reformatting is performed based on the curvature of the maxillary or mandibular arches. Generation of specific multiplanar reconstructions in curved arches and cross-sectional views that are perpendicular to the potential implant site is imperative for accurate linear bone measurement of the available alveolar ridge height and width. Other advantages of CBCT are the high spatial resolution and relatively lower radiation doses when compared to Multi-Slice CT scans.

One of the biggest limitations of CBCT in imaging diagnosis is the poor soft tissue contrast that limits accurate visualization of soft tissue structures such as salivary glands, muscles, neurovascular structures, as well as soft tissue pathologies. Poor soft tissue contrast also hinders potential soft tissue integration in presurgical implant planning. Another limitation of the CBCT modality is limited bone density measurement as the lack of standardized measurements and inconsistent HU values are challenging. The presence of beam hardening and volume averaging artifacts around implants and metallic restorations have a significant impact on implant dentistry. These artifacts prevent and limit the visualization and accurate diagnosis of bone quality and quantity within the peri-implant areas. These limitations are significant for the post-surgical evaluation of areas surrounding implants: the evaluation of peri-implantitis and bone loss, the assessment of thin buccal or lingual bone quantity for possible dehiscence or fenestration of the implant. Moreover, the presence of artifacts degrades image quality that may affect the digital workflow and image fusion of CBCT with other digital modalities such as extra-oral facial or intraoral optical data. A summary of the advantages and limitations of CBCT is shown in Table 4.2.

4.2.3   Applications of CBCT for Diagnosis and Treatment Planning

Recommendations for the applications of radiography and CBCT imaging for dental implant patient are detailed below by the position statement of the American Academy of Oral and Maxillofacial Radiology, Table 4.3 [11]:

Basic principles in radiology should be applied in imaging for implant evaluations. The clinician should have appropriate training in operating the CBCT unit and have competency interpreting the 3D images. Knowledge of the normal anatomy of the oral and maxillofacial complex, the capability of identifying anatomic variations, abnormalities, and potential pathologies within the scan are

Table 4.2 Advantages and limitations of CBCT

Advantages	Limitations
Size and cost—the availability to dental offices	Poor soft tissue contrast
Multiplanar reconstruction	Image noise
Short time for data acquisition	Limited bone density measurement (HU)
High spatial resolution	Beam hardening artifacts created by metal
Relatively low radiation dose (compared with MDCT)	Increased radiation dose compared with 2D radiographs-dependent on CBCT unit and FOV selection
Virtual and interactive treatment planning	Technique sensitive to motion
Reliable linear and volumetric measurements	

responsibilities expected from the professional who ordered the scans [2]. The selection of appropriate FOV should be based on the patient's selection criteria. Nevertheless, it is important to consider that the bigger the FOV the more likelihood of having incidental findings due to more anatomical structures included within the volume. The practitioner is responsible for interpreting the entire volume captured and is liable for any missed diagnosis. Consultation with a qualified oral maxillofacial or medical radiologist should be considered if the practitioner is not familiar or is not willing to accept the responsibilities to review the entire CBCT volume.

CBCT data is exported in a medical diagnostic standard imaging format called Digital Imaging and Communications in Medicine (DICOM) file. DICOM files can be imported into third-party application-specific software, providing visualization and virtual simulations of the volumetric data for treatment planning and diagnosis. Several software programs are available for task-specific applications. The clinician should be comfortable in 3D diagnosis and become familiar with the available software applications for image interpretation and interactive treatment planning.

4.2.4 Anatomic Considerations in Implant Planning

CBCT imaging is a great diagnostic tool in implant planning to exclude the presence of incidental findings such as pathology, foreign bodies, and bone defects in the specific implant area or adjacent surrounding structures. For that, the clinician should be familiar with the normal oral and maxillofacial anatomy and be able to identify possible anatomy variants and predict future complications that may influence in the planning for the implant placement. Different minimal space requirements are necessary for safe implant placement, with at least 1.5 mm of a distance of the implant to an adjacent tooth, at least 3 mm of distance from the implant to an adjacent implant, and at least 2 mm of buffer space to vital anatomic structures such as the Inferior alveolar canal (Table 4.4).

Table **4.3** Recommendations for CBCT use in implant surgery per the position statement of the American Academy of Oral and Maxillofacial Radiology [12]

Recommendation 1	Panoramic radiography should be used as the imaging modality of choice in the initial evaluation of the dental implant patient
Recommendation 2	Use intraoral periapical radiography to supplement the preliminary information from panoramic radiography
Recommendation 3	Do not use cross-sectional imaging, including CBCT, as an initial diagnostic imaging examination
Recommendation 4	The radiographic examination of any potential implant site should include cross-sectional imaging orthogonal to the site of interest. This reaffirms the previously stated position of the AAOMR
Recommendation 5	CBCT should be considered as the imaging modality of choice for preoperative cross-sectional imaging of potential implant sites
Recommendation 6	CBCT should be considered when clinical conditions indicate a need for augmentation procedures or site development before placement of dental implants: (1) sinus augmentation, (2) block or particulate bone grafting, (3) ramus or symphysis grafting, (4) assessment of impacted teeth in the field of interest, and (5) evaluation of prior traumatic injury
Recommendation 7	CBCT imaging should be considered if bone reconstruction and augmentation procedures (e.g., ridge preservation or bone grafting) have been performed to treat bone volume deficiencies before implant placement
Recommendation 8	In the absence of clinical signs or symptoms, use intraoral periapical radiography for the postoperative assessment of implants. Panoramic radiographs may be indicated for more extensive implant therapy cases
Recommendation 9	Use cross-sectional imaging (particularly CBCT) immediately postoperatively only if the patient presents with implant mobility or altered sensation, especially if the fixture is in the posterior mandible
Recommendation 10	Do not use CBCT imaging for periodic review of clinically asymptomatic implants. Finally, implant failure, owing to either biological or mechanical causes, requires a complete assessment to characterize the existing defect, plan for surgical removal and corrective procedures, such as ridge preservation or bone augmentation, and identify the effect of surgery or the defect on adjacent structures
Recommendation 11	Cross-sectional imaging, optimally CBCT, should be considered if implant retrieval is anticipated

4.2.4.1 Anterior Maxilla

A common limitation in the anterior maxilla is buccal bone atrophy and associated prominent buccal concavity resulting in a limited residual ridge. Anatomic structures that should be evaluated within the anterior maxilla are the floor of the nasal cavity, evaluation of the morphology, and size of the nasopalatine canals and incisal foramen that may limit the available bone width depending on the size, location, and the overall trajectory of the canals [9].

Table 4.4 Minimal distances from implant to adjacent structures and anatomic considerations for implant planning

Anatomical structure	Consideration
Implant distance to adjacent teeth	At least 1.5 mm
Implant distance adjacent implant	At least 3 mm
Implant distance to vital anatomic structures	At least 2 mm
Anterior maxilla	Floor of the nasal cavity
	Prominent buccal concavity and limited residual ridge
	Variable width of nasopalatine canals
Posterior maxilla	Sinus pneumatization
	Antral septa
	Sinus disease
	Prominent posterior superior alveolar artery
Anterior mandible	Prominent buccal concavity and limited residual ridge
	Anterior loop and mandibular incisive canal
	Mental foramen
	Lingual canal
Posterior mandible	Mental foramen
	Inferior alveolar canal
	Lingual inclined alveolar ridge and lingual undercut

4.2.4.2 Posterior Maxilla

The sinus floor position and morphology are important anatomic structures within the posterior maxilla. The sinus floor is a limiting factor for the available bone height, especially in cases of severe pneumatization and the presence of antral septum that may result in the variability of height measurements (Fig. 4.2). It is important to identify any potential inflammatory sinus disease such as sinusitis, or prominent neurovascular canals when sinus lift procedure is planned (Fig. 4.3). Recommendation for further evaluation by an otorhinolaryngologist is suggested in case the pathology of sinuses is identified prior to implant-related surgical procedures [13].

4.2.4.3 Anterior Mandible

Buccal concavity and limited residual ridges are also limitations for available bone height and width in the anterior mandible. The identification of prominent neurovascular structures within the anterior mandible that includes the presence of mandibular incisive foramen, prominent lingual canal, mental foramen position, and the possibility of the anterior loop is valuable to predict possible neurovascular damage and exacerbated bleeding [14] (Fig. 4.4).

4.2.4.4 Posterior Mandible

The inferior alveolar canal may be the reference for available bone height measurements in the posterior mandible. Visualization of the inferior alveolar canal cortices

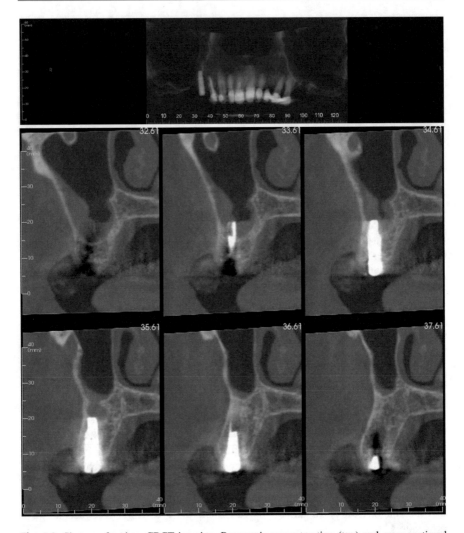

Fig. 4.2 Sinus perforation. CBCT imaging: Panoramic reconstruction (top) and cross-sectional reconstructions (bottom) of the right maxillary sinus show sinus perforation by implant at the edentulous site #4. Associated mucosal thickening is noted along with the implant and the sinus floor

may not be very clear in some patients and caution should be considered to avoid nerve damage. The mental foramen is usually positioned within the premolars sites and limits the available height and width depending on the foramen morphology. The posterior mandible also may present anatomical limitations when the alveolar crest has lingual inclination or in cases where there is a prominent submandibular gland depression resulting in a prominent lingual undercut. These may limit the available bone height and width and affect the position of the potential implant towards the lingual plate. Caution to not perforate the lingual cortex in the areas of lingual undercut should be considered [15–17] (Fig. 4.5).

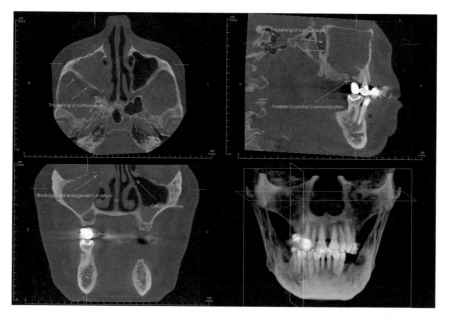

Fig. 4.3 Maxillary sinus disease. CBCT image in axial (top left), sagittal (top right), coronal (bottom left), and volume rendering reconstruction (bottom right). The right maxillary sinus is completely filled and the ostiomeatal complex is obstructed (coronal view). There is a surgical defect with likely oroantral communication in the edentulous site of #4. The right maxillary sinus also has soft tissue density along the floor, but the ostiomeatal complex is patent

4.2.5   Assessment of Bone Quality

Quality of bone is crucial for successful implant treatment providing ideally primary stability and conducive osseointegration. Because of a lack of reliable and consistent bone density measuring capabilities in CBCT owing the geometric beam shape, increased scatter radiation, lower contrast resolution, and lack of standardization among CBCT units [18, 19], radiographic validation of the bone quality for implant planning is based on subjective radiological observations of the cortical thickness and trabeculation density and appearance. Significant research advancement warrants promise in the areas for the quantitative CBCT method that would allow structural and quantitative bone analysis [20, 21]. Beneficial outcomes of bone assessment include presurgical assessment of bone quality, especially considering vascularization potential for conducive osseointegration [22]. Additional research is needed for further technology development in this area.

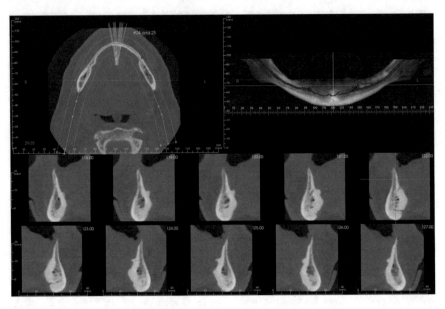

Fig. 4.4 Anterior mandibular anatomic challenges. CBCT image in axial (top left), reconstructed panoramic (top right) with tracing of Inferior alveolar canal (red lines) and multiple cross-sections (bottom). There is significant buccolingual bone atrophy with limited alveolar bone width. IAC tracing was performed showing anterior loop and extension of the mandibular incisive canal and lingual canal

4.2.6   Computer-Guided Implant Planning

CBCT permits reliable and consistent evaluation of the bone to determine suitability for implant placement, thickness of the cortical plate, quality of the bone trabeculation, anatomical characterization of the bone morphology as well as the relationship with the surrounding anatomical structures. Technology advances in CBCT resulted in a shift of treatment planning from a surgical driven approach based on the availability of bone that would dictate the implant positioning to a prosthetically driven approach, where final results based on functionality and aesthetics are great considerations for surgical decision and implant positioning [23].

There are numerous specialized software available for implant treatment planning. The software will provide an implant library with a variety of commercially available implants, with different sizes and dimensions, as well as customized corresponding overlays for ideal virtual implant placement and prosthetic rehabilitation. Optimal virtual implant planning is achieved by implant parallelism, considering individual anatomy, prosthetic functionality, and aesthetics. Therefore, CBCT volumetric imaging provides information on bone availability and anatomy, angulation of the implant relative to adjacent teeth, and available distance to key structures. Moreover, virtual implant planning assesses the needs for bone augmentation and the suitable timing of the augmentation if it can be accomplished

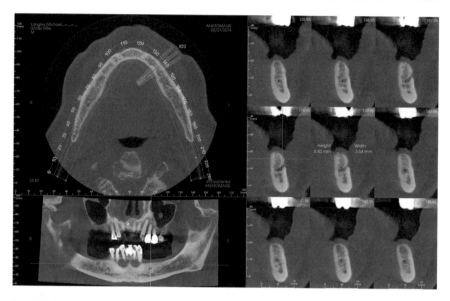

Fig. 4.5 Posterior mandibular anatomic challenges. CBCT image in axial (top left), slice panoramic view (bottom left) and cross-sections (right). Cross-sections shows limited bone height in the edentulous area of #20, where mental foramen is positioned

during implant placement or prior to. Possibility of combining the virtual planning with other technology with CAD/CAM -design surgical guide fabrication, intraoral scans, and computer-guided dental implant placement is a great quality of multiple 3D assets. The limitations with virtual implant planning are the need for transferring of data from presurgical planning to surgery. This is a multistep approach, which requires CBCT data acquisition, image interpretation, volume segmentation for preparation of models, surgical guides, registration of 3D impression scan on top of the 3D model so that it can lastly be transferred into a surgical setting. Therefore, minimizing errors in each step to avoid discrepancies from the virtual planning to the implant surgery is crucial for a successful virtual treatment planning and execution [24]. Optimization of the CBCT scan acquisition for better resolution and image quality will be key for a successful surgery outcome [25]. Box 1 lists CBCT image acquisition considerations for image optimization.

Box 1 Clinical suggestions for optimal CBCT acquisition when virtual planning is indicated

- Select the smallest FOV possible to avoid the inclusion of unnecessary areas that may contain metallic restorations.
- Minimize the presence of artifacts.

(continued)

- Minimize patient movement.
- Selection of optimal scanning resolution to control the noise and artifacts
- Confirm perfect occlusal/ridge fit when images are acquired with radiographic scanning templates.
- Separation of upper and lower jaws is recommended when bone segmentation is necessary
- Utilize cotton rolls to separate the cheek and lips when visualization of the gingiva outline at the facial site is necessary.

4.2.7   CBCT and Post-Surgical Evaluation

Two-dimensional periapical radiographs are still the recommended image modality for post-surgical evaluation of implant placement assessment and osseointegration evaluation. Bitewings may be used during the prosthetic phase when implant abutment and restoration fit confirmation are necessary, as well as adequate bone level evaluation. CBCT images application for post-surgical evaluation are indicated for the assessment of bone graft healing and morphology, or when clinical complications are suspected, such as neurovascular damage, incorrect implant placement or intrusion into the sinus, or obvious perforation of bone plates. CBCT also may be a useful resource for evaluation of alveolar dimension changes during the post-surgery healing time. CBCT limitations from metal-derived artifacts such as beam hardening and volume averaging result in darkening, overestimation of implant width, and equivocal bone-implant interface. Therefore, CBCT imaging may not be reliable when bone loss and peri-implantitis are considered. A similar problem occurs when thin bone cortication is present surrounding the implant or dehiscence is considered. Visualization and accuracy of bone content are challenging in areas surrounding implant and metallic restorations. Ongoing research is being done to reduce or overcome metal-derived artifacts in CBCT imaging [23, 26–28]. Metal artifact reduction (MAR) correction algorithms are being implemented in commercially available machines and have potential improvement of image quality with artifact reduction. However, more research is warranted for the evaluation of the effectiveness of technology development and implementation in this area, especially considering the great variability and inconsistencies of parameters among the different CBCT units.

4.3   Digital Workflow for Implant Therapy

The implementation of digital technologies in implant dentistry goes beyond the fascinating computerized world and should be focused in what the technology can offer by simplifying the workflow and improving patient satisfaction. Therefore, the digital workflow can be adapted to user preference and logistics, and different levels

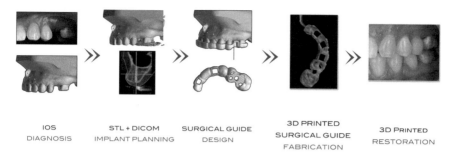

IOS
DIAGNOSIS

STL + DICOM
IMPLANT PLANNING

SURGICAL GUIDE
DESIGN

3D PRINTED
SURGICAL GUIDE
FABRICATION

3D PRINTED
RESTORATION

Fig. 4.6 An example of the complete digital workflow: from the treatment planning phase to surgical phase and prosthetic rehabilitation

of implementation can be achieved with the interchangeable combinations with analogue steps. The digital workflow for implant surgery can be either fully digital (direct acquisition of the virtual image from the oral cavity with an IOS device) or partially-digital (digitalization of a dental stone cast with an IOS or extra-oral scanner device, commonly referred as a bench or laboratory scanner). The acquired imaging data is then outputted in .STL (an abbreviation of "stereolithography" or backronyms such as "Standard Triangle Language" and "Standard Tessellation Language") file (Fig. 4.6). The .STL file is combined with the .DICOM (Digital Imaging and Communications in Medicine data) CBCT file in a treatment planning software for a computer-guided surgery (CGS). With the software, the implants can be virtually placed and surgical guides can be designed and exported in .STL files that will be utilized for milling or 3D printing fabrication. Further details regarding techniques and materials for implant surgery will be discussed in this chapter.

4.3.1 Intraoral Digital Acquisition

Intraoral scanners (IOS) are devices for capturing non-contact digital impressions through projection of a light source (laser, or more recently, structured light) onto the object to be scanned, in this case the intraoral structures. Dental and gingival tissue surfaces captured by the imaging sensors are processed by the scanning software, which generates point clouds that will be then triangulated by the same software, creating a three-dimensional (3D) surface model (mesh). Intraoral digital scanners allow clinicians to record the surface of the teeth, implant scan bodies, and surrounding soft tissues in 3D. The images enable clinicians with instant visualization and evaluation of the structure of interest, and seamless communication with the laboratory personnel. They can also be exported to a 3D-printer, or a chairside milling unit for prosthesis manufacturing [29–31]. Intraoral digital impression has progressed beyond single tooth preparations and quadrants scanning to full-arch scanning with more user-friendly features in the past few years (Fig. 4.7).

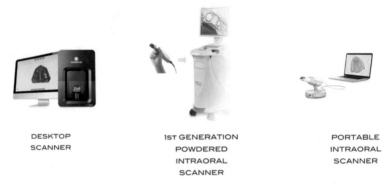

DESKTOP SCANNER	1ST GENERATION POWDERED INTRAORAL SCANNER	PORTABLE INTRAORAL SCANNER
Shining 3D scanner source: https://www.3dnatives.com	Cerec Bluecam, Dentsply Sirona http://www.sunshinedentalcare.com/cerec	Trios intraoral scanner, 3shape https://bitemagazine.com.au

Fig. 4.7 The different generations of scanners utilized in dentistry. The powder-free intraoral scanners gained in popularity in the last decade and the most recent models are more accurate, smaller and faster

Several studies have compared digital impressions to conventional methods; most recent published data suggest optical impression has higher accuracy, improved patient satisfaction, working time reduction, dentists' preference and provides a platform for interdisciplinary communication [19, 32, 33]. There are many devices currently commercially available with different features, e.g., powder use, scanning speed, tip size, and ability to detect in-color impressions [29]. The first generation of scanning systems frequently needs powder use, is monochromatic and is a closed system, i.e., only proprietary files as output or semi-closed (pay per .STL file) [31, 34]. The latest devices are generally powder-free, faster and allow in-color impressions. They are mostly open systems (free. STL and .PLY [Polygon File Format or the Stanford Triangle Format] files). The currently available IOS is constructed on one of the three main principles: confocal laser scanner, active wave front sampling, and optical triangulation technique. Table 4.5 provides a summary of commonly used commercially available intraoral scanners.

4.3.2   Digital Versus Conventional Impressions

The ultimate goal of a dental impression is to accurately reproduce teeth surface and surrounding soft tissue contours. Conventional impression techniques are still considered the gold standard [35] and the most widely used. However, the use of digital impressions has been increasing significantly. Recently, many laboratory and clinical studies comparing both approaches have been conducted and are summarized below.

Table 4.5 Comparisons of the features of commonly used intraoral scanners

Digital intraoral scanning systems						
Intraoral scanner	Company	Working principle	Light source	Powder free	Output format	Website
Midmark Mobile True Definition[a]	Midmark	Active wave front sampling	Pulsating blue light	No	Proprietary or STL	Midmark.com/truedef
TRIOS	3Shape A/S	Confocal laser scanner	Blue LED light	Yes	Proprietary or STL	3shape.com
iTero Element	Align Technology	Confocal laser scanner	Red Laser	Yes	Proprietary and STL	Itero.com
Carestream Dental 3700	Carestream Dental	Optical triangulation	Light	Yes	Proprietary and STL	Carestreamdental.com
CEREC Bluecam	Dentsply Sirona	Optical triangulation	White light	No	Proprietary	Dentsplysirona.com
CEREC Omnicam	Dentsply Sirona	Optical triangulation	White light	Yes	Proprietary and STL	Dentsplysirona.com
Primescan	Dentsply Sirona	Optical triangulation	Blue light	Yes	Proprietary and STL	Dentsplysirona.com
Virtuo Vivo	Dental Wings	Blue Laser-Multiscan Imaging™ technology	Blue laser	Yes	Proprietary and STL	Dentalwings.com
Medit I500	Medit	Optical triangulation	Blue laser	Yes	STL, OBJ or PLY	Medit.com

[a]Previous 3M

4.3.2.1 Laboratory Studies

Milled models fabricated from digital impression images were comparable to gypsum models obtained from conventional impression [36]. Dies generated from IOS did not present clinical difference compared to those generated from conventional polyvinyl siloxane (PVS) [37]. Two IOS systems (Omnicam and True Definition) were tested and found their accuracy being clinically acceptable [39]. One study simulating full edentulous ridge impression found no difference between digital and conventional impressions, and an implant angulation of up to 15° did not affect the accuracy [40]. Limitations of complete arch scanning, e.g., mobile tissues, a lack of landmarks, and a long-distance between implants reduce the accuracy [8, 26]. Artificial landmarks [41] and an auxiliary geometric device (AGD) [42] were recently used to improve accuracy. However, a recent systematic review reported that the available data on the accuracy of digital impressions have a low evidence level and do not include sufficient data on in-vivo application to derive further clinical recommendations [25].

4.3.2.2 Clinical Studies

Single implant impression with IOS is in general more accurate than a long span partial edentulous ridge or complete edentulous ridge impression. One study showed only 1 of the 21 scans demonstrated an acceptable interimplant distance ($<100\,\mu m$) and an acceptable angulation error ($<0.4°$) [8]. Another study using IOS found angulation errors ranging from 5.0° to 8.5°, interimplant distance errors ranging from 160 to 270 μm, and linear displacement errors ranging from 270 to 450 μm in edentulous patients [6]. These results indicated that it is possible to perform a digital impression of multiple implants, however, further clinical investigations are still needed to approve the predictability of the results [43, 44].

4.3.2.3 Accuracy Comparison Between Different Intraoral Scanners

Accuracy refers to the trueness and precision. Trueness describes the closeness of a measurement to the actual value, and precision describes the closeness of multiple measurements (see Fig. 4.8) [23, 33].

Five systems were compared with the True Definition (3M ESPE Dental Products, Seefeld, Germany) showing the highest overall "trueness," followed by CS 3500 intraoral scanner (Dental Imaging software 6.14.0; Carestream Health Inc., Brunn am Gebirge, Austria). Zfx IntraScan (software version 5.02; Zfx GmbH, Dachau, Germany), CEREC AC Bluecam (software version 4.2.4.72893; Sirona, Bensheim, Germany), and CEREC AC Omnicam (software version 4.2.3.68181; Sirona, Bensheim, Germany) showed higher differences from the reference data set than the control group. Nevertheless, all tested IOS technologies seemed to be able to reproduce a single quadrant within clinical acceptable accuracy [45].

A similar comparison of 7 systems was performed [33]. PlanScan (Planmeca Group, Helsinki, Finland) had the best trueness and precision, while the 3Shape Trios was the poorest for sextant scanning. For complete-arch scanning, the Carestream 3500 (CS) (Carestream Dental) had the best performance, while the powdered scanning system CEREC Bluecam (CB) (Dentsply Sirona) showed the

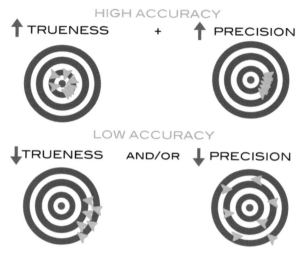

Fig. 4.8 Accuracy, combination of trueness and precision; illustratively described

least precision. 3Shape TRIOS 3 provided the best combination of speed, trueness, and precision.

Eight different IOS systems were compared and concluded that 2 systems (Dental Wings and 3D Progress) demonstrated a low performance showing average deviations between 148 and 344 µm, while 2 systems (True Definition and Trios 3) presented the best performance with only 31 and 32 µm of average deviation, which is clinically insignificant [21].

It is known that scanners differ regarding the speed, trueness, and precision of sextant or complete-arch scans and the results of studies comparing different scanning systems should be interpreted with caution, since they were performed without a standardized method to evaluate and compare multiple IOS systems.

4.3.2.4 Time-Efficiency of Intraoral Scanners

There is a learning curve with the use of new devices and techniques, as reported in a clinical study that the average scanning time decreased from 16.7 min for each of the first 40 patients to 9.5 min for each of the last 20 cases [46]. Garino et al. used the iTero powderless scanner and after 328 scans, the mean scanning time was 11 min and 58 s [47]. Yuzbasioglu et al. tested the CEREC Omnicam in a sample of 24 adults and found that the mean scanning time was significantly lower than the time required for conventional impression with a polyether material [48]. Similar findings were reported from other groups that there was a significantly reduced chair time for the digital workflow for implant crowns (14.8 min) compared to the conventional approach (17.9 min) [32]. A recent clinical trial also reported a significantly reduced time for digital impression technique (10.9 min) compared to the conventional method (14.3 min) [49]. Table 4.6 provides a summary of working time for IOS compared to conventional impressions reported in clinical studies.

Table 4.6 Time operating of intraoral scanning reported in clinical trials

Study/design	Patients/implants	Prosthesis	Intraoral scanner	Area of scanning	Conventional impression material	Digital impression time started	Impression technique	Number of procedures evaluated	Procedure time (min) Mean ± SD[a]
Joda and Bragger [32] RCT[b]	20/40	Single implant-supported crowns	iTero; Align Tech	Quadrant scan	Polyether (Impregum Penta; 3M)	Removal of cover screwed and insertion of scan body	Digital	20	14.8 ± 2.2
						Removal of cover screwed and insertion of transfer post	Conventional	20	17.9 ± 1.1
Schepke et al. [50] Prospective	50/50	Single implant-supported crowns	Omnicam; Dentsply Sirona	Complete-arch	Polyether (Impregum Penta; 3M)	Removal of intraoral scanner from scan unit	Digital	50	6.39 ± 1.85
						Removal Beginning of mixing procedure	Conventional	20	12.13 ± 1.4
Wismeijer et al. [51] Prospective	27/38	Single and partial fixed implant-supported prosthesis	iTero; Align Tech	Quadrant scan	Polyether (Impregum Penta; 3M)	Removal of cover screwed and insertion of scan body	Digital	27	23.44 ± 9.08
						Removal of cover screwed and fabrication of individual tray	Conventional	27	15.18 ± 5.46
Pan et al. [49] Prospective	20/40	Single implant-supported crowns	3Shape Trios Standard ® 11, 3Shape A/S	Complete-arch	Polyether (Impregum Penta; 3M)	Tray selection to color determination	Digital	20	10.9 ± 2.1
						Removal of healing abutment to color determination	Conventional	20	14.3 ± 3.0

[a]SD, standard deviation
[b]RCT, randomized clinical trial

4.3.2.5 Patient Reported Outcomes

There was an overall patient preference for the digital impression, compared to the conventional method, even though the patients had perceived the duration of IO scan more negatively than conventional approach [51]. More recent studies showed the benefits of IOS, even for patients who had no experience with either conventional or digital impressions previously. [32, 48].

The overall patient experience evaluated with the visual analogue scale (VAS) questionnaires favored the digital technique. All patients would select the digital workflow if they need future implant prosthetic treatments [52]. A recent study reported the comfort, anxiety, and taste were significantly better with the IOS [19]. Table 4.7 is a summary of recent clinical trials reporting patient experience to digital impression compared to conventional technique for implant-supported restorations.

4.3.2.6 Operator Experience

A pilot study revealed that the digital technique was preferred by 60% of the second-year dental students, while 7% preferred conventional impressions and 33% were satisfied with either technique [54]. Overall, the participants' perceptions of difficulty and applicability tended to favor digital impressions. Students expressed an expectation that digital technologies being a time-saving procedure [4] will become the predominant impression technique in their future careers [55]. On the other hand, experienced dentists favored the conventional method, indicating that this group was reluctant to adopt this new technology [56]. Repeated experience can affect the trueness of the scanned images [57, 58].

4.3.2.7 Limitations of Intraoral Scanning

As good as it is, IOS only capture the surfaces of the oral structures. There is no depth information and the dynamic function of soft tissues cannot be evaluated. The presence of saliva, patient movement during scanning, mobile mucosa, highly reflecting surfaces, or access difficulties are the major limitations [59, 60]. Patient and saliva control rely on operator execution and teamwork. Geometric devices have been utilized to overcome areas with mobile mucosa and long distance between teeth and/or implant scan bodies. The initial cost seems to be an important challenge for the introduction of the digital workflow. At the same time, a recent published article showed that digital impressions are more efficient and cost effective than standard impressions, and implementation costs can be offset within the first year [61].

4.4 Computer-Aided Design (CAD)

Computer-aided design comprises of software which allows the integration of the digital data and provides tools for dental appliance manufacturing. A transition from closed to open-source CAD/CAM technologies has created greater flexibility in the digital workflow. Various data acquisition sources, e.g., IOS, laboratory cast scanner, and CBCT, can be combined with different compatible software programs

Table 4.7 Patients preferences evaluated in clinical trials when digital impression is compared to conventional impressions for implant-supported rehabilitations

Study design	Patients implants	Prosthesis	Intraoral scanner	Area of scanning	Evaluation method outcome reported	Result
Wismeijer et al. [51] Clinical observational	27/38	Single and partial fixed implant-supported prosthesis	(iTero; Align Tech)	Quadrant scan	Self-developed questionnaire/treatment time taste nausea sensation comfort	Digital impression overall experience significantly more favorable than conventional impression technique ($P = 0.026$). Negative correlations found between patient satisfaction and time involved for digital impression technique
Schepke et al. [50] prospective	50/50	Single implant-supported crowns	(Omnicam; Dentsply Sirona)	Complete-arch	VAS/comfort and anxiety	During conventional impression technique participants experienced more discomfort, more feelings of helplessness, and more shortness of breath than during digital impression ($P < 0.001$)
Joda and Bragger [32] RCT	20/40	Single implant-supported crowns	(iTero; Align Tech)	Quadrant scan	VAS/convenience, anxiety taste, nausea sensation and pain	Overall patient preference for digital impression higher than conventional impression technique ($P < 0.001$)
Delize et al. [19] Clinical, non-randomized	31/31	Single implant-supported crowns	IOS (TRIOS® second generation, 3Shape)—newly experienced operators	Quadrant scan	VAS/pain, comfort, nausea, taste, anxiety	No difference was found for pain ($p = 0.99$) and treatment duration ($p = 0.71$). However, the comfort ($p = 0.0087$), anxiety ($p = 0.031$), and taste ($p = 0.014$) domain results were significantly better with the IOS. A trend was observed for nausea ($p = 0.074$)
Guo et al. [53] prospective	20/20	Single implant-supported crowns	(Trios 1, 3Shape Trios Standard-P11, 3Shape A/S, Copenhagen, Denmark)	Complete-arch + refined area after implant placement	VAS/overall convenience, anxiety, taste, nausea, difficulty breathing and the possible sensation of pain	Among the 20 patients, 17 showed a preference for the immediate digital impression technique (85%), and three expressed indifference regarding the impression methods

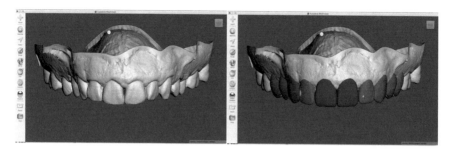

Fig. 4.9 Wax-up designed in a free 3D sculpting-based CAD software (Computer-Assisted Design), Meshmixer—Autodesk

[43]. A trend in today's digital dentistry is the push for "open systems" and the CAD software does not necessarily need to be dental specific. As an example, Meshmixer is a powerful 3-D design software that can be used to create 3-D models, wax-ups, occlusal splints, or even dentures (Fig. 4.9). Use of open-source software may reduce the cost and gain more acceptance.

Certainly, the learning curve for the use of an open-source system, especially those not dental specific, is more difficult. Table 4.8 presents examples of CAD software and their principal features. Intriguingly, a recent study confirmed that as the number of repetitions increased to digitally design the abutment, the skill increased and the time spent to complete the task decreased [62].

4.5 Computer-Aided Manufacturing (CAM)

Computer-aided manufacturing (CAM) refers to the final step on the "digital workflow" when the data created using CAD is used for manufacturing of structures with the desired material. There are two methods of CAM currently available: addictive manufacturing (AM) and subtractive manufacturing (SM). Subtractive manufacturing is a process that removes or grinds a specific material to form the final object. This technology has dominated the fabrication of dental prosthesis and other dental devices in the past three decades; however, it involves higher costs and a significant waste of material. AM or 3D printing is based on the addition of consecutive two-dimensional (2D) layers of material to form the customized 3D object of interest. Being at a lower cost, 3D printing has become the preferred method to produce models, surgical templates, and interim prosthesis fabrication.

4.5.1 Additive Manufacturing: 3D Printing

Additive manufacturing and 3D printing are becoming increasingly important in many surgical fields, e.g., neurosurgery, heart surgery, craniomaxillofacial surgery, and implant dentistry [63]. There are numerous advantages in the area of computer-

Table 4.8 Examples of CAD software and their major characteristics

Digital intraoral scanning systems

CAD software frequently used in dentistry

Software name	Company	Major indication	User friendliness	Cost
Simplant	Dentsply Sirona	Implant planning software	Company executes planning and clinician reviews it	$$[a]
NobelClinician	Nobel Biocare	Implant planning software	Easy to use	$$
coDiagnostiX	Dental Wings	Implant planning software	Easy to use	$$[a]
Blue Sky Plan	Blue Sky Bio	Implant planning and orthodontics software	Easy to use	$[b]
Implant Studio	3shape	Implant planning software	Easy to use	$$[a]
Exoplan	Exocad	Implant planning software	Easy to use	$$
Galileos Implant	Dentsply Sirona	Implant planning software	Easy to use	$$
Meshmixer	Autodesk, Inc	3D CAD software	Not user friendly for dental	$
Geomagic Freeforms	3dsystems	Engineering software	Not user friendly for dental	$$
Blender Dental	Blender foundation	3D CAD software with dental module	Relatively user friendly with dental add-on	$$

[a]$$—license required for software usage or free software + fee for guide fabrication from company
[b]$—free software (might need to pay to export data)

assisted surgery, such as treatment time reduction, high accuracy, and overall cost reduction. Today a large number of 3D printers with different printing technologies along with resin materials are available. The most utilized 3D-printers in implant dentistry will be briefly described in this chapter.

4.5.1.1 Fused Deposition Modelling (FDM)

In the fused deposition modelling (FDM) machines, filaments of a thermoplastic material, e.g., polylactic acid (PLA) polymers, are heated and then extruded through the nozzle to build precise structures. Favorable properties, e.g., strong and stiff, make PLA polymers suitable for use in the oral cavity. Some studies have added biological compounds into the build filaments. Thermoplastics-infused biodegradable polyester with bioactive tri-calcium phosphate has been shown to be a promising prospect for use in building tissue scaffold structures in dentistry [10].

4.5.1.2 Stereolithography (SLA)

SLA printers create structures layer by layer using ultraviolet light or laser to solidify a liquid photopolymerizing resin. These polymers (resin) offer a flexibility in color, rigidity, and modification of components. Light-cured resins may be used for a variety of purposes such as: dental casts, wax-ups, surgical template guides, temporary crowns, dentures, etc.

4.5.1.3 Selective Laser Sintering (SLS)

SLS constructs scaffolds from 3D digital data by sequentially fusing regions in a powder bed, layer by layer, via a computer-controlled scanning laser beam. Layer-by-layer additive fabrication in SLS allows construction of scaffolds with complex internal and external geometries. Any powdered biomaterial that will fuse but not decompose under a laser beam can be used to fabricate scaffolds. Additionally, SLS does not require the use of organic solvents, can be used to make intricate biphasic scaffold geometries, and does not require the use of a filament (as in FDM). It may be easier to incorporate multiple materials. It is fast and cost effective [64, 65].

4.5.1.4 Digital Light Processing (DLP)

The DLP printer operates in a similar way compared to the SLA, except that it uses projector technology for photopolymerization and then presents significantly faster printing time. However, the resolution may be reduced, depending on the quality of the projector and the material used.

4.6   Computer-Guided Implant Surgery Workflow

Correct implant positioning is essential to obtain favorable esthetic and prosthetic outcomes as well as long-term stability of peri-implant hard and soft tissues. Moreover, optimal implant position allows for a screw-retained prosthesis that are retrievable and together with an adequate design will improve patient ability to perform home care [66].

The use of CBCT and IOS revolutionized the way we practice implant treatment planning. The superimposed images enable virtual implant planning, while taking the surrounding anatomic structures and future prosthetic needs into consideration [67]. The virtual implant locations can be translated into a surgical guide [16, 68]. Recent studies demonstrated that computer-guided surgery (CGS) should be considered to improve accuracy for multiple-implant cases in complete or partial edentulism [15]. CGS may result in a higher implant survival rate and comparable long-term cost to non-guided implant placement [69]. CGS can facilitate flapless implant surgeries for patient satisfaction, a reduction in treatment time, and decreased postoperative discomfort [70, 71].

4.6.1 Double CBCT Scan Technique

This method requires 2 CBCT scans for treatment planning [24, 72]. The first scan is taken when the patient wears the radiographic guide and the second scan is taken only on the radiographic guide (Fig. 4.10 top panel). The guide, representing the ideal future prosthesis, must contain radiopaque marks, e.g., gutta-percha (Fig. 4.10 middle panel). A planning software is then used for virtual implant placement (Fig. 4.10 bottom panel). Once the implants are virtually placed a surgical guide can be made.

At the surgical site, the guide is fixated with specific pins and screws in the patient jaw (top row in Fig. 4.11). With the surgical template in place, a guided surgical implant kit of the implant system selected is used for osteotomy and implant placement (bottom row in Fig. 4.11). In the fully guided protocol, implant placement is also guided and stops in the screwdriver allow precise implant placement also in the corono-apical direction (Fig. 4.12).

4.6.2 Limitations of the Double CBCT Scan Technique

The limitations pertain to the extra cost, increased radiation exposure and time when a new radiopaque template has to be made and the degree of accuracy to match the 2 scans [7, 27].

4.6.3 Optical Scanning Technique

Image fusion of the STL data, obtained from the optical scanning, with the DICOM data, obtained from the CBCT, is performed by matching the common reference points (Fig. 4.13) [9, 28]. The STL data can be obtained either from casts, wax-ups, or directly with the use of IOS. STL data provide prosthesis locations plus surface of surrounding tissues and DICOM data provide bone locations. Optimal implant positioning is then planned on software accordingly. Utilizing this digital application eliminates analogue preoperative waxing-up since a virtual/digital wax-up can be designed (Fig. 4.14).

The guide can then be virtually fabricated and exported in .STL file to be manufactured by 3D printing or milling. The introduction of optical scanning

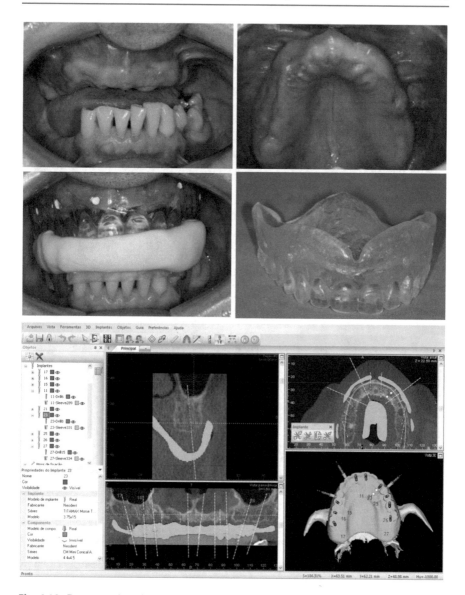

Fig. 4.10 Demonstration of the double scan technique. Top row: the maxillary edentulous arch to be restored. Middle row: a template guide in mouth and extra-orally for dual CBCT scans. Bottom row: screenshots of the prosthetically driven implant planning on software at different view planes

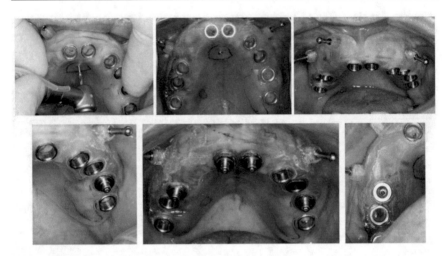

Fig. 4.11 Guide fixation using fixation screws and pins (top row, left and middle panel); surgical guided fixated for flapless implant surgery (top row, right panel); stops in the surgical template to avoid movements of the surgical guide and consequently deviations (bottom row, left and middle panel); implant in position after fully guided placement (bottom row, right panel)

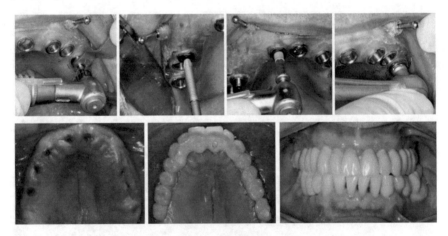

Fig. 4.12 Demonstration of the fully guided protocol. Top: osteotomy and implant placement are assisted by the guide. Bottom: immediate interim prosthesis is delivered

images was then a remarkable step to eliminate a radiographic template fabrication and a second CBCT scan. The steps are summarized below [18]:

1. Take intraoral digital scans of the maxilla, mandible, and maximal intercuspal position with an intraoral scanner. Save the digital impression as *example.stl*.
2. Open *example.stl* into a Guided Treatment Planning Software (e.g., Blue Sky Plan v.4.0; Blue Sky Bio) and align with the digital file in .DICOM including the hard tissue information (Fig. 4.13).

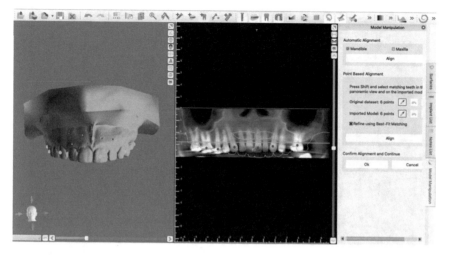

Fig. 4.13 Matching the STL with the DICOM data in specific implant planning software

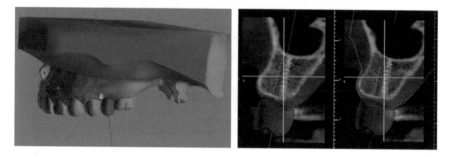

Fig. 4.14 An example of virtual wax-up on software. After merging the STL and DICOM data sets, a virtual restoration at tooth #13 location is placed and the implant position is planned accordingly

3. Virtually place the implant in optimal 3D position and create a virtual guide on software (Fig. 4.14).
4. Export the *example.stl* of the guide to be 3D printed or milled.
5. Verify the guide accuracy in the oral cavity and use in the surgery (Fig. 4.15).

4.6.4   Limitations of the Optical Scanning Technique

Previous reports stated that patients must have at least 6 remaining teeth distributed in 2 quadrants to allow for accurate imaging matching [73, 74]. In complete edentulous cases, a tomographic guide or the existing denture might be used [7,75]. The high introductory costs of intraoral scanners could be potentially a barrier. Soft tissue features cannot be evaluated with this method.

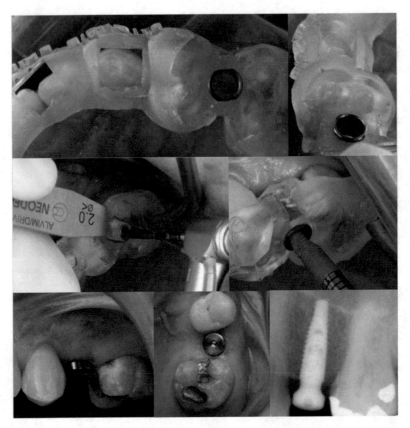

Fig. 4.15 Surgical steps using a tooth-supported guide in a fully digital workflow. Windows in the surgical guide allows better visualization of template adaptation on teeth (top row). Guided drilling sequence and implant placement (middle row) and final implant position clinically and radiographically (bottom row)

4.6.5 Accuracy of Computer-Guided Implant Surgery

Recent literature [38] shows encouraging outcomes for the CGS accuracy using a complete digital workflow for tooth-supported guides and are summarized in Table 4.9. Bone-supported guides showed a statistically significant greater deviation [76] and therefore was excluded from the analysis in this chapter. Some factors may influence the accuracy, including the number of unrestored teeth, implant location, implant diameter, and cortical interference [20].

Table 4.9 Summary of the accuracy of CGS using tooth-supported guides in a fully digital workflow

Digital intraoral scanning systems

Author	Study design	Number of implants/patients	Implant system	IOS utilized	Accuracy evaluation method	Results Angular deviation	Global deviation (shoulder)	Global deviation (apex)	Corono-apical deviation
Tallarico et al. [78]	RCT	28 implants/10 patients	Osstem TSIII, Osstem, Seoul, South Korea	CS 3600 intraoral scanner (Carestream Dental, Atlanta, GA, USA)	Comparison[a]	2.25±1.41°	N/A	N/A	0.58±0.44 mm
Tallarico et al. [77]	Prospective	119 implants/39 patients	Osstem TSIII, Osstem, Seoul, South Korea	3M true definition scanner	Comparison	1.43±1.98°	N/A	N/A	0.42±0.37 mm
Derksen et al. [20]	Prospective	145 implants/66 patients	Straumann tissue level	3M true definition scanner	Comparison	2.72±1.42°	0.75±0.34 mm	1.06±0.44 mm	N/A
Smikarn et al. [79]	RCT	30 implants/patients	Bone level Straumann	TRIOS (3Shape)	Superposition[b]	3.1±2.3°	1+0.6 mm	1.3±0.6 mm	0.7±0.6 mm
Skjerven et al. [80]	Prospective	27 implants/20 patients	19 Astra Tech EV (Dentsply implants) and 8 Straumann bone level	TRIOS (3Shape)	Comparison	3.85±1.83°	1.05±0.59 mm	1.63±1.05 mm	N/A
Kiatkroekkrai et al. [81]	RCT	30 implants/20 patients	Bone Level Straumann	TRIOS (3Shape)	Superposition	2.41°±1.47°	0.87±0.49 mm	1.10±0.53 mm	0.58±0.47 mm

RCT, randomized clinical trial
[a]Comparison of .STL files from planned position and final position (obtained with IOS)
[b]Superimposing post CBCT images with planned positions

References

1. Kapos T, Evans C. CAD/CAM technology for implant abutments, crowns, and superstructures. Int J Oral Maxillofac Implants. 2014;29 Suppl:117–36. ISSN: 1942-4434 (Electronic) 0882-2786 (Linking). https://doi.org/10.11607/jomi.2014suppl.g2.3. https://www.ncbi.nlm.nih.gov/pubmed/24660194

2. Strub JR, Rekow ED, Witkowski S. Computer-aided design and fabrication of dental restorations: current systems and future possibilities. J Am Dent Assoc. 2006;137(9):1289–96. ISSN: 0002-8177 (Print) 0002-8177 (Linking). https://doi.org/10.14219/jada.archive.2006.0389. https://www.ncbi.nlm.nih.gov/pubmed/16946436

3. Abduo J, Lyons K. Rationale for the use of CAD/CAM technology in implant prosthodontics. Int J Dent. 2013;2013:768121. ISSN: 1687-8728 (Print) 1687-8728 (Linking). https://doi.org/10.1155/2013/768121. https://www.ncbi.nlm.nih.gov/pubmed/23690778

4. Ahmed KE, et al. Performance and perception of dental students using three intraoral CAD/CAM scanners for full-arch scanning. J Prosthodont Res. 2019;632:167–72. ISSN: 2212-4632 (Electronic) 1883-1958 (Linking). https://doi.org/10.1016/j.jpor.2018.11.003. https://www.ncbi.nlm.nih.gov/pubmed/30528397

5. Al-Moraissi E, et al. Does intraoperative perforation of Schneiderian membrane during sinus lift surgery causes an increased the risk of implants failure?: a systematic review and meta regression analysis. Clin Implant Dent Relat Res. 2018;20(5):882–9. ISSN: 1523-0899. https://doi.org/10.1111/cid.12660.

6. Alsharbaty MHM, et al. A clinical comparative study of 3-dimensional accuracy between digital and conventional implant impression techniques. J Prosthodont. 2019;28(4):e902–8. ISSN: 1532-849X (Electronic) 1059-941X (Linking). https://doi.org/10.1111/jopr.12764. https://www.ncbi.nlm.nih.gov/pubmed/29423969

7. An X, Yang HW, Choi BH. Digital workflow for computer-guided implant surgery in edentulous patients with an intraoral scanner and old complete denture. J Prosthodont. 2019;28(6):715–8. ISSN: 1532-849X (Electronic) 1059-941X (Linking). https://doi.org/10.1111/jopr.13073. https://www.ncbi.nlm.nih.gov/ubmed/31087422

8. Andriessen FS, et al. Applicability and accuracy of an intraoral scanner for scanning multiple implants in edentulous mandibles: a pilot study. J Prosthet Dent. 2017;111(3):186–94. ISSN: 1097-6841 (Electronic) 0022-3913 (Linking). https://doi.org/10.1016/j.prosdent.2013.07.010. https://www.ncbi.nlm.nih.gov/pubmed/24210732

9. Arcuri L, et al. Full digital workflow for implant-prosthetic rehabilitations: a case report. Oral Implantol (Rome) 2015;8(4):114–21. ISSN: 1974-5648 (Print) 1974-5648 (Linking). https://doi.org/10.11138/orl/2015.8.4.114. https://www.ncbi.nlm.nih.gov/pubmed/28042423

10. Barazanchi A, et al. Additive technology: update on current materials and applications in dentistry. J Prosthodont. 2017;26(2):156–63. ISSN: 1532-849X (Electronic) 1059-941X (Linking). https://doi.org/10.1111/jopr.12510. https://www.ncbi.nlm.nih.gov/pubmed/27662423

11. Rios HF, Borgnakke WS, Benavides E. The use of cone-beam computed tomography in management of patients requiring dental implants: an American Academy of Periodontology best evidence review. J Periodontol. 2017;88(10):946–59

12. Tyndall DA, et al. Position statement of the American Academy of Oral and Maxillofacial Radiology on selection criteria for the use of radiology in dental implantology with emphasis on cone beam computed tomography. Oral Surg Oral Med Oral Pathol Oral Radiol. 2012;113(6):817–26. ISSN: 2212-4411 (Electronic). https://doi.org/10.1016/j.oooo.2012.03.005. http://www.ncbi.nlm.nih.gov/pubmed/22668710

13. Boyne PJ, James RA. Grafting of the maxillary sinus floor with autogenous marrow and bone. J Oral Surg. 1980;38(8):613–6. ISSN: 0022-3255 (Print) 0022-3255 (Linking). https://www.ncbi.nlm.nih.gov/pubmed/6993637

14. Chan HL, Wang HL. Sinus pathology and anatomy in relation to complications in lateral window sinus augmentation. Implant Dent. 2011;20(6):406–12. ISSN: 1538-2982 (Electronic) 1056-6163 (Linking). https://doi.org/10.1097/ID.0b013e3182341f79. https://www.ncbi.nlm.nih.gov/pubmed/21986451

15. Choi W, et al. Freehand versus guided surgery: factors influencing accuracy of dental implant placement. Implant Dent. 2017;26(4):500–9. ISSN: 1538-2982 (Electronic) 1056-6163 (Linking). https://doi.org/10.1097/ID.0000000000000620. https://www.ncbi.nlm.nih.gov/pubmed/28731896

16. D'Haese J, et al. Current state of the art of computer-guided implant surgery. Periodontol 2000. 2017;73(1):121–33. ISSN: 1600-0757 (Electronic) 0906-6713 (Linking). https://doi.org/10.1111/prd.12175. https://www.ncbi.nlm.nih.gov/pubmed/28000275

17. Dawood A, et al. 3D printing in dentistry. Br Dent J. 2015;219(11):521–9. ISSN: 1476-5373 (Electronic) 0007-0610 (Linking). https://doi.org/10.1038/sj.bdj.2015.914. https://www.ncbi.nlm.nih.gov/pubmed/26657435

18. de Siqueira RAC, et al. Using digital technique to obtain the ideal soft tissue contour in immediate implants with provisionalization. Implant Dent. 2019;28(4):411–6. ISSN: 1538-2982 (Electronic) 1056-6163 (Linking). https://doi.org/10.1097/ID.0000000000000914. https://www.ncbi.nlm.nih.gov/pubmed/31157756

19. Delize V, et al. Intrasubject comparison of digital vs. conventional workflow for screw-retained single-implant crowns: Prosthodontic and patient-centered outcomes. Clin Oral Implants Res. 2019. ISSN: 1600-0501 (Electronic) 0905-7161 (Linking). https://doi.org/10.1111/clr.13494. https://www.ncbi.nlm.nih.gov/pubmed/31183902

20. Derksen W, et al. The accuracy of computer guided implant surgery with tooth supported, digitally designed drill guides based on CBCT and intraoral scanning. A prospective cohort study. Clin Oral Implants Res. 2019. ISSN: 1600-0501 (Electronic) 0905-7161 (Linking). https://doi.org/10.1111/clr.13514. https://www.ncbi.nlm.nih.gov/pubmed/31330566

21. Di Fiore A, et al. Full arch digital scanning systems performances for implant-supported fixed dental prostheses: a comparative study of 8 intraoral scanners. J Prosthodont Res. (2019). ISSN: 2212-4632 (Electronic) 1883-1958 (Linking). https://doi.org/10.1016/j.jpor.2019.04.002. https://www.ncbi.nlm.nih.gov/pubmed/31072730

22. Elian N, et al. Distribution of the maxillary artery as it relates to sinus floor augmentation. Int J Oral Maxillofac Implants. 2005;20(5):784–7. ISSN: 0882-2786 (Print) 0882-2786 (Linking). https://www.ncbi.nlm.nih.gov/pubmed/16274154

23. Ender A, Mehl A. Accuracy of complete-arch dental impressions: a new method of measuring trueness and precision. J Prosthet Dent. 2013;109(2):121–8. ISSN: 1097-6841 (Electronic) 0022-3913 (Linking). https://doi.org/10.1016/S0022-3913(13)60028-1. https://www.ncbi.nlm.nih.gov/pubmed/23395338

24. Ersoy AE, et al. Reliability of implant placement with stereolithographic surgical guides generated from computed tomography: clinical data from 94 implants. J Periodontol. 2008;79(8):1339–45. ISSN: 0022-3492 (Print) 0022-3492 (Linking). https://doi.org/10.1902/jop.2008.080059. https://www.ncbi.nlm.nih.gov/pubmed/18672982

25. Flugge T, et al. The accuracy of different dental impression techniques for implant-supported dental prostheses: a systematic review and meta4.7 References 113 analysis. Clin Oral Implants Res. 2018;29 Suppl 16:374–92. ISSN: 0905-7161. https://doi.org/10.1111/clr.13273

26. Flugge TV, et al. Precision of dental implant digitization using intraoral scanners. Int J Prosthodont. 2016;29(3):277–83. ISSN: 0893-2174 (Print) 0893-2174 (Linking). https://doi.org/10.11607/ijp.4417. https://www.ncbi.nlm.nih.gov/pubmed/27148990

27. Flugge TV, et al. Three-dimensional plotting and printing of an implant drilling guide: simplifying guided implant surgery. J Oral Maxillofac Surg. 2013;71(8):1340–6. ISSN: 1531-5053 (Electronic) 0278-2391 (Linking). https://doi.org/10.1016/j.joms.2013.04.010. https://www.ncbi.nlm.nih.gov/pubmed/23866950

28. De Vico G, et al. A novel workflow for computer guided implant surgery matching digital dental casts and CBCT scan. Oral Implantol. 2016;9(1):33–48. ISSN: 1974-5648 (Print) 1974-5648 (Linking). https://doi.org/10.11138/orl/2016.9.1.033. https://www.ncbi.nlm.nih.gov/pubmed/28042429

29. Mangano F, et al. Intraoral scanners in dentistry: a review of the current literature. BMC Oral Health. 2017;17(1):149. ISSN: 1472-6831 (Electronic) 1472-6831 (Linking). https://doi.org/10.1186/s12903-017-0442-x. https://www.ncbi.nlm.nih.gov/pubmed/29233132

30. Ting-Shu S, Jian S. Intraoral digital impression technique: a review. J Prosthodont. 2015;24(4):313–21. ISSN: 1059-941x. https://doi.org/10.1111/jopr.12218
31. Zimmermann M, et al. Intraoral scanning systems – a current overview. Int J Comput Dent. 2015;18(2):101–29. ISSN: 1463-4201 (Print) 1463-4201 (Linking). https://www.ncbi.nlm.nih.gov/pubmed/26110925
32. Joda T, Bragger U. Time-efficiency analysis comparing digital and conventional workflows for implant crowns: a prospective clinical crossover trial. Int J Oral Maxillofac Implants. 2015;30(5):1047–53. ISSN: 1942-4434 (Electronic) 0882-2786 (Linking). https://doi.org/10.11607/jomi.3963. https://www.ncbi.nlm.nih.gov/pubmed/26394340
33. Renne W, et al. Evaluation of the accuracy of 7 digital scanners: an in vitro analysis based on 3-dimensional comparisons. J Prosthet Dent. 2017;118(1):36–42. ISSN: 1097-6841 (Electronic) 0022-3913 (Linking). https://doi.org/10.1016/j.prosdent.2016.09.024. https://www.ncbi.nlm.nih.gov/pubmed/28024822
34. Prudente MS, et al. Influence of scanner, powder application, and adjustments on CAD-CAM crown misfit. J Prosthet Dent. 2018;119(3):377–383. ISSN: 1097-6841 (Electronic) 0022-3913 (Linking). https://doi.org/10.1016/j.prosdent.2017.03.024. https://www.ncbi.nlm.nih.gov/pubmed/28689912
35. Kapos T, et al. Computer-aided design and computer-assisted manufacturing in prosthetic implant dentistry. Int J Oral Maxillofac Implants. 2009;24 Suppl:110–7. ISSN: 0882-2786 (Print) 0882-2786 (Linking). https://www.ncbi.nlm.nih.gov/pubmed/19885438
36. Lee SJ, et al. Accuracy of digital versus conventional implant impressions. Clin Oral Implants Res. 2015;26(6):715–9. ISSN: 1600-0501 (Electronic) 0905-7161 (Linking). https://doi.org/10.1111/clr.12375. https://www.ncbi.nlm.nih.gov/pubmed/24720423
37. Serag M, et al. A comparative study of the accuracy of dies made from digital intraoral scanning vs. elastic impressions: an in vitro study. J Prosthodont. 2018;27(1):88–93. ISSN: 1532-849X (Electronic) 1059-941X (Linking). https://doi.org/10.1111/jopr.12481. https://www.ncbi.nlm.nih.gov/pubmed/27149542
38. Siqueira R, Chen Z, Galli M, Saleh I, Wang H-L, Chan H-L. Does a fully digital workflow improve the accuracy of computer-assisted implant surgery in partially edentulous patients? A systematic review of clinical trials. Clin Implant Dent Relat Res. 2020;1–12. https://doi.org/10.1111/cid.12937
39. Marghalani A, et al. Digital versus conventional implant impressions for partially edentulous arches: an evaluation of accuracy. J Prosthet Dent. 2018;119(4):574–9. ISSN: 1097-6841 (Electronic) 0022-3913 (Linking). https://doi.org/10.1016/j.prosdent.2017.07.002. https://www.ncbi.nlm.nih.gov/pubmed/28927923
40. Papaspyridakos P, et al. Digital versus conventional implant impressions for edentulous patients: accuracy outcomes. Clin Oral Implants Res. 2016;27(4):465–72. ISSN: n (Electronic) 0905-7161 (Linking). https://doi.org/10.1111/clr.12567. https://www.ncbi.nlm.nih.gov/pubmed/25682892
41. Kim JE, et al. Accuracy of intraoral digital impressions using an artificial landmark. J Prosthet Dent. 2017;117(6):755–61. ISSN: 1097-6841 (Electronic) 0022-3913 (Linking). https://doi.org/10.1016/j.prosdent.2016.09.016. https://www.ncbi.nlm.nih.gov/pubmed/27863856
42. Iturrate M, et al. Accuracy analysis of complete-arch digital scans in edentulous arches when using an auxiliary geometric device". J Prosthet Dent. 2019;121(3):447–54. ISSN: 1097-6841 (Electronic) 0022-3913 (Linking). https://doi.org/10.1016/j.prosdent.2018.09.017. https://www.ncbi.nlm.nih.gov/pubmed/30554826
43. Lin WS, et al. Use of intraoral digital scanning for a CAD/CAM-fabricated milled bar and superstructure framework for an implant-supported, removable complete dental prosthesis. J Prosthet Dent. 2015;113(6):509–15. ISSN: 1097-6841 (Electronic) 0022-3913 (Linking). https://doi.org/10.1016/j.prosdent.2015.01.014. https://www.ncbi.nlm.nih.gov/pubmed/25862270
44. Lin WS, et al. Use of digital data acquisition and CAD/CAM technology for the fabrication of a fixed complete dental prosthesis on dental implants. J Prosthet Dent. 2014;111(1):1–5. ISSN: 1097-6841 (Electronic) 0022-3913 (Linking). https://doi.org/10.1016/j.prosdent.2013.04.010. https://www.ncbi.nlm.nih.gov/pubmed/24189115

45. Güth J-F, et al. Accuracy of digital models obtained by direct and indirect data capturing. Clin Oral Investig. 2013;17(4):1201–8
46. Garino F, Garino B. The OrthoCAD iOC intraoral scanner: a six-month user report. J Clin Orthod. 2011;45(3):161–4. ISSN: 0022-3875 (Print) 0022-3875 (Linking). https://www.ncbi.nlm.nih.gov/pubmed/21785200
47. Garino F, Garino GB, Castroflorio T. The iTero intraoral scanner in Invisalign treatment: a two-year report. J Clin Orthod. 2014;48(2):98–106. ISSN: 0022-3875 (Print) 0022-3875 (Linking). https://www.ncbi.nlm.nih.gov/pubmed/24763683
48. Yuzbasioglu E, et al. Comparison of digital and conventional impression techniques: evaluation of patients' perception, treatment comfort, effectiveness and clinical outcomes. BMC Oral Health. 2014;14:10. ISSN: 1472-6831 (Electronic) 1472-6831 (Linking). https://doi.org/10.1186/1472-6831-14-10. https://www.ncbi.nlm.nih.gov/pubmed/24479892
49. Pan S, et al. Time efficiency and quality of outcomes in a model-free digital workflow using digital impression immediately after implant placement: a double-blind self-controlled clinical trial. Clin Oral Implants Res. 2019;30(7):617–26. ISSN: 1600-0501 (Electronic) 0905-7161 (Linking). https://doi.org/10.1111/clr.13447. https://www.ncbi.nlm.nih.gov/pubmed/31021451
50. Schepke U, et al. Digital versus analog complete-arch impressions for single-unit premolar implant crowns: Operating time and patient preference. J Prosthet Dent. 2015;114(3):403–406 e401. doi:10.1016/j.prosdent.2015.04.003
51. Wismeijer D, et al. Patients' preferences when comparing analogue implant impressions using a polyether impression material versus digital impressions (Intraoral Scan) of dental implants. Clin Oral Implants Res. 2014;25(10):1113–8. ISSN: 1600-0501 (Electronic) 0905-7161 (Linking). https://doi.org/10.1111/clr.12234. https://www.ncbi.nlm.nih.gov/pubmed/23941118
52. Joda T, Bragger U. Patient-centered outcomes comparing digital and conventional implant impression procedures: a randomized crossover trial.Clin Oral Implants Res. 2016;27(12):e185–9. ISSN: 1600-0501 (Electronic) 0905-7161 (Linking). https://doi.org/10.1111/clr.12600. https://www.ncbi.nlm.nih.gov/pubmed/25864771
53. Guo DN, et al. Clinical Efficiency and Patient Preference of Immediate Digital Impression after Implant Placement for Single Implant-Supported Crown. Chin J Dent Res. 2019;22(1):21–28. doi:10.3290/j.cjdr.a41771
54. Lee SJ, Gallucci GO. Digital vs. conventional implant impressions: efficiency outcomes. Clin Oral Implants Res. 2013;24(1):111–5. ISSN: 1600-0501 (Electronic) 0905-7161 (Linking). https://doi.org/10.1111/j.1600-0501.2012.02430.x. https://www.ncbi.nlm.nih.gov/pubmed/22353208
55. Marti AM, et al. Comparison of digital scanning and polyvinyl siloxane impression techniques by dental students: instructional efficiency and attitudes towards technology. Eur J Dent Educ. 2017;21(3):200–5. ISSN: 1600-0579 (Electronic) 1396-5883 (Linking). https://doi.org/10.1111/eje.12201. https://www.ncbi.nlm.nih.gov/pubmed/26960967
56. Joda T, et al. Time efficiency, difficulty, and operator's preference comparing digital and conventional implant impressions: a randomized controlled trial. Clin Oral Implants Res. 2017;28(10):1318–1323. ISSN: 1600-0501 (Electronic) 0905-7161 (Linking). https://doi.org/10.1111/clr.12982. https://www.ncbi.nlm.nih.gov/pubmed/27596805
57. Kim J, et al. Comparison of experience curves between two 3-dimensional intraoral scanners. J Prosthet Dent. 2016;116(2):221–30. ISSN: 1097-6841 (Electronic) 0022-3913 (Linking). https://doi.org/10.1016/j.prosdent.2015.12.018. https://www.ncbi.nlm.nih.gov/pubmed/27061634
58. Lim JH, et al. Comparison of digital intraoral scanner reproducibility and image trueness considering repetitive experience. J Prosthet Dent. 2018;119(2):225–32. ISSN: 1097-6841 (Electronic) 0022-3913 (Linking). https://doi.org/10.1016/j.prosdent.2017.05.002. https://www.ncbi.nlm.nih.gov/pubmed/28689906
59. Patzelt SB, et al. Assessing the feasibility and accuracy of digitizing edentulous jaws. J Am Dent Assoc. 2013;144(8):914–20. ISSN: 1943-4723 (Electronic) 0002-8177 (Linking). https://doi.org/10.14219/jada.archive.2013.0209. https://www.ncbi.nlm.nih.gov/pubmed/23904578

60. Runkel C, et al. Digital impressions in dentistry-accuracy of impression digitalisation by desktop scanners. Clin Oral Investig. 2019. ISSN: 1436-3771 (Electronic) 1432-6981 (Linking). https://doi.org/10.1007/s00784-019-02995-w. https://www.ncbi.nlm.nih.gov/pubmed/31302771

61. Resnick CM, et al. Is it cost effective to add an intraoral scanner to an oral and maxillofacial surgery practice? J Oral Maxillofac Surg. 2019;77(8):1687–94. ISSN: 1531-5053 (Electronic) 0278-2391 (Linking). https://doi.org/10.1016/j.joms.2019.03.011. https://www.ncbi.nlm.nih.gov/pubmed/30991020

62. Son K, Lee WS, Lee KB. Prediction of the learning curves of 2 dental CAD software programs. J Prosthet Dent. 2019;121(1):95–100. ISSN: 1097-6841 (Electronic) 0022-3913 (Linking). https://doi.org/10.1016/j.prosdent.2018.01.004. https://www.ncbi.nlm.nih.gov/pubmed/30017157

63. Sommacal B, et al. Evaluation of two 3D printers for guided implant surgery. Int J Oral Maxillofac Implants. 2018;33(4):743–6. ISSN: 1942-4434 (Electronic) 0882-2786 (Linking). https://doi.org/10.11607/jomi.6074. https://www.ncbi.nlm.nih.gov/pubmed/29543930

64. Berry E, et al. Preliminary experience with medical applications of rapid prototyping by selective laser sintering. Med Eng Phys. 1997;19(1):90–6. ISSN: 1350-4533 (Print) 1350-4533 (Linking). https://www.ncbi.nlm.nih.gov/pubmed/9140877

65. Tan KH, et al. Scaffold development using selective laser sintering of polyetheretherketone-hydroxyapatite biocomposite blends. Biomaterials. 2003;24(18):3115–23. ISSN: 0142-9612 (Print) 0142-9612 (Linking). https://doi.org/10.1016/s0142-9612(03)00131-5. https://www.ncbi.nlm.nih.gov/pubmed/12895584

66. Lambert FE, et al. Descriptive analysis of implant and prosthodontic survival rates with fixed implant-supported rehabilitations in the edentulous maxilla. J Periodontol. 2009;80(8):1220–30. ISSN: 0022-3492 (Print) 0022-3492 (Linking). https://doi.org/10.1902/jop.2009.090109. https://www.ncbi.nlm.nih.gov/pubmed/19656021

67. Ganz SD. Presurgical planning with CT-derived fabrication of surgical guides. J Oral Maxillofac Surg. 2005;63(9 Suppl 2):59–71. ISSN: 0278-2391 (Print) 0278-2391 (Linking). https://doi.org/10.1016/j.joms.2005.05.156. https://www.ncbi.nlm.nih.gov/pubmed/16125016

68. Vercruyssen M, et al. Computer-supported implant planning and guided surgery: a narrative review. Clin Oral Implants Res. 2015;26(Suppl 11):69–76. ISSN: 1600-0501 (Electronic) 0905-7161 (Linking). https://doi.org/10.1111/clr.12638. https://www.ncbi.nlm.nih.gov/pubmed/26385623

69. Ravida A, et al. Clinical outcomes and cost effectiveness of computer-guided versus conventional implant-retained hybrid prostheses: a long-term retrospective analysis of treatment protocols. J Periodontol. 2018;89(9):1015–24. ISSN: 1943-3670 (Electronic) 0022-3492 (Linking). https://doi.org/10.1002/JPER.18-0015. https://www.ncbi.nlm.nih.gov/pubmed/29761505

70. Hammerle CH, et al. Consensus statements and recommended clinical procedures regarding computer-assisted implant dentistry. Int J Oral Maxillofac Implants. 2009;24 Suppl:126–31. ISSN: 0882-2786 (Print) 0882-2786 (Linking). https://www.ncbi.nlm.nih.gov/pubmed/19885440

71. Moraschini V, et al. Implant survival rates, marginal bone level changes, and complications in full-mouth rehabilitation with flapless computer-guided surgery: a systematic review and meta-analysis. Int J Oral Maxillofac Surg. 2015;44(7):892–901. ISSN: 1399-0020 (Electronic) 0901-5027 (Linking). https://doi.org/10.1016/j.ijom.2015.02.013. https://www.ncbi.nlm.nih.gov/pubmed/25790741

72. Ramasamy M, et al. Implant surgical guides: From the past to the present. J Pharm Bioallied Sci. 2013;5(Suppl 1):S98–102. ISSN: 0976-4879 (Print) 0975-7406 (Linking). https://doi.org/10.4103/0975-7406.113306. https://www.ncbi.nlm.nih.gov/pubmed/23946587

73. De Vico G, et al. Computer-assisted virtual treatment planning combined with flapless surgery and immediate loading in the rehabilitation of partial edentulies. Oral Implantol. 2012;5(1):3–10. ISSN: 1974-5648 (Print) 1974-5648 (Linking). https://www.ncbi.nlm.nih.gov/pubmed/23285400

74. van Steenberghe D, et al. A custom template and definitive prosthesis allowing immediate implant loading in the maxilla: a clinical report. Int J Oral Maxillofac Implants. 2002;17(5):663–70. ISSN: 0882-2786 (Print) 0882-2786 (Linking). https://www.ncbi.nlm.nih.gov/pubmed/12381066
75. Oh JH, et al. Digital workflow for computer-guided implant surgery in edentulous patients: a case report. J Oral Maxillofac Surg. 2017;75(12):2541–9. ISSN: 1531-5053 (Electronic) 0278-2391 (Linking). https://doi.org/10.1016/j.joms.2017.08.008. https://www.ncbi.nlm.nih.gov/pubmed/28881181
76. Raico Gallardo YN, et al. Accuracy comparison of guided surgery for dental implants according to the tissue of support: a systematic review and meta-analysis. Clin Oral Implants Res. 2017;28(5):602–12. ISSN: 1600-0501 (Electronic) 0905-7161 (Linking). https://doi.org/10.1111/clr.12841. https://www.ncbi.nlm.nih.gov/pubmed/27062555
77. Tallarico, M. et al. Accuracy of computer-assisted template-based implant placement using conventional impression and scan model or intraoral digital impression: A randomised controlled trial with 1 year of follow-up. Int J Oral Implantol (Berl). 2019;12(2):197–206.
78. Tallarico M, et al. Accuracy of newly developed sleeve-designed templates for insertion of dental implants: A prospective multicenters clinical trial. Clin Implant Dent Relat Res. 2019;21:108–13. https://doi.org/10.1111/cid.12704
79. Smitkarn P, et al. The accuracy of single-tooth implants placed using fully digital-guided surgery and freehand implant surgery. J Clin Periodontol. 2019;46:949–57. https://doi.org/10.1111/jcpe.13160.
80. Skjerven H, et al. In vivo accuracy of implant placement using a full digital planning modality and stereolithographic guides. Int J Oral Maxillofac Implants. 2019;34:124–32. https://doi.org/110.11607/jomi.16939.
81. Kiatkroekkrai P, et al. Accuracy of implant position when placed using static computer-assisted implant surgical guides manufactured with two different optical scanning techniques: a randomized clinical trial. Int J Oral Maxillofac Surg. 2020;49:377–83.

Ultrasound for Periodontal Imaging

5

Lawrence H. Le, Kim-Cuong T. Nguyen, Neelambar R. Kaipatur, and Paul W. Major

5.1   Periodontium

The periodontal complex has four main entities: the gingiva, cementum, periodontal ligament, and alveolar bone (Fig. 5.1). Although the uniqueness of each structure helps distinguish them from each other, the periodontium as one entity helps provide the necessary support for the teeth in which they are embedded. The gingiva forms the collar around the tooth and the alveolar bone covering, and is divided into unattached, marginal, or free gingiva, and attached gingiva [1]. The keratin in the attached gingiva gives its strength and toughness to adhere to the tooth and alveolar bone [2]. The attached gingiva functions to protect the tissue from receding and to protect the periodontal ligament from bacterial invasion [3]. The cementum is the outermost layer of the tooth root covering the root dentin and serves to anchor the periodontal ligament fibers. It is broadly classified into acellular and cellular cementum [4]. The periodontal ligament is a thin layer of connective tissue that surrounds the tooth, and attaches the cementum of the tooth root to the alveolar bone. The periodontal fibers are strong and oriented in different directions

L. H. Le (✉)
Department of Radiology and Diagnostic Imaging, University of Alberta, Edmonton, AB, Canada

School of Dentistry, University of Alberta, Edmonton, AB, Canada

Department of Biomedical Engineering, University of Alberta, Edmonton, AB, Canada
e-mail: lawrence.le@ualberta.ca

K.-C. T. Nguyen
Department of Radiology and Diagnostic Imaging, University of Alberta, Edmonton, AB, Canada

Department of Biomedical Engineering, University of Alberta, Edmonton, AB, Canada
e-mail: cuong1@ualberta.ca

N. R. Kaipatur · P. W. Major
School of Dentistry, University of Alberta, Edmonton, AB, Canada
e-mail: kaipatur@ualberta.ca; major@ualberta.ca

© Springer Nature Switzerland AG 2021
H.-L. (Albert) Chan, O. D. Kripfgans (eds.), *Dental Ultrasound in Periodontology and Implantology*, https://doi.org/10.1007/978-3-030-51288-0_5

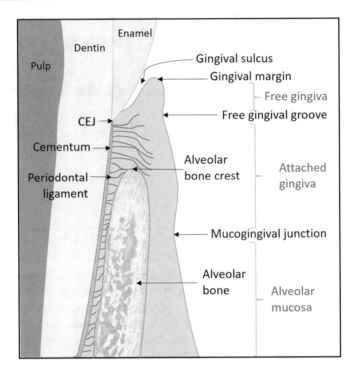

Fig. 5.1 The periodontium

to withstand loading forces during chewing [5]. Alveolar bone development and preservation are dependent on the presence of teeth and are subject to remodeling. It comprises the alveolar process of the jaws that houses the developing tooth buds during growth and later becomes the alveolar bone proper that forms the tooth socket and supports the tooth. The alveolar process provides attachment for periodontal ligament and the associated tooth root [6]. Alveolar bone loss can be due to numerous reasons. Dental caries is a common cause for alveolar bone loss as a result of bacterial infection extending to the root apex leading to a periapical abscess and apical bone loss [7, 8]. Other local causes include periodontitis and residual ridge resorption due to tooth loss [9, 10]. Systemic causes of alveolar bone loss include Chediak-Higashi syndrome (CHS), osteoporosis, Down syndrome, Papillon-Lefevre syndrome (PLS), HIV infection, and neutropenia [11, 12].

5.2   Current Clinical Methods to Assess Periodontium

Periodontitis or periodontal (gum) disease (Fig. 5.2) is one of the most common oral health problems. Prevalence increases with age and it affects a significant percentage of the world population [13]. 15% of the middle-aged adults and twice as many seniors suffer from periodontal disease [14]. The most common signs

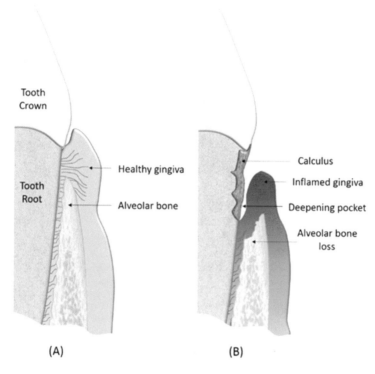

Fig. 5.2 Periodontal disease: (a) healthy and (b) diseased

include inflammation, bleeding on probing, increased pocket depth, and clinical attachment loss, culminating in alveolar bone loss and eventual tooth loss [1]. Periodontal probing is one of the most common diagnostic tools used by dentists to measure pocket depth and clinical attachment level [15]. Two inherent drawbacks associated with periodontal probing include the invasiveness of the procedure and lack of measurement accuracy in individuals with extensive gingival inflammation and low pain threshold. In addition, periodontal probing does not accurately measure alveolar bone level, which is an important measure of disease state [16].

Consistent and accurate measurement requires a reliable identification landmark. The cementoenamel junction (CEJ) or cervical line is defined as a line on the surface of a tooth where the enamel on the crown meets the cementum on the root. The CEJ is considered a stable landmark and is used as a reference marker to evaluate alveolar bone level and accurately measure gingival recession and clinical attachment loss [17]. A periodontal probe (Fig. 5.3) reliably measures the distance from the CEJ to the bottom of the gingival sulcus [18], but the drawbacks include challenges with tactile visualization of the CEJ and invasiveness of the procedure as described above.

Due to the inherent difficulties with alveolar crest identification using the traditional clinical probing method, radiography was until recently considered

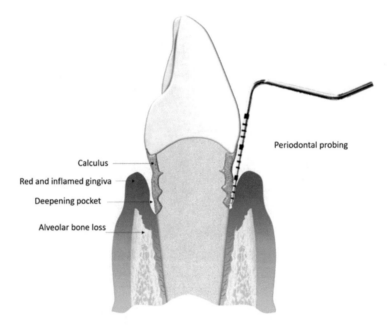

Calculus

Red and inflamed gingiva

Deepening pocket

Alveolar bone loss

Periodontal probing

Fig. 5.3 Periodontal probing

the gold standard and a non-invasive method to detect CEJ and alveolar bone crest. Panoramic radiograph (Fig. 5.4a) is useful as an overall screening image to identify the dentoalveolar structures but does not provide the accuracy or sufficient resolution for periodontal diagnosis and treatment planning. Intraoral radiographs (Fig. 5.4b) have the resolution and structural detail to locate alveolar crest on the mesial and distal aspects of tooth roots, but the overlapping tooth structures render it hard to visualize on the buccal and lingual surfaces of the teeth in the two-dimensional (2D) periapical image [19].

Innovative methods using computer-assisted localization (CAL) of CEJ in digital radiographs were introduced in 1989 [20]. Although digital radiographs led to faster acquisition and instant identification, the inherent drawback of inability to locate the buccal and palatal CEJ lines in periapical films was still evident. Cone-beam computerized tomography (CBCT) has been shown to make available, fast, and accurate 3D volumetric image reconstruction and visualization of internal anatomical features that 2D intraoral and panoramic images have had difficulty to display [21–23] (Fig. 5.5). CBCT images have been used to measure the distance from a reference landmark such as CEJ to alveolar bone crest. Accuracy of the CBCT measurements has been demonstrated in a number of peer-reviewed articles. In an in vitro study on dry human skulls, Leung et al. [24] reported a measurement error of 0.4 mm for CEJ and 0.6 mm for alveolar bone crest identification from a known reference point as compared to direct measurement as the gold standard. The accuracy of CBCT with respect to intraoral radiography was also established

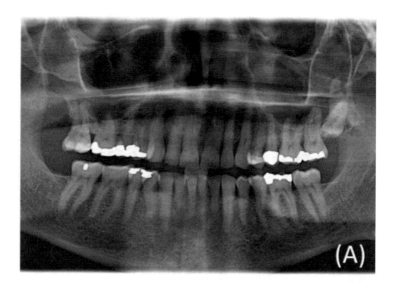

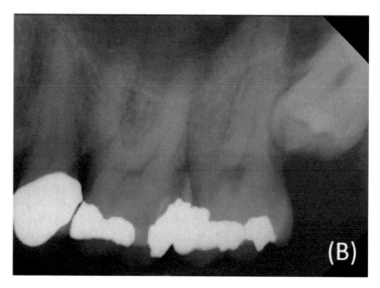

Fig. 5.4 Examples of 2D radiographs: (**a**) panoramic and (**b**) periapical

for identification of vertical bony defects in an in vivo study involving human subjects [25]. The biggest advantage of a CBCT image is the 3D visualization of the structures on the buccal (cheek), labial (lip), and lingual (tongue) sides, without any overlap from other hard tissues such as teeth [26]. Unfortunately, CBCT has increased radiation dose, which is 5–74 times higher than a single panoramic radiograph. The added dose accumulation with repeated imaging that is necessary to track progression of periodontal disease is unwarranted [27]. Although recent

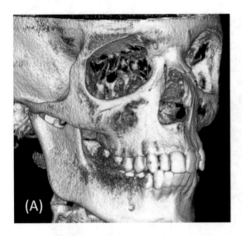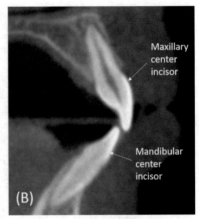

Fig. 5.5 CBCT imaging: (**a**) 3D reconstruction of a human skull and (**b**) cross-section of upper and lower incisor teeth

systematic reviews [21, 26] concluded that CBCT is the standard of care to identify intra-bony periodontal defects and furcation defects, the authors also emphasized that the financial burden of procuring a dental CBCT unit and the excessive radiation dose preclude the routine use of CBCT. The radiation risk is much higher in pediatric population due to its impact on growth potential and early development of cancer [28]. Low and medium resolution CBCT does not have sufficient spatial resolution to accurately identify the CEJ and alveolar crest [29]. Figure 5.6 displays CBCT and μCT images of a porcine incisor for comparison. The image was scanned by an i-CAT 17-19 dental CBCT unit (Imaging Sciences International, Hatfield, PA, USA) with a voxel size of 200-μm and a 16 cm $\times$ 56 cm field-of-view (FOV). As seen from Fig. 5.6a, the edges of the hard tissues are not well defined, and it is difficult to identify the CEJ and alveolar bone accurately. Achieving better resolution using small FOV imaging and smaller voxel size can result in higher radiation dose [30].

For comparison, the μCT image (Fig. 5.6b), which was scanned by a MILABS U-SPECT4 CT system (Utrecht, The Netherlands) with an 18-μm voxel, shows a distinct enamel layer that is in contrast to underlying dentin and the cementum with a clearly identifiable alveolar bone crest. This leads us to believe that the μCT can be considered a gold standard for accuracy in identifying key periodontal landmarks, but the miniaturization of the equipment limits its application for in vitro studies or small animal research.

5.3   Ultrasound Imaging

Ultrasound is a mechanical wave with frequency higher than 20 kHz. It is generated and detected by a transducer, comprised of one or more crystal elements of dipole-like piezoelectric material. The elements convert electrical energy into mechanical deformation of the crystals and conversely generate electrical signals by the defor-

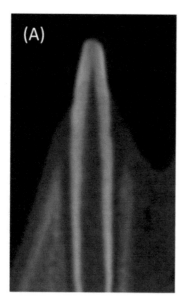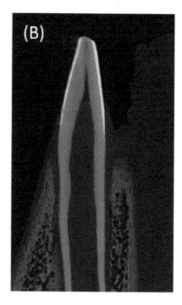

Fig. 5.6 Imaging of a porcine incisor: (**a**) a CBCT image and (**b**) a μCT image

mation of the elements due to external pressure. The passing of ultrasound through the tissue shakes the tissue particles around their neighborhood. The vibrating particles initiate the motion of their neighboring particles, thus transmitting the ultrasound energy from one place to another without the migration of the particles. However, the particles must expend energy to overcome the frictional forces among particles to pass the energy, and the amount of energy loss is characterized by the attenuation coefficient of the tissue. In the context of ultrasound imaging, the tissue is characterized by the density, speed of ultrasound, and attenuation coefficient, where the product of density and velocity is known as acoustic impedance. The generation and propagation of ultrasound within the tissue is strictly mechanical without involvement of ionizing radiation.

Ultrasonography is an imaging technique to use the reflections or echoes of the ultrasound signals to image the internal structures of the tissues. The strength of the returning echoes is governed by the acoustic impedance contrast of the interface separating the media. Energy partition will take place at the interface, i.e., part of the energy will be reflected, while the rest will be transmitted across the interface, which is an ideal situation when scattering and attenuation of ultrasound energy are ignored. Ultrasound is a non-invasive, ionizing-radiation free, economical, and painless diagnostic tool for hard and soft material imaging, and is used in many fields, especially in medicine and engineering. Medical ultrasound has been routinely used to image soft tissues with frequencies ranging from 2 to 15 MHz. Ultrasound has also been applied to characterize bone tissue [31], to estimate the cortical thickness [32], and to image scoliotic spine in children [33]. The bone/soft tissue interface strongly reflects ultrasound energy, thus making bone tissue imaging possible.

The use of ultrasound in dentistry, primarily in periodontics, has been the subject of research for many years but has not been adopted for routine imaging. Ultrasound has been considered a promising tool for imaging hard dental structures. In early 1960s, Baum et al. [34] claimed to identify enamel-dentin and dentin-pulp interfaces using freshly extracted teeth and 15-MHz pulse-echo ultrasound. Subsequent research effort has mainly been focused on ex vivo studies of hard tissues using radio-frequency data instead of images [35]. Although imaging studies of the dento-periodontium are limited, recent literature suggests the potential use of ultrasound imaging in periodontal diagnosis as a good alternative to radiographic imaging due to the increased radiation dose associated with the latter and potential harmful effect on an individual's health. Interpretation of ultrasound images requires specific expertise and is a major challenge for dental clinicians. This may represent a significant barrier for adoption as a routine diagnostic tool in the field of dentistry.

5.3.1   Ex Vivo Imaging

Tsiolis et al. [36] used a 20-MHz ultrasonic scanner, designed for dermatological use, to image the porcine periodontium. The scanner was equipped with a single transducer translated by a motor to produce a 15-mm B-mode image of the internal periodontal structures. By comparing linear measurements between a manually created notch in the enamel and the alveolar crest, they found the ultrasound measurements had better repeatability than the direct measurement and transgingival probing. Chifor et al. [37] also used a similar ultrasonic scanner to study pig mandibles and found accurate measurements of periodontal space width, alveolar bone thickness, and gingiva thickness. Their results also demonstrated a much higher positive correlation between ultrasound and CBCT ($R = 0.98$, $p < 0.01$) than that between ultrasound and microscopy ($R = 0.79$, $p < 0.0001$). Nguyen et al. [38] used a single 20-MHz transducer to image six porcine lower central incisors and found unambiguous identification of the CEJ, enamel, dentin, and cementum. They also found μCT and ultrasound measurements were in strong agreement. Nguyen et al. [39] also imaged hard dental tissues and periodontal attachment apparatus using a 20-MHz portable medical diagnostic SonixTablet ultrasound phase array system (Analogic, Vancouver, BC, Canada). The system had an 8–40 MHz array transducer comprised of 128 elements of 0.1-mm pitch with a small 4 mm $\times$ 13 mm array footprint. The scanner was capable to operate up to 40 MHz with hardware upgrade. The lateral and axial resolutions of the ultrasound probe were 0.50 mm and 0.20 mm, respectively. Further, they analyzed the echoes coming from the interfaces and interpreted their existence in terms of traveling time and signal simulation.

Figure 5.7a shows the center incisors of a mandible from a 4-month-old piglet [39]. The experimental setup is shown in Fig. 5.7b, where the transducer straddled the tooth and gingiva on the labial side. A piece of 4-mm gel pad was placed between

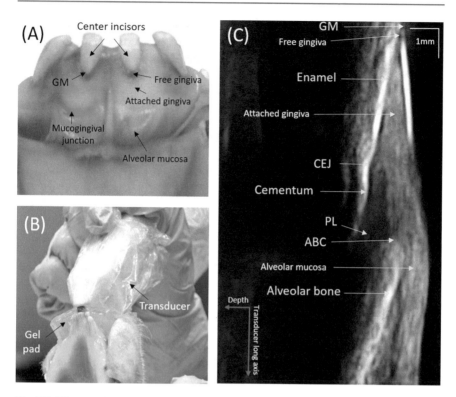

Fig. 5.7 Ultrasound scan of a porcine incisor: (**a**) the mandible, (**b**) the transducer aligned with the long axis of a center incisor, and (**c**) the corresponding ultrasound image of the center incisor

the transducer and the tooth tissue to ensure good coupling between the contact areas. Another purpose of the gel pad was to keep the region of interest within the focal zone of the ultrasound beam. The presence of the gel pad also created echoes from the gel pad-enamel and gel pad-gingiva interfaces, which makes measurement of the gingival thickness possible. The scanning started with the transducer over the enamel and ended with the transducer over the gingiva by sliding the transducer slowly along the long axis of the tooth.

A frame of a video clip, showing the cross-section of a B-mode ultrasound image, is shown in Fig. 5.7c. The interfaces of the enamel and cementum are sharp and well defined as they are strong reflectors and have high acoustic impedance contrast with gingiva [39]. The alveolar bone layer is porous and the pores scatter ultrasound energy. Therefore, the image of the bone layer is blurred but visible and the alveolar crest is clearly identified. The section of gingiva close to the gingival margin has strong reflection as compared to the rest of the gingiva. This happens in most cases for porcine samples because this part of gingiva is denser. In contrast to the CBCT image, the CEJ can be visually recognized. The enamel has much higher speed of ultrasound and density than the gingiva. As the enamel becomes thinner when it approaches the CEJ, more low-speed gingiva fills in the place. Ultrasound takes longer to reach the CEJ area and therefore the image shows a concave region with "the peak of the hump" toward left. The image does not show a continuation of the cementum beyond the alveolar crest. This is because ultrasound cannot penetrate through thick alveolar process. Thickness of the gingiva can be measured from the ultrasonograph, which is impossible in the CBCT image. Nguyen et al. [39] further compared the measurements from ultrasound and CBCT images and found the difference between these measurements were within 10%, showing ultrasound is as good as CBCT in providing clinically relevant information. The gel pad-enamel and gingiva-enamel interfaces have large acoustic impedance contrast, resulting in strong reflection. Therefore, strong hyper-echoic signals are expected, as evidenced by the enamel reflector.

5.3.2   In Vivo Imaging

Fukukita et al. [40] appear to be the first group to produce early in vivo B-scan images of the tooth and alveolar bone using a single 20-MHz transducer with a mechanical driving motor. Salmon and Le Denmat [41] developed a 25-MHz single transducer ultrasound prototype system to perform ultrasound imaging on healthy volunteers. The transducer was linearly translated to provide continuous scanning for a B-mode image, which showed the cementum and the alveolar process. Zimbran et al. [42] imaged periodontal structures of human premolars in vivo using a very high frequency (40 MHz) Ultrasonix SonoTouch scanner. While the scanning set up was not provided, it was expected that the transducer was placed extra-orally on the cheek to image the premolars. In a recent study, Chan et al. [43] studied 144 teeth from 6 fresh cadavers by means of 14-MHz ultrasound, CBCT with 80 μm resolution, and direct measurement. By comparing the alveolar bone level with respect to CEJ and the thickness of the bone crest, they found the ultrasound measurements were as accurate as CBCT and direct measurements.

The scanning setup for human incisors is shown in Fig. 5.8a. The subject was a 15-year-old male volunteer. The long axis of the transducer lined up with the long axis of the tooth. The transducer had a clip at its front to hold a small piece of gel pad. Figure 5.8b shows an ultrasound B-mode image. The image shows clearly enamel boundary, CEJ, gingival margin (GM), gingiva, cementum, alveolar bone crest (ABC), alveolar bone, and periodontal ligament (PL). The portion of cementum underlying the alveolar bone cannot be seen as expected because ultrasound cannot penetrate through thick bone.

5.4   Discussion

CBCT is a valuable clinical imaging tool for assessing alveolar bone and providing evidence-based treatment. It allows reconstruction of any sectional views without overlying tissue obstruction, thus allowing a clear visualization of the alveolar structures on the lingual and buccal sides. However, the identification of CEJ on

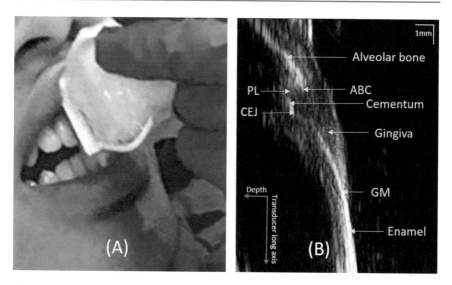

Fig. 5.8 Ultrasound scan of a human incisor: (**a**) scanning configuration and (**b**) ultrasound image

CBCT images is still a challenge [39] unless high-resolution CBCT is employed, which will require much higher radiation exposure to patients. Furthermore, dental CBCT is not suitable for soft tissue imaging such as gingival characterization and measurement. Development of diagnostic high-quality imaging modality without ionizing radiation is highly desirable. Reports on recent research have demonstrated that high frequency ultrasound is ionizing radiation-free and has the potential to visualize alveolar bone on the buccal and lingual surfaces, diagnose periapical inflammatory lesions [44, 45], and measure sulcus depth and gingival thickness [42]. The use of multi-element array transducer has significantly reduced the data acquisition time to few seconds, thereby decreasing patient chair time and minimizing the impact of patient motion to degrade the image quality. A phase array ultrasound equipped with multi-element transducer is preferable to a single transducer translated by a motor to generate a B-mode image. The former system will steer all elements electronically to focus on a depth point to generate one A-line, which greatly enhances the signal-to-nose ratio. The image, which is made up of many A-lines, can be obtained by sweeping the beam across the target. The quality of the image is much superior to that of a single element transducer with translation. However, one current drawback is the size of the transducer, which presently restricts intraoral use to incisors or canines. Small, compact, and flexible transducers need to be designed to study premolars and molars intraorally.

Periodontal tissues are complex with tissues of different scales such as gingiva, alveolar bone, cementum, and periodontal ligament. Imaging these hard and soft tissues require different ultrasound frequency or wavelength as their speeds span from 1540 m/s (gingiva) to 3200 m/s (cementum). In principle, using high frequency will increase imaging resolution to see small details or scales. However, the intrinsic attenuation characteristics of oral tissues have preferential filtering to remove high frequencies faster than low frequencies as the signal travels through the tissues. As high frequency components are removed, the wavelength of the probing signal becomes larger and the signal becomes less sharp, thus losing the originally required resolution to look at small scales. Acoustic attenuation usually increases with frequency [46] and places a limitation to depth penetration of the ultrasound signal. Thus, a compromise must be made to choose a center frequency to balance between imaging depth and imaging details.

Alveolar bone is cancellous bone covered by a thin cortical bone. Assuming that the acoustic impedances of gingiva and cortical bone are 1.63 MRayl [39] and 7.38 MRayl [47], respectively, the echoes carry approximately 41% of the incident energy but delineate a good estimation of the gingiva-alveolar bone interface. The bone surface is neither regular nor smooth. The rough surfaces of the pores tend to scatter ultrasound in all directions. The scattering process has two negative impacts. First, the scattered energy will not be received by the transducer, thus creating an apparent loss of the signal's energy; second, the scattered signals are considered noise, generating speckle characteristics in the image, which reduces image contrast and thus the diagnostic quality of the image. Due to scattering, the gingiva-alveolar bone interface is blurred and fuzzy. This is also a reason why most of the ultrasound images published so far lack good diagnostic quality and clarity. Even though in theory, there is about 59% incident energy transmitted across the gingiva-alveolar bone interface into the alveolar bone, the actual amount of incident energy striking the bottom of the alveolar layer is less due to scattering and attenuation within the alveolar bone composition. Therefore, the corresponding echoes are less likely to be detected. For this reason, the thickness of the alveolar bone could not be determined [37, 41]. Löst et al. [48] recognized the cancellous bone as the limiting factor to prevent the identification of the underlying periodontal space in the ultrasound images.

Overall, high frequency ultrasound is desirable as it generates signals of smaller wavelength, which can be used to study small-scale structures. However, high frequency signals cannot propagate greater depth due to intrinsic attenuation of the tissue and being easily scattered by small inhomogeneities, thus affecting the image quality. A study using a range of center frequencies should be investigated to find an optimal frequency for intraoral applications such as identification of soft tissue thickness for non-invasive implant placements including orthodontic mini-implants (temporary anchorage devices), fenestration and dehiscence defects, furcation and bony defects, periapical pathology including identification of cysts and granulomas, submerged and ectopic teeth localization, and sutural width. Ultrasound can potentially be used for evaluating disease progression and treatment effects especially in periodontal regeneration procedures and orthodontics. In contrast to radiography, ultrasound imaging demands more technical skills from the operator in addition to an understanding of ultrasound physics, which can be a barrier entailing slow adoption of the imaging technique in dentistry. Training in image acquisition and image interpretation is important for dental professionals to understand the technique and its capabilities in order to adopt the new technology.

Application of image processing techniques is important to enhance signal-to-noise ratio and contrast of the images. Pattern recognition algorithms and machine learning will also play a pivotal role in aiding clinicians to automatically identify anatomic structures and diagnostic features in ultrasound images [49–52].

Though the feasibility of using ultrasound to study dento-periodontal tissues has been confirmed, the accuracy and validity of ultrasound imaging as a diagnostic tool have not been adequately studied due to small number of published reports and small sample size used for the studies [39, 53]. Further studies using sufficiently large sample sizes of ex vivo and especially in vivo data are warranted to establish satisfactory level of confidence for ultrasound imaging.

5.5   Conclusion

Although ultrasound research is in its infancy, it has shown significant potential as a diagnostic tool in dentistry. Since ultrasound does not expose the patient to ionizing radiation, imaging can be done routinely on children and can be repeated at regular intervals to assess change over time. The potential of ultrasound to be a routine diagnostic tool in every dental office, like an intraoral X-ray unit, is in the near future.

Acknowledgments The authors thank the Women and Children's Health Research Institute (WCHRI), Canada for the financial support of a Seed Grant. The work was partly supported by LH Le's NSERC Discovery Grant. KCT Nguyen acknowledges the support from Alberta Innovates for the PhD fellowship.

References

1. Newman MG, et al. Newman and Carranza's clinical periodontology e-book. Elsevier Health Sciences; 2018. ISBN:032353323X.
2. Cohen L. Keratinization of the gingivae. Dent Pract Dent Rec. 1967;18.4:134–8. ISSN:0011-8729.
3. Ainamo J, Löe H. Anatomical characteristics of gingiva. A clinical and microscopic study of the free and attached gingiva. J Periodontol. 1966;37.1:5–13. ISSN:1943-3670.
4. Foster BL. On the discovery of cementum. J Periodontal Res. 2017;52.4:666–85. ISSN:0022-3484.
5. De Jong T, et al. The intricate anatomy of the periodontal ligament and its development: lessons for periodontal regeneration. J Periodontal Res. 2017;52.6:965–74. ISSN:0022-3484.
6. Goldman HM. Alveolar bone in health and disease, possibilities of reattachment. J Dent Med. 1948;3.2:30. ISSN:0096-0241.
7. Stashenko P, Yu SM, Wang C-Y. Kinetics of immune cell and bone resorptive responses to endodontic infections. J Endod. 1992;18.9:422–6. ISSN:0099-2399.
8. Chu T-MG, Liu SS-Y, Babler WJ. Craniofacial biology, orthodontics, and implants. In: Basic and applied bone biology. Amsterdam: Elsevier; 2014. p. 225–42.
9. Manson JD. Bone morphology and bone loss in periodontal disease. J Clin Periodontol. 1976;3.1:14–22. ISSN:0303-6979.
10. Beube FE. Correlation of degree of alveolar bone loss with other factors for determining the removal or retention of teeth. Dent Clin North Am. 1969;13.4:801. ISSN:0011-8532.

11. Kinane DF, Marshall GJ. Periodontal manifestations of systemic disease. Aust Dent J. 2001;46.1:2–12. ISSN:0045-0421.
12. Jeffcoat MK. Bone loss in the oral cavity. J Bone Miner Res. 1993;8.S2:S467–73. ISSN:0884-0431.
13. Pihlstrom BL, Michalowicz BS, Johnson NW. Periodontal diseases. Lancet. 2005;366.9499:1809–20. ISSN:0140-6736.
14. Web Page. 2014. http://www.cda-adc.ca/_files/about/news_events/health_month/PDFs/dentist_questions_answers.pdf.
15. Listgarten MA. Periodontal probing: what does it mean? J Clin Periodontol. 1980;7.3:165–76. ISSN:0303-6979.
16. Xiang X, et al. An update on novel non-invasive approaches for periodontal diagnosis. J Periodontol. 2010;81.2:186–98. ISSN:0022-3492.
17. Preshaw PM, et al. Measurement of clinical attachment levels using a constant-force periodontal probe modified to detect the cementoenamel junction. J Clin Periodontol. 1999;26.7:434–40. ISSN:0303-6979.
18. Hug HU, et al. Validity of clinical assessments related to the cementoenamel junction. J Dent Res. 1983;62.7:825–9. ISSN:0022-0345.
19. Misch KA, Erica SY, Sarment DP. Accuracy of cone beam computed tomography for periodontal defect measurements. J Periodontol. 2006;77.7:1261–6. ISSN:1943-3670.
20. Haralick RM, Ramesh V, Hausmann E, Allen K. Computerized detection of cemento-enamel junctions in digitized dental radiographs. In: Images of the Twenty-First Century. Proceedings of the Annual International Engineering in Medicine and Biology Society, 1989 Nov 9: p. 1652–54. IEEE.
21. Walter C, et al. Cone beam computed tomography (CBCT) for diagnosis and treatment planning in periodontology: a systematic review. Quintessence Int. 2016;47.1:25–37.
22. K de Faria Vasconcelos, et al. Detection of periodontal bone loss using cone beam CT and intraoral radiography. Dentomaxillofac Radiol. 2012;41.1:64–9. ISSN:0250-832X.
23. Sun L, et al. Accuracy of cone-beam computed tomography in detecting alveolar bone dehiscences and fenestrations. Am J Orthod Dentofacial Orthop. 2015;147.3:313–23. ISSN:0889-5406.
24. Leung CC, et al. Accuracy and reliability of cone-beam computed tomography for measuring alveolar bone height and detecting bony dehiscences and fenestrations. Am J Orthod Dentofacial Orthop. 2010;137.4:S109–19. ISSN:0889-5406.
25. Grimard BA, et al. Comparison of clinical, periapical radiograph, and cone-beam volume tomography measurement techniques for assessing bone level changes following regenerative periodontal therapy. J Periodontol. 2009;80.1:48–55. ISSN:0022-3492.
26. Haas LF, et al. Precision of cone beam CT to assess periodontal bone defects: a systematic review and meta-analysis. Dentomaxillofac Radiol. 2017;47.2:20170084. ISSN:0250-832X.
27. Scarfe WC, Farman AG. What is cone-beam CT and how does it work? Dent Clin North Am. 2008;52.4:707–30. ISSN:0011-8532.
28. Theodorakou C, et al. Estimation of paediatric organ and effective doses from dental cone beam CT using anthropomorphic phantoms. Br J Radiol. 2012;85.1010:153–60. ISSN:0007-1285.
29. Brüllmann D, Schulze RKW. Spatial resolution in CBCT machines for dental/maxillofacial applications—what do we know today? Dentomaxillofac Radiol. 2014;44.1:20140204. ISSN:0250-832X.
30. Li G. Patient radiation dose and protection from cone-beam computed tomography. Imaging Sci Dent. 2013;43.2:63–9. ISSN:2233-7822.
31. Nguyen K-CT, Le LH, Tran TNHT, Sacchi MD, Lou EHM. Excitation of ultrasonic Lamb waves using a phased array system with two array probes: phantom and in-vitro bone studies. Ultrason. 2014;54.5:1178–85.
32. Zheng R, Le LH, Sacchi MD, Lou E. Imaging internal structure of long bones using wave scattering theory. Ultrasound Med Biol. 2015;40.11:2955–65.
33. Chen W, Le LH, Lou E. Reliability of the axial vertebral rotation measurements of adolescent idiopathic scoliosis using the center of lamina method on ultrasound images: in-vitro and in-vivo study. J Euro Spine. 2016;25.10:3265–73.

34. Baum G, et al. Observation of internal structures of teeth by ultrasonography. Science. 1963;139.3554:495–6. ISSN:0036-8075.
35. Barber FE, Lees S, Lobene RR. Ultrasonic pulse-echo measurements in teeth. Arch Oral Biol. 1969;14.7:745, IN3. ISSN:0003-9969.
36. Tsiolis FI, Needleman IG, Griffiths GS. Periodontal ultrasonography. J Clin Periodontol. 2003;30.10:849–54. ISSN:1600-051X.
37. Chifor R, et al. The evaluation of 20 MHz ultrasonography, computed tomography scans as compared to direct microscopy for periodontal system assessment. Med Ultrason. 2011;13.2:120–6.
38. Nguyen K-CT, Le LH, Kaipatur NR, Major PW. Imaging cemento-enamel junction using a 20-MHz ultrasonic transducer. Ultrasound Med Biol. 2016;42.1:333–8.
39. Nguyen K-CT, Le LH, Kaipatur NR, Zheng R, Lou EH, Major PW. High-resolution ultrasonic imaging of dento-periodontal tissues using a multi-element phased array system. Ann Biomed Eng. 2016; 44(10):2874-86. ISSN:0090-6964.
40. Fukukita H, et al. Development and application of an ultrasonic imaging system for dental diagnosis. J Clin Ultrasound. 1985;13.8:597–600. ISSN:1097-0096.
41. Salmon B, Le Denmat D. Intraoral ultrasonography: development of a specific high-frequency probe and clinical pilot study. Clin Oral Investig. 2012;16.2:643–9. ISSN:1432-6981.
42. Zimbran A, Dudea S, Dudea D. Evaluation of periodontal tissues using 40MHz ultrasonography. Preliminary report. Med Ultrason. 2013;15.1:6–9. ISSN:1844-4172.
43. Chan H-L, et al. Non-invasive evaluation of facial crestal bone with ultrasonography. PLoS One. 2017;12.2:e0171237. ISSN:1932-6203.
44. Cotti E, et al. A new technique for the study of periapical bone lesions: ultrasound real time imaging. Int Endod J. 2002;35.2:148–52. ISSN:0143-2885.
45. Musu D, et al. Ultrasonography in the diagnosis of bone lesions of the jaws: a systematic review. Oral Surg Oral Med Oral Pathol Oral Radiol 2016;122.1:e19–29. ISSN:2212-4403.
46. Tole NM, Ostensen H. Basic physics of ultrasonographic imaging. World Health Organization; 2005. ISBN:9241592990.
47. Culjat MO, et al. A review of tissue substitutes for ultrasound imaging. Ultrasound Med Biol. 2010;36.6:861–73. ISSN:0301-5629.
48. Löst C, Irion K-M, Nüssie W. Determination of the facial/oral alveolar crest using RF-echograms. J Clin Periodontol. 1989;16.8:539–44. ISSN:1600-051X.
49. Nguyen K-CT, Shi D, Kaipatur NR, LOU HM, Major PW, Punithakumar K, Le LH. Graph cuts-based segmentation of alveolar bone in ultrasound imaging. In: 2018 IEEE international conference on bioinformatics and biomedicine (BIBM). Piscataway: IEEE; 2018 Dec 3: p. 2049–55. ISBN:1538654881.
50. Nguyen K-CT, Kaipatur NR, Lou EH, Major PW, Punithakumar K, Le LH. Registration of ultrasound and CBCT images for enhancing tooth-periodontium visualization: a feasibility study. In: 2019 International Conference on Multimedia Analysis and Pattern Recognition (MAPR) 2019 May 9: p. 1–5. IEEE. ISBN:1728118298.
51. Duong DQ, Nguyen K-CT, Kaipatur NR, Lou EH, Noga M, Major PW, Punithakumar K, Le LH. Fully automated segmentation of alveolar bone using deep convolutional neural networks from intraoral ultrasound images. In: 2019 41st Annual International Conference of the IEEE Engineering in Medicine and Biology Society (EMBC) 2019 Jul 23: p. 6632–35. IEEE.
52. Nguyen K-CT, Duong DQ, Almeida FT, Major PW, Pham T-T, Kaipatur NR, Lou EHM, Noga M, Punithakumar K, Le LH. Machine learning-based segmentation of alveolar bone in intraoral ultrasonographs. J Dental Res. May 11, 2020. http://doi.org/10.1177/0022034520920593.
53. Nguyen K-CT, Pacheco-Pŭreira C, Kaipatur NR, Cheung J, Major PW, Le LH. Comparison of ultrasound imaging and cone-beam computed tomography for examination of the alveolar bone level: a systematic review. PloS ONE 2018;13.10:e0200596. http://doi.org/10.1371/journal.pone.0200596.

Ultrasonic Imaging for Estimating the Risk of Peri-Implant Esthetic Complications

6

Hsun-Liang (Albert) Chan and Oliver D. Kripfgans

6.1 Introduction

The central goal of implant therapy has evolved from merely survival, i.e. presence of the implant in-situ and free of symptoms, to functional and esthetic success. Although "beauty is in the eye of the beholder" and the assessment is subjective, certain criteria exist to evaluate implant esthetics. A widely applied method to assess implant esthetics is the White and Pink Esthetic Scores [1]. While the White Esthetic Score is pertinent to the shade, shape, and texture of the restoration, the Pink Esthetic Score assesses soft tissue harmony surrounding the examined implant(s). More specifically, the facial mucosal level, papillae height, mucosal color, contour, and texture in comparison to the adjacent tissues are evaluated. Among these esthetic characters, the mucosal level is probably the most significant because it is eye catching to the patients. Mucosal recession results in longer crown, show-up of the metal hue, and is very dissatisfactory to both patients and clinicians (Fig. 6.1).

Many risk factors have been mentioned in the literature that are associated with mucosal recession, and among them are improper implant positioning, thin tissue phenotype, including both soft and hard tissues, and restorative factors, etc. Regarding the restorative factors, the three designs of importance to the mucosal level are abutment design and associated angles, the cervical crown contour, and the overall emergence angle formed by the abutment-to-crown relationship. According to the prosthodontic glossary of terms (2017) [2], the emergence angle is the angle

H.-L. (Albert) Chan
Department of Periodontics and Oral Medicine, School of Dentistry, University of Michigan, Ann Arbor, MI, USA
e-mail: hlchan@umich.edu

O. D. Kripfgans (✉)
Department of Radiology, Medical School, University of Michigan, Ann Arbor, MI, USA
e-mail: greentom@umich.edu

© Springer Nature Switzerland AG 2021
H.-L. (Albert) Chan, O. D. Kripfgans (eds.), *Dental Ultrasound in Periodontology and Implantology*, https://doi.org/10.1007/978-3-030-51288-0_6

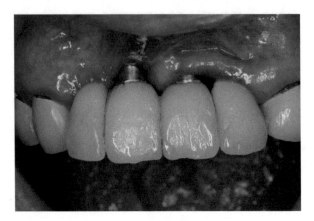

Fig. 6.1 Clinical image of an implant with of a live human subject. There is mucosal recession on two implants located at the right (#8) and left (#9) central incisor sites. The recession is unaesthetic and causes exposure of implant threads, which is more prone for dental plaque accumulation

between the average tangent of the transitional contour relative to the long axis of a tooth, dental implant, or dental implant abutment. Therefore, the emergency angle can be measured at both the implant-abutment and abutment-crown interface. In 2010, Su et al. classified the implant abutment and crown contour into two zones, namely the critical and subcritical contours [3]. The critical zone is comparable to the abutment-crown area, whereas the subcritical zone is similar to the implant-abutment area. These zones are hypothesized to influence tissue infiltration and maturation, as well as the generation of tension that modifies tissue growth. The emergence angle of an implant crown has been documented to impact on facial bone remodeling [4,5], soft tissue thickness [6], the amount of undetected cement [7], and the fracture strength of the implant-supported superstructure [8]. The emergence profile is essentially the prosthetic contour [9, 10].

Although many factors pertinent to mucosal recession were identified in the literature, they were mentioned or studied individually rather than collectively. Ultrasound can provide cross-sectional images of the implant, peri-implant tissues, crown, and abutment with superior soft tissue contrast without radiation. Therefore, it is currently the most optimal imaging method to study mucosal level in relation to these factors. This chapter will focus on ultrasound to image implant prosthetic components and the application of this useful imaging modality to study risk factors associate with mucosal recession around implants in a longitudinal study.

6.1.1 Scanning Modes

6.1.1.1 Still and Cine Images

Still image refers to a single 2D frame image, while Cine images are a video of a collection of still images. A still image gives a snapshot of the region of interest.

Cine images are recorded when a probe is either manually or mechanically moved cross an area of interest. The number of frames obtained is determined by the "frame rate." Cine images are especially useful when tracing of an anatomical structure is necessary between frames to confirm this particular structure. Both image types are saved in Digital Imaging and Communications in Medicine (DICOM) format by default.

6.1.1.2 B-Mode Scan

B-mode is a two-dimensional image composed of dots of various degree of brightness representing ultrasound echoes. The brightness is determined by the amplitude of the returned echo signal. B-mode images allow for visualization and quantification of soft–hard tissue boundaries, various tooth and implant structures, and characterization of soft tissues.

6.1.1.3 Color Flow Scan

A color flow scan can detect blood flow direction and relative velocity and displayed in a color (blue and red) encoded display from throughout the ultrasound image. The velocity is quantifiable and may indicate blood vessel density and the degree of inflammation, based on the colored pixel density.

6.1.1.4 Power Doppler Scan

Power Doppler scan displays the strength of the Doppler signal in color, rather than the speed and direction information. It is particularly useful for small vessels and those with low-velocity flow. The signal is quantifiable and its increase indicates higher blood volume and may suggest inflammation. All the 3 scanning modes can be saved as "Still" or "Cine" images.

6.1.2   The Scanning Protocol

The scanning starts with a B-mode cross-sectional scan at the mid-facial site of an implant because important anatomical landmarks can be identified and used to orient the examiner. Due to use of a high frequency transducer, the implant fixture that is intraosseous cannot been imaged unless the overlying bone is very thin. Figure 6.2 demonstrates such a scan on a healthy implant of a live human. The US image is compared to the clinical and CBCT images. On the US image, the implant (I), abutment (A), and crown (C) are well delineated. The arrows show the junctions between the different implant components. Additionally, the alveolar bone surface and soft tissue are clearly seen as well.

Another clinical case demonstrates mid-facial peri-implant structures, in comparison to the corresponding CBCT image and clinical photos before and after a soft tissue flap elevation (see Fig. 6.3). As can be seen, the cross-sectional CBCT image may not be diagnostic due to artifacts surrounding the implant. CBCT cannot differentiate the thin facial bone, which can be delineated on the ultrasound image.

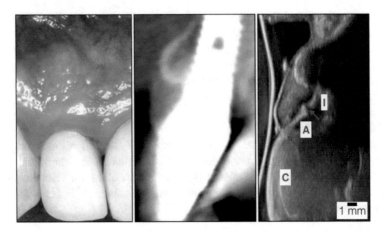

Fig. 6.2 Ultrasound image of a healthy implant in a live human subject, in comparison to a clinical and cross-sectional CBCT image. On the ultrasound image, the implant (I), abutment (A), and crown (C) surface are clearly delineated. Soft tissue characteristics (speckle) are clearly seen

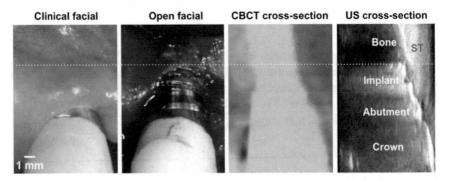

Fig. 6.3 Ultrasound image of an implant with recession in a live human, in comparison to the clinical photos and a CBCT scan. Ultrasound can clearly delineate bone, implant, abutment, and crown. On the other hand, CBCT is inferior in providing surface details due to inherent limitations

Other peri-implant structures and restorative components can also be evaluated on the ultrasound image.

If necessary, the interproximal tissues can also be evaluated with ultrasound by relocating the ultrasound probe mesially and distally until the implant fixture/abutment complex is about to disappear on the image. After the still scans, a Cine scan across the width of the peri-implant space from the mesial to distal sites may be taken. The B-mode scan is adequate for anatomical peri-implant structure evaluation. For functional evaluation, color flow and power Doppler are needed. More details in interproximal tissue evaluation and functional analysis can be found in Chap. 8.

6.1.3   Benchtop Characteristics of Implant Restorations with Ultrasound

Evaluation of the implant fixture, abutment, and crown is an integral part of studying peri-implant structures because these landmarks are the boundaries with which soft- and hard-tissues are measured. However, because of the convexity of abutment and crown, and implant axis in relation to the alveolar ridge, ultrasound might not reflect well to form well-delineated images. Experiences from live human clinical scans suggested these findings; sometimes the abutment contour cannot be fully captured by ultrasound and cause uncertainties in imaging interpretation. The ultrasound's "look" direction will dictate the signal intensity from these structures. Additionally, image modes, e.g. compound and harmonic, etc., will create noticeable differences in images. Therefore, a laboratory experiment was set up to characterize various implant components and to study optimal scanning angles and the image mode. Figure 6.4 shows the setup of the benchtop experiments. A sterilized temporary crown/abutment complex and a commercially available implant was studied. After the complex was screwed onto the implant (Fig. 6.4a), a piece of porcine gingival tissue was sutured on the complex to mimic the clinical scenario (Fig. 6.4b). Then the sample was secured to a mechanical rotary system and placed in a tank filled with water that served for sound coupling (Fig. 6.4c). An ultrasound probe prototype (L25-8), paired with a commercially available scanner, was used to scan the sample.

Three scan modes were selected, namely F24, CSH24 (compound spatial harmonics), and SH24 (spatial harmonics). The in-plane angle of the probe was calibrated to the long axis of the implant as such at $0°$ the ultrasound wave was propagated in perpendicular to the implant. Once calibrated, the sample was moved to $+30°$ and imaged with the 3 modes, rotated in $5°$ increments and imaged each time until $-30°$ was reached. Figure 6.5 shows the 3 image modes when

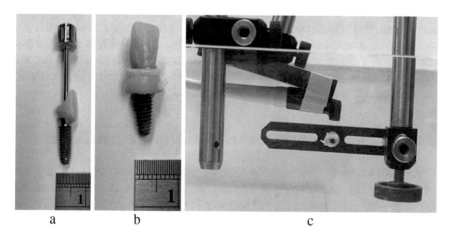

a   b   c

Fig. 6.4 Laboratory setup for studying the influence of the scanning modes and angles on ultrasound image quality

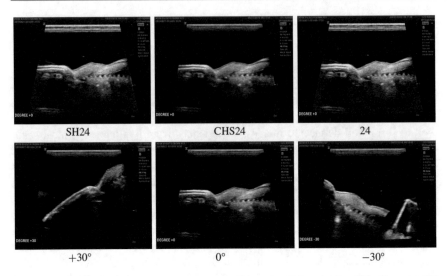

Fig. 6.5 Images of the 3 scanning modes at 0° (top row) and images at +30°, 0°, and −30° (bottom row). There were subtle differences in soft and hard tissue delineation between the 3 image modes at the 0° position, but overall the crown contour, abutment surface, and implant surface could be differentiated clearly. Extreme scanning angles (+30 and −30) may not be able to capture all anatomical structures

the specimen was set at 0° (top row) and the images at 3 different angles, +30, 0, and −30° (bottom row). As can be seen, all the 3 modes could image the crown, abutment, implant surface, and soft tissue. However, subtle image intensity differences were evident and might be clinically significant for distinguishing different structures. Larger positive angle can image the cervical ⅓ of the crown very well but at the same time lose the abutment outline. The 0° angle image provides adequate delineation of the abutment and implant surfaces but less so for the cervical ⅓ of the crown. In general, a negative angle might not be advisable because most structures become less clear. Therefore, in the clinical setting, a few still images at different angles might be taken to capture all important implant structures that may not be in the same imaging plane. Sometimes a cineloop image will be helpful to capture all the required anatomical information.

6.1.4 Risk Assessment of Mucosal Recession with Ultrasound

To take advantage of this versatile imaging modality, a longitudinal study was executed to study the influence of hard tissue, soft tissue, and restoration-related factors on mucosal recession around implants. Most information in this session was partially derived from Dr. Ali Bushahri's master thesis project at the University of Michigan School of Dentistry, entitled *Facial Mucosal Level Determinants for Single Immediately Placed Implants Evaluated Clinically, Radiographically and*

Ultrasonographically. Drs. Chan and Kripfgans served on his thesis committee, and Dr. Chan was the committee Chair.

A cohort of 15 subjects who had been treated with single immediate implant placement with or without immediate provisionalization in the maxillary anterior area in another clinical trial (Chan et al. 2019 JCP) were re-examined. The average follow-up time from final crown restoration visit across the study population was 18.0 ± 4.4 months (range: 11.5 to 26.5). These subjects had previous calibrated clinical readings, including the mucosal margin level. The margin was determined by first positioning a periodontal probe as a tangent to the gingival zeniths of both adjacent teeth (Fig. 6.6). Subsequently, the mucosal margin level was then measured (in millimeters) as the distance between the first probe and the implant of interest's gingival zenith using a second periodontal probe to the closest 0.5 mm. The margin level differences between the final crown placement visit and the final visit were calculated. Two groups were then categorized, the recession group (R) and non-recession (NR) group using a threshold of 1 mm mucosal level change.

A custom-made ultrasound probe prototype (L25-8, Mindray, Mountain View, CUSA) and an off-shelf scanner (ZS-3, Mindray, Mountain View, CA, USA) operating on the sonography technology software (ZS-3, Mindray, Mountain View, CA, USA) were used for ultrasonography of the implant-supported restoration and peri-implant soft and hard tissue. On mid-facial ultrasound images, the following parameters were measured (Fig. 6.7): (1) mucosal margin angle—i.e., the acute angle of the mucosal margin, between the external and sulcular wall of the free mucosa; (2) mid-facial tissue thickness measured at 1, 2, and 5 mm from the mucosal margin; (3) mid-facial soft tissue height (STH)—i.e., the vertical distance between the free mucosal margin and the corresponding bone crest, and the crestal bone thickness (CBT). All parameters assessed on ultrasonographic scans were measured in millimeters accurate to 0.01 mm. Ultrasound crestal bone thickness was measured at 0.5 mm from the crest.

The restorative features, i.e. the implant-abutment angle and abutment-crown angle were determined as well (Fig. 6.7). The former was defined as the outer angle (in degrees) corresponding to the junction between the implant and the abutment.

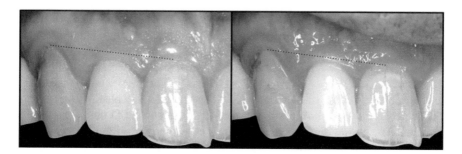

Fig. 6.6 Illustration of the mucosal level changes between the final crown visit (Right) and the final visit (Left). The dotted line serves as the reference. It is evident that the mucosal level receded during this period of time

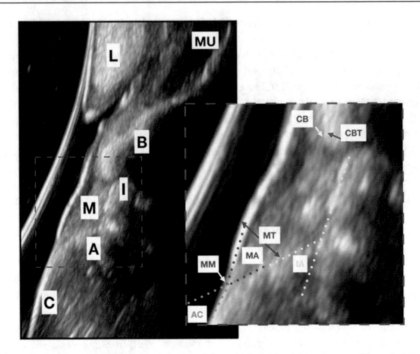

Fig. 6.7 A representative ultrasound image of the mid-facial implant structures. The red dotted area is magnified to further explain the structures and parameters of interest. L: lip; MU: muscle; B: bone; I: implant; A: abutment; C: crown; M: mucosa; CB: crestal bone; CBT: crestal bone thickness; MT: mucosal thickness at 1 mm, MM: mucosal margin; MA: mucosal angle; IA: implant-abutment angle; AC: abutment-crown angle

Similarly, the latter was defined as the outer angle (in degrees) corresponding to the junction between the abutment and the crown.

Table 6.1 summarizes the mean values of the various measured parameters. Comparisons of the soft tissue parameters between the R and NR group reveal 2 interesting and yet expected findings. There was a statistically significant difference in mucosal marginal angle between group R and NR ($p = 0.005$), where the resultant mean angles were 38.78±9.48 (median: 39.43) and 72.01±22.55 (median: 73.05), respectively (Fig. 6.8). The cutoff point for this angle to differentiate implants with recession from non-recession implants seems to be **50°**. Tissue thickness at 1 mm in group R was 0.84 ± 0.16, versus 1.84 ± 0.75 in group NR. The difference between these two groups was highly significant ($p = 0.001$) (Fig. 6.9). Tissue thickness of at least **1–1.5 mm** might be needed for a stable mucosal margin. The mean crestal bone thickness, measured at 0.5 mm apical to the bone crest, is 1.47 mm. The crestal bone thickness of the 3 cases in the R group is 0, 0.84, and 1.35 mm, with the mean value of 0.73 ± 0.68 mm, compared to and 1.65 ± 0.86 mm in the NR group (Fig. 6.10). The difference is approaching statistical significance ($p = 0.10$).

Table 6.1 Summary of proposed ultrasonic measurements for clinical diagnostics

	Implant-abutment angle	Abutment-crown angle	Mucosal angle	Mucosal thickness at 1 mm	Crestal bone thickness at 0.5 mm
Mean ($N = 15$)	36.8	35.0	61.3	1.4	1.47
Standard deviation	18.4	15.1	21.8	0.4	0.9

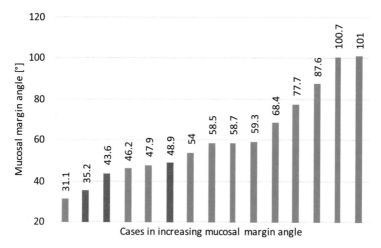

Fig. 6.8 Mucosal angle distribution among the studied subjects. The red bars represent the recession group

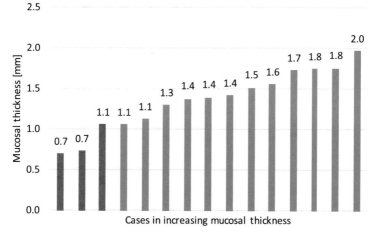

Fig. 6.9 Mucosal thickness distribution among the studied subjects. The red bars represent the recession group

As for restorative-related parameters, although the sample size is small, the bar graph with distributions of the implant-abutment angle shows **20°–50°** may be the optimal angle range for a stable mucosal margin (Fig. 6.11). The 3 cases in the R

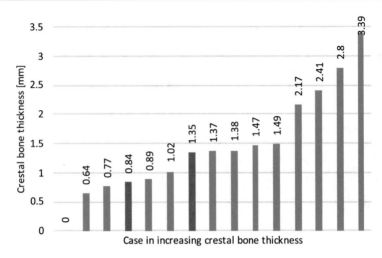

Fig. 6.10 Crestal bone thickness distribution among the studied subjects. The red bars represent the recession group

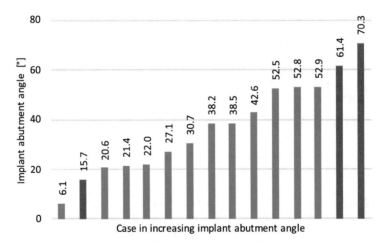

Fig. 6.11 Distribution of the implant-abutment angle. The recession group is marked with red color

group either fall below or beyond that range. In the same token, the **15°–40°** range for the abutment-crown angle might be considered favorable (Fig. 6.12). Table 6.2 summarizes the optimal dimension of the soft tissue and angle range of the implant restorations based on the results of this preliminary study.

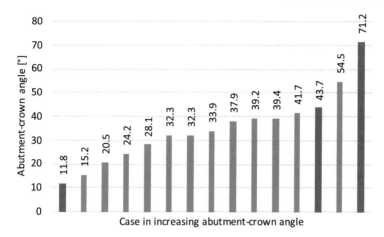

Fig. 6.12 Distribution of the abutment-crown angle. The recession group is marked with red color

Table 6.2 Summary of proposed clinical parameters for stable implant mucosal margins

Parameters	Optimal number or range	Measurement site
Mucosal angle	>= 50 degrees	At the mucosal margin
Mucosal thickness	>= 1 − 1.5 mm	At 1 mm apical to the mucosal margin
Crestal bone thickness	>= 1.5 mm	At 0.5 mm apical to the crest
Implant-abutment angle	20°−50°	Implant-abutment interface
Abutment-crown angle	15°−40°	Abutment-crown interface

6.1.5   Clinical Implications and Conclusion

The mucosal margin angle is a novel marker that represents the interface between the implant restoration and soft tissue. It is also an indicator of soft tissue thickness. A minimal angle (50°) seems required for mucosal margin stability. For soft tissue thickness, 1–1.5 mm might be needed to reduce the incidence of recession. Both soft tissue thickness and mucosal angle are statistically significantly associated with the occurrence of mucosal recession. The crestal bone is 2-times thicker in the non-recession group than in the recession group; however, the difference does not reach statistical significance. It is possible the bone thickness is a late recession indicator; while soft tissue features are an early indicator. With longer follow-up time, crestal bone thickness may become more important in maintaining soft tissue margin level. The presence of optimal implant-abutment and abutment-crown angles reaffirms the importance of implant positioning. Improper implant positioning will result in bizarre restoration angles, which adversely affect tissue level. Table 6.2 summarizes proposed clinical parameters for stable implant mucosal margins. Once confirmed by clinical trials of larger sample size, these ultrasound parameters can be used to evaluate risks of mucosal recession and provide decision-making criteria in the clinics.

References

1. Furhauser R, et al. Evaluation of soft tissue around single-tooth implant crowns: the pink esthetic score. Clin Oral Implants Res. 2005;16(6):639–44. ISSN: 0905-7161 (Print) 0905-7161 (Linking). https://doi.org/10.1111/j.1600-0501.2005.01193.x. https://www.ncbi.nlm.nih.gov/pubmed/16307569
2. The glossary of prosthodontic terms: ninth edition. J Prosthet Dent. 2017;117(5S):e1–105. ISSN: 1097-6841 (Electronic) 0022-3913 (Linking). https://doi.org/10.1016/j.prosdent.2016.12.001. https://www.ncbi.nlm.nih.gov/pubmed/28418832
3. Su H, et al. Considerations of implant abutment and crown contour: critical contour and subcritical contour. Int J Periodontics Restorative Dent. 2010;30(4):335–43. ISSN: 0198-7569 (Print) 0198-7569 (Linking). https://www.ncbi.nlm.nih.gov/pubmed/20664835
4. Funato A, et al. Timing, positioning, and sequential staging in esthetic implant therapy: a four-dimensional perspective. Int J Periodontics Restorative Dent. 2007;27(4):313–23. ISSN: 0198-7569 (Print) 0198-7569 (Linking). https://www.ncbi.nlm.nih.gov/pubmed/17726987
5. Grunder U, Gracis S, Capelli M. Influence of the 3-D bone-to-implant relationship on esthetics. Int J Periodontics Restorative Dent. 2005;25(2):113–9. ISSN: 0198-7569 (Print) 0198-7569 (Linking). https://www.ncbi.nlm.nih.gov/pubmed/15839587
6. Le BT, Borzabadi-Farahani A, Pluemsakunthai W. Is buccolingual angulation of maxillary anterior implants associated with the crestal labial soft tissue thickness? Int J Oral Maxillofac Surg. 2014;43(7):874–8. ISSN: 1399-0020 (Electronic) 0901-5027 (Linking). https://doi.org/10.1016/j.ijom.2014.02.009. https://www.ncbi.nlm.nih.gov/pubmed/24637160
7. Linkevicius T, et al. The influence of margin location on the amount of undetected cement excess after delivery of cement-retained implant restorations Clin Oral Implants Res. 2011;22(12):1379–84. ISSN: 1600-0501 (Electronic) 0905-7161 (Linking). https://doi.org/10.1111/j.1600-0501.2010.02119.x. https://www.ncbi.nlm.nih.gov/pubmed/21382089
8. Saker S, El-Shahat S, Ghazy M. Fracture resistance of straight and angulated zirconia implant abutments supporting anterior three-unit lithium disilicate fixed dental prostheses. Int J Oral Maxillofac Implants. 2016;31(6):1240–6. ISSN: 1942-4434 (Electronic) 0882-2786 (Linking). https://doi.org/10.11607/jomi.4131. https://www.ncbi.nlm.nih.gov/pubmed/27861648
9. Lee EA. Transitional custom abutments: optimizing aesthetic treatment in implant-supported restorations. Pract Periodontics Aesthet Dent. 1999;11(9):1027–34, quiz 1036. ISSN: 1042-2722 (Print) 1042-2722 (Linking). https://www.ncbi.nlm.nih.gov/pubmed/10853587
10. Bichacho N, Landsberg CJ. Single implant restorations: prosthetically induced soft tissue topography. Pract Periodontics Aesthet Dent. 1997;9(7):745–52, quiz 754. ISSN: 1042-2722 (Print) 1042-2722 (Linking). https://www.ncbi.nlm.nih.gov/pubmed/9743681

Ultrasound Indications in Implant Related and Other Oral Surgery

7

Hsun-Liang (Albert) Chan and Oliver D. Kripfgans

7.1 Introduction

The number of dental implant procedures to replace missing dentition is rapidly increasing and has become the standard of care owing to the high survival rate [1, 2]. Successful implant treatment requires prudent evaluation of the surgical site and comprehensive treatment planning, including use of imaging. Features of an ideal imaging modality include: accurate, versatile, no harm, user-friendly, and cost efficiency, etc. [3]. Currently, two-dimensional (2D) imaging modalities, e.g. intra-oral radiographs and panoramic films, are the most commonly used. Nevertheless, image magnification/distortion and the lack of cross-sectional information, etc. are among the major disadvantages [4]. The use of Cone-Beam Computed Tomography (CBCT) is on a rise in recent years [5]. The American Academy of Oral and Maxillofacial Radiology (AAOMR) recommends that evaluation of a potential implant site should include cross-sectional imaging [6]. As useful as CBCT can be, certain disadvantages limit its routine use, i.e. inferior soft tissue contrast, higher cost, higher radiation exposure, and suboptimal imaging quality from interfering artifacts created by metal objects [7, 8]. In medicine, ultrasound always precedes use of CT scans. A systematic review [9] was conducted by our research group to understand the current status of dental ultrasonography research and its potential for clinical use in implant therapy. Table 7.1 summarizes the search results categorized by the

H.-L. (Albert) Chan
Department of Periodontics and Oral Medicine, School of Dentistry, University of Michigan, Ann Arbor, MI, USA
e-mail: hlchan@umich.edu

O. D. Kripfgans (✉)
Department of Radiology, Medical School, University of Michigan, Ann Arbor, MI, USA
e-mail: greentom@umich.edu

© Springer Nature Switzerland AG 2021
H.-L. (Albert) Chan, O. D. Kripfgans (eds.), *Dental Ultrasound in Periodontology and Implantology*, https://doi.org/10.1007/978-3-030-51288-0_7

Table 7.1 Potential clinical indications of ultrasonography for different phases of implant therapy [5] (modified from Bhaskar et al. [9] with permission)

Treatment phase	Potential indications
Planning phase	• Evaluate soft and hard tissue phenotype • Identify vital structures • Evaluate ridge width • Indicate bone density
Surgical phase	• Evaluate cortical bone • Identify vital structures • Evaluate drill bit-bone boundary distances
Follow-up phase	• Indicate primary stability (Chap. 10) • Evaluate marginal bone level around implants (Chap. 8) • Indicate implant-bone stability (Chap. 10)

implant treatment timing, i.e. treatment planning, intraoperative, and postoperative phases.

Table 7.2 summarizes the research and development status of ultrasound imaging, ranging from benchtop studies, preclinical and clinical studies for all possible implant related indications. This review demonstrated a continuous interest in ultrasound imaging in dental research, reflected by published studies proposing numerous indications with which ultrasound can be applied during the three phases of implant treatment. This chapter will focus on indications during pre-surgical treatment planning and during the surgery. Evaluation of marginal bone level after implants are placed will be discussed in detail in Chap. 8. Chapter 10 will specifically focus on ultrasound-based assessment of implant-bone stability. Wound healing evaluated by ultrasound will be discussed in Chap. 9. Peri-implant structure evaluation using ultrasound will be described in Chap. 6.

7.2   Pre-Surgical Treatment Planning

7.2.1   Tissue Phenotype Evaluation

Soft tissue phenotype is relevant to soft tissue strength for resisting mechanical trauma, tissue recession tendency, implant esthetics, and peri-implant bone remodeling, etc. It is in part determined by soft tissue thickness. Several authors investigated the accuracy of using ultrasound to measure soft tissue thickness [10–12, 14]. These validation studies used either human cadavers or porcine cadavers, with ultrasound frequencies at 5, 10, and 16.1 MHz. The mean difference between ultrasound and direct soft tissue thickness readings was 0.13 mm [14], 0.2 mm [10], 0.3 mm [12], and 0.5 mm [11]. In the last two studies, the measured tissue thickness was approximately 5 mm; therefore, the measurement deviation was approximately 10%. One study [14] found a strong correlation ($r = 0.89$) between ultrasound and direct measurements. Two studies [13, 14] applied ultrasound to measure soft

Table 7.2 Summary of the studies classified by the main indications and study designs (modified from Bhasker et al. [9] with permission)

Indication category	Specific parameter to measure	First author (year)	Study design Preclinical/ simulation	Clinical human
Soft tissue evaluation	Tissue thickness	Traxler [10]	V	
		Culjat [11]	V	
		Culjat [12]	V	
		De Bruyckere [13]		V
		Eghbali [14]	V	V
		Chan [14]	V	
		Tattan [15]		V
Hard tissue evaluation	Ridge Width	Traxler [16]	V	
	Peri-implant bone level	Bertram [17]		V
		Chan [14]	V	
	Bone density	Klein [18]		V
		Kammeler [19]	V	
	Crestal bone level	Salmon [20]		V
	Cortical bone thickness	Degen [21]	V	
	Crestal bone level and thickness	Chan [22]	V	
		Tattan [15]		V
Vital structure evaluation	Sublingual a.	Lustig [23]		V
	Inferior alveolar canal & maxillary sinus	Machtei [24]		V
	Bone boundaries	Rosenberg [25]	V	V
	Inferior alveolar canal	Zigdon-Giladi [26]		V
	Greater palatine foreman, mental foramen and lingual n.	Chan [27]	V	
	Lingual structures	Barootchi [28]	V	V
Implant stability evaluation	Transmission sound velocity	Veltri [29]	V	
		Kumar [30]	V	
	Transmission sound energy	Ossi [31]	V	
		Ossi [32]	V	
		Mathieu [33]	V	
		Mathieu [34]	V	
	Reflection sound amplitude pattern	Vayron [35]	V	
		Vayron [36]	V	
		Mathieu [37]	V	
		Vayron [38]	V	
		Vayron [39]	V	

tissue dimensional changes after a grafting procedure around implants in humans. A reduction of approximately 0.1 mm in soft tissue thickness was found at 1 year. These studies demonstrate the accuracy of ultrasound in estimating oral soft tissue thickness.

Hard tissue phenotype, i.e. crestal bone thickness, is another important parameter because it is related to the amount of ridge resorption after tooth extraction, peri-implant bone volume, and implant success. A descriptive study [20] suggested the crestal bone level was detectable in at least 90% of the studied sites (162 sites from three patients) on ultrasound images obtained by using a 25 MHz probe and a newly designed ultrasound system. Our group showed an accurate estimation of crestal bone height and thickness on human cadavers by using a commercially available ultrasound scanner (ZS3, Mindray) [27]. The correlations of the ultrasound readings to CBCT and direct measures were between 0.78 and 0.88, respectively. The mean absolute differences in crestal bone height and thickness between ultrasound and CBCT were 0.09 mm (95% CI: −1.20–1.00 mm) and 0.03 mm (95% CI: −0.48–0.54 mm), respectively. Figure 7.1 showed evaluation of tissue phenotype with ultrasound. In addition to soft tissue thickness, B-mode ultrasound imaging can provide useful anatomical information about the muscle attachment level, tissue characteristics (pixel brightness) that may be related to tissue elasticity, supracrestal soft tissue height, and mucosal margin angle, etc. Figure 7.2 illustrated ultrasound

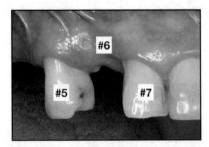

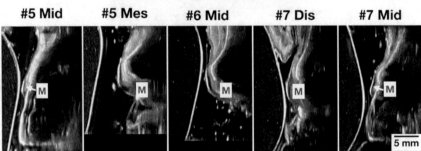

Fig. 7.1 The periodontal tissue around teeth #5 and #7 and edentulous tissue dimensions around tooth #6 location were evaluated with ultrasound. The mucosal (M) thickness, the supracrestal tissue dimension (including sulcus), and the interdental papilla height, etc. can be measured from these images

Fig. 7.2 A color-flow image of periodontal tissues. In addition to soft tissue dimensions, this type of ultrasound image can evaluate the blood flow, which could be very valuable for periodontal disease diagnosis and wound healing evaluation

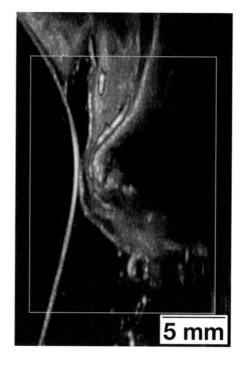

5 mm

can quantify blood flow in periodontal tissue that could be of a great diagnostic value in periodontal disease diagnostics and wound healing evaluation. The vessel shown immediately adjacent to the alveolar bone is a supraperiosteal vessel with a size of $100-200\mu$.

7.2.2 Jawbone Density

Jawbone density has also been evaluated by ultrasound [18]. A 1.2 MHz ultrasound scanner (DBMSonic 1200 instrument, IGEA, Carpi, Italy) was used to measure the ultrasound transmission velocity (UTV) values at different anatomical jaw locations on 108 patients. It was composed of 2 transducers, which were placed on the facial and lingual/palatal side of the jaw. The device recorded the period of the fastest signal conducted through the bone as an indicator of bone density. Similar technology had been applied to orthopedic medicine. Significantly higher UTV was found in maxillary anterior and mandibular posterior regions than in maxillary posterior regions. It was concluded that assessment of alveolar ridge using UTV might offer the possibility to identify bone quality before implant surgery or to monitor bone healing after augmentation procedures. A subsequent study using the same device correlated UTV to bone density measured from histomorphometry, CBCT, and micro-CT [40]. Bone quality of ex vivo cortical, cancellous, and mixed bone blocks were measured and compared. Amplitude-dependent UTV values were obtained. UTV values were 1945.17, 1266.9, and 1472.2 m/s for cortical, cancellous, and mixed samples. There was a high correlation ($r > 0.9$) between UTV values and those from histomorphometry and radiography. Cortical bone thickness, another important clinical parameter, was determined with a combination of low (5 MHz) and high (50 MHz) frequency ultrasound set up [21]. The cortical bone thickness was measured at specific sites around implants using ultrasound, CBCT, and stereomicroscopy. Ultrasound and CBCT measurements deviated from the true bone thickness by approximately 10%. The authors concluded that ultrasound has a high potential to supplement CBCT in measurement of cortical bone thickness.

7.2.3 Edentulous Ridge Width

Ridge width is among the most important clinical parameters for implant therapy. It primarily determines the implant diameter and if a bone augmentation procedure is required. Residual ridge width was measured with ultrasound on 11 sites from 4 patients and compared to open bone measurements [16]. An ultrasound device with a 10 MHz mechanical sector and linear transducers was used. This study concluded that the ultrasound measurement produced nearly the same data as ridge mapping. Figure 7.3 illustrated the accuracy of ultrasound in imaging crestal bone ridge width. It can also image the integrity of cortical bone. With normal bone ridge, the ultrasound image of the crestal bone is a continuous and hyperechoic line. When there is soft tissue invagination or impaired bone healing, the cortical bone surface shows irregularity or discontinuous and less hyperechoic. Ultrasound can potentially become a screen tool for assessing ridge width and cortical bone quality before implant surgery.

7.2.4 Maxillary Palate Anatomy

The maxillary nerve (CNV2), the 2nd branch of the trigeminal nerve, innervates the mid-third of the face. After leaving the trigeminal ganglion, the nerve passes through the foramen rotundum before leaving the skull and gives rise to many sensory branches. Some branches that are relevant to dentistry are (1) superior alveolar nerve, (2) infraorbital nerve, (3) greater and lesser palatine nerves and nasopalatine nerve. While infiltration of anesthetic injections is usually sufficient for short surgical procedures in the maxilla, advanced procedures, e.g. quadrant osseous periodontal flap surgery, bone regeneration, lateral sinus augmentation, and full arch rehabilitation, may require block anesthesia of CNV2. Intraorally, anesthesia of CNV2 can be achieved from the greater palatine canal (GPC), through which the greater palatine nerve travel after it is branched off from the maxillary nerve. Therefore, it is important to identify the canal and its opening in the oral cavity, the greater palatine foramen (GPF). In the literature, landmarks, e.g. molar teeth, midline maxillary suture, the posterior border of the hard palate, etc., have been used but are not satisfactory to locate the GPF [41]. In general, it is located at

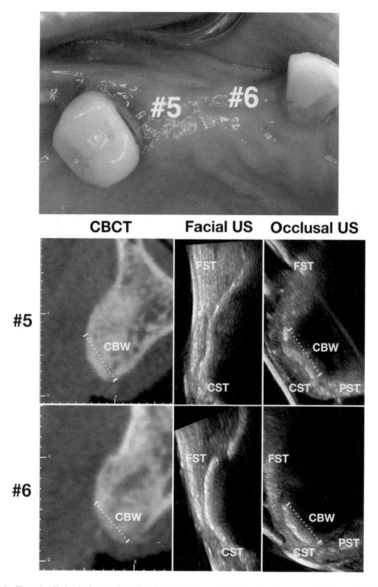

Fig. 7.3 Top, A clinical photo of teeth #5 and #6 planned for implant surgery. Bottom, Facial and occlusal ultrasound scans, with CBCT as a reference, to show crestal bone width (CBW) measures. The red arrow indicates a step between native and newly formed bone, which is also shown on the ultrasound image. FST: facial soft tissue; CST: crestal soft tissue; PST: palatal soft tissue

the junction of the hard palate process and the maxillary alveolar process, mesial or opposite to the 3rd molar; however, the exact location varies from individual to individual [42]. Therefore, imaging-guided block anesthesia of the maxillary

B-mode   Color

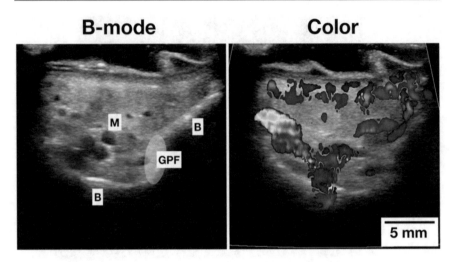

Fig. 7.4 B-mode and color-flow images of the greater palatine foramen (GPF). The bright line is the maxillary bone (B). The discontinuous line is the GPF location. The Color flow shows the greater palatine vessels in the region. M: mucosa

nerve is needed. Ultrasound can provide GPF location in real time during injection. Figure 7.4 illustrates an image of the GPF in a live human. The white line is the maxillary bone surface. Discontinuity of the white line indicates the foramen. B-mode may already show the foramen. Sometimes the Color mode can be used to confirm its location by showing the course of the blood flow in the greater palatine artery/vein, which travel together with the nerve in the canal.

Once the canal is identified, a standard dental long needle (32 mm long) is inserted almost to the end and 1.8 cc of lidocaine is administered slowly after aspiration. CBCT can be helpful to gauge the length of the canal. On average the canal length is 32 mm. Injection beyond the canal into the pterygopalatine fossa and even into the cranium will lead to serious complications, e.g. direct nerve damage, hematoma, diplopia (double vision), transient ophthalmoplegia, ptosis, temporary blindness, and unconsciousness, etc. Therefore, it is important not to pass the needle over the total length of the canal.

Periodontal/peri-implant plastic surgery to cover exposed roots/implants and correct other soft tissue deficiencies is a common procedure. Autogenous tissue harvested from the palate is still the gold standard for this type of procedures. Therefore, knowledge about the quality and quantity of the palatal mucosa is key. The area adjacent to the premolars is a common donor site. Ultrasound can accurately measure tissue thickness and vascularity so the surgeon will know at chairside if there is adequate soft tissue thickness for harvest or allograft will have to be used. Knowing the vascularity can help the surgeon to expect the bleeding tendency, which often time complicates the surgery (Fig. 7.5).

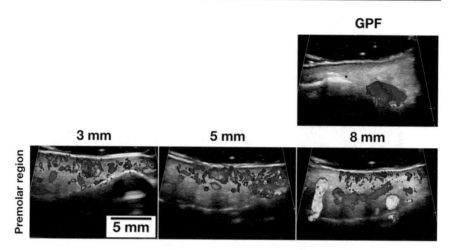

Fig. 7.5 The vessels in the GPF (top) and the palate at the premolar region at 3, 5, and 8 mm from the cementoenamel junction (CEJ). The palatal thickness and vascularization can be evaluated and measured before the grafting harvesting surgery

Box 1
Ultrasonography can image the greater palatine canal, which is a gateway for block anesthesia of the maxillary nerve. Anesthesia of this nerve is often needed for major surgical procedures, e.g. lateral window sinus augmentation.

7.2.5   Mandibular Lingual Anatomy

The lingual nerve is a branch of the mandibular nerve, the 3rd branch of the trigeminal nerve. This nerve provides sensory innervation to the mucous membranes of the anterior two-thirds of the tongue and the lingual tissues. It also accompanies chorda tympani nerve to provide taste sensation of the anterior two-thirds of the tongue. After branching off from the mandibular nerve, it travels in the pterygomandibular space along with the inferior alveolar nerve (IAN). While the IAN goes into the mandible through the mandibular foramen, the lingual nerve stays in soft tissue, running beyond the anterior edge of the medial pterygoid muscle and descend toward the distal side of the third molar. It is located at a mean 3 mm apical to the osseous crest and 2 mm horizontally from the lingual cortical plate in the third molar area [43]. Nevertheless, the nerve may be situated at or above the crest of bone in 15–20% cases [44]. Furthermore, 22% of the time the nerve may contact the lingual cortical plate [43]. Once passing the 3rd molar, it travels mesially, apically, and medially toward the tongue. Seventy-five percent of lingual nerves turned toward the tongue at first and second molar region. The vertical distance

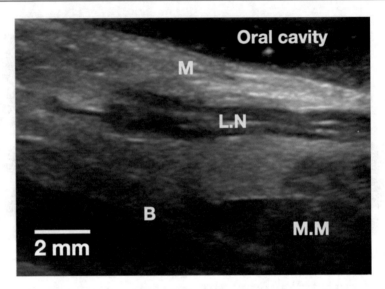

Fig. 7.6 Illustration of the lingual nerve (L.N) and the adjacent structures. M: mucosa; M.M: mylohyoid muscle; B: Lingual plate of the mandible

between the nerve and the cementoenamel junction (CEJ) of the second molar, first molar, and the second premolar was 9.6, 13, and 14.8 mm, respectively [45]. Because its superficial location in general in the 3rd molar region, precaution has to be exercised when performing a flap surgery in this area, e.g. 3rd molar extraction, bone augmentation surgery, and periodontal surgery. A 0.6–2% incidence of lingual nerve injury has been reported following third molar extraction [46–50]. One way to avoid traumatizing this nerve is to know its location. Ultrasound may be the most ideal imaging modality for this nerve because it cannot be seen on radiographs. Our group published a proof-of-principle study [45] and a subsequent study showing ultrasound can image the lingual nerve [28]. Figure 7.6 illustrates the lingual nerve. The nerve is shown as a hypoechoic linear structure with hyperechoic streaks, a character of many other nerves in the body composed of fascicles (a group of nerve fibers in the main nerve).

Another clinical indication for locating the lingual nerve is for its block anesthesia. The most common target for local anesthesia of the lingual nerve is the pterygomandibular space. Once the inferior alveolar nerve is anesthetized, the long needle is withdrawn half way where the lingual nerve is anesthetized. However, inadequate anesthesia of the lingual nerve is common because of the unreliable landmarks. Exclusive lingual nerve block at the 3rd molar region can be an effective alternative because of the following advantages: (1) greater success rate due to easier and closer access, (2) aspiration is not required because of no major vessels in this area, and (3) less chance of post-injection trismus (limited mouth opening). Blind injection in the lingual mucosa of the 3rd molar may already have profound anesthesia of the lingual nerve. Visualization of the nerve with ultrasound can

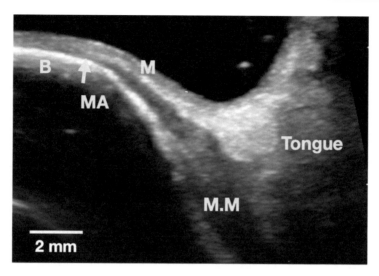

Fig. 7.7 Ultrasound illustration of the lingual structures, including the lingual plate of the mandible (B), the mucosa (M), the mylohyoid muscle (M.M), and the attachment of the mylohyoid muscle (MA)

improve clinician confidence, increase anesthesia success rate and working time, and reduce injection quantity. Moreover, ultrasound can be a learning tool for dental students to practice lingual nerve anesthesia.

Anatomy of the mandibular lingual region has becoming more important because of the popularity of performing bone regeneration for implant placement in this region. Lingual flap releasing requires detachment of the lingual mucosa from the underlying mylohyoid muscle. Knowledge of relevant anatomy besides the above mentioned lingual nerve, i.e. the lingual mucosa thickness, sublingual salivary glands, and mylohyoid muscle attachment is key to successful lingual flap management. Our recent ultrasound cadaver study showed that the mean mucosal thickness is 1.45±0.5 and 1.54±0.5 mm, measured at 5 and 10 mm from the mucosal margin, respectively [28]. Histology showed similar dimension, 1.40±0.51 and 1.37±0.50 mm, without statistical significance. The mean mylohyoid muscle dimension is 2.32±0.56 and 2.47±0.57 mm, respectively at 5 and 10 mm from the muscle attachment. Again, similar dimension was measured on histology, without statistical significance (Fig. 7.7). Regarding the lingual nerve dimension, the cross-sectional diameter was 2.38 ± 0.44 and 2.5 ± 0.35 mm at the 3rd molar and retromolar sites, compared to 2.43 ± 0.42 and 2.54 ± 0.34 mm on the histology, respectively, without statistical significance.

7.2.6 Mental Foramen Evaluation

The mental foramen is the pathway for the mental nerve, the terminal branch of the inferior nerve, and its accompanying vascular bundles. There are three nervous branches emerging from this foramen, providing sensations to the skin, lower lip, gingiva, and mucous membrane mesial to the second premolar to the midline. According to our retrospective cone-beam computed tomography study [51], the mental foramen is located either below the apex of second premolar or between the first and second premolars in 82% of the cases. Its vertical location is halfway between the CEJ and the lower border of the mandible with a range from 13.3 to 23.6 mm from the CEJ and between 12.2 and 20.7 mm from the inferior border of the mandible. Injury to this important nerve can result in temporary or permanent paresthesia, with an incidence rate of up to 7% of cases [52–54]. Therefore, knowledge of the mental foramen location is necessary when performing surgery in this area. Before and during a surgery in this area, ultrasound can provide mental foramen location in real time; therefore, it will be of great value in minimally invasive procedures, e.g. flapless implant surgery. Our group demonstrates ultrasound can image mental foramen in a cadaver study [22]. Figure 7.8 shows features of mental foramen on ultrasound image in a live human.

7.2.7 Other Anatomical Structures

The sublingual artery is another important structure in the anterior lingual mandible that can be identified by ultrasound [23]. Although rare, injury of this vessel can result in massive hemorrhage in the sublingual and submandibular spaces, which in turn can cause fatal airway obstruction. The diameter, direction of blood flow, and blood volume were evaluated in 20 subjects by using a 10-MHz superficial transducer. In all subjects, blood flow was identified and directed into the bone. The average diameter of the artery was $1.41(\pm 0.34\,\text{mm})$ and the average blood flow $2.92 \pm 3.19\,\text{mL/min}$. The ultrasound/Doppler is a reliable tool to visualize and measure the blood supply to the anterior mandible.

7.2.8 Intra-Surgical Evaluation

During osteotomy ultrasound waves can be sent into bone through the osteotomy site. Sound impedance differences between cancellous bone and more dense cortical bone surrounding important structures could then locate these structures, e.g. the inferior alveolar nerve (IAN) and the maxillary sinus. A novel ultrasound device was used to identify IAN and the maxillary sinus intraoperatively on 14 patients [24]. The ultrasound readings were compared to measurements made from panoramic radiographs. The overall differences between the ultrasound and radiographic measurements were minor (0.4 mm), with positive correlation ($r = 0.57$). After

Fig. 7.8 B-mode image of
the mental foramen with
color flow indicating the
mental artery and vein

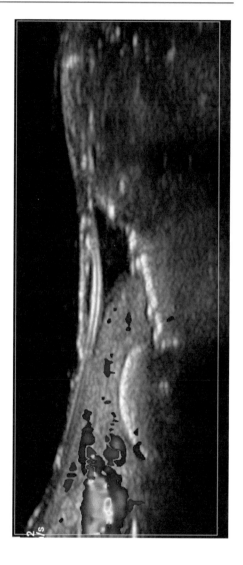

stratifying the data, the differences in IAC readings were 0.1 mm, with high
correlation (0.967). On the other hand, the correlations of maxillary sinus floor
readings were weak ($r = 0.19$). Subsequently, a follow-up with larger sample
size study was conducted by the same group [26]. The accuracy of ultrasound for
identifying IAC was tested on ten patients with 18 implant osteotomies. The mean
differences in residual bone height were 0.18 mm, with good correlation ($r = 0.61$).
Therefore, this tested ultrasound device might be a useful alternative to locate IAC
for implant surgeries in posterior mandible intraoperatively.

Bone boundaries should not be violated during implant surgery else, soft tissue
damage and surgical complications may occur. Therefore, one study [25] aimed to

measure bone boundaries using a device that propagates 5 MHz ultrasonic waves through an aqueous milieu. Two parameters were measured: the depth of drill penetration into bone (drilled tract), and the distance between the drill tip to the bone boundary (residual depth). The correlations of ultrasound and mechanical measurements in the preclinical settings were ~0.99, with mean differences between 0.27 and 1.1 mm. In a clinical setting, the correlation between ultrasound and mechanical measurements was 0.78, with a mean difference of 0.05 mm. Radiographic and ultrasound measurements had correlations of 0.705 and 0.975 for the drilled tract and residual depth measures, respectively. The corresponding mean differences were 0.38 and 0.31 mm, respectively. Therefore, the study concluded this ultrasound method could be useful to monitor intraosseous drilling.

7.2.9 Conclusions

Ultrasound is versatile to identify clinically relevant anatomical structures during the treatment phase. It has been confirmed by clinical studies to accurately measure soft tissue phenotype and hard tissue morphotype, crestal ridge width and quality, mental foramen, greater palatine foramen, lingual nerve, lingual structures, etc. Therefore, ultrasound can already become an initial screening device at chairside for measuring ridge width and the other above mentioned anatomical landmarks during the treatment planning phase. During the surgery, it is fundamental to place an implant in an ideal position without disrupting vital structures in vicinity. Ultrasound can detect the impedance differences between the cancellous bone and the cortical bone that surrounds important structures; therefore, it has been shown to correctly identify IAN and maxillary sinus floor in lieu of radiographs to avoid surgical complications. Flapless implant surgery is becoming more popular because of tissue preservation, faster healing, and reduced morbidity. Cross-sectional drill-bit location could be imaged in real time with ultrasound to provide surgical feedback. There is no doubt ultrasound will be used in a conceivable future provided the device can be built more ergonomic, user friendly, more affordable, and more easily integrated into the current clinical workflow.

References

1. Branemark PI, et al. Osseointegrated implants in the treatment of the edentulous jaw experience from a 10-year period. Scand J Plast Reconstr Surg Suppl.1977;16:1–132. http://www.ncbi. nlm.nih.gov/pubmed/356184. ISSN: 0581-9474 (Print) 0581-9474 (Linking)
2. Lambrecht, JT et al. Long-term evaluation of submerged and nonsubmerged ITI solid-screw titanium implants: a 10-year life table analysis of 468 implants. Int J Oral Maxillofac Implants 2003;18 6:826–34. http://www.ncbi.nlm.nih.gov/pubmed/14696658. ISSN: 0882-2786 (Print) 0882-2786 (Linking).
3. Vandenberghe B, Jacobs R, Bosmans H. Modern dental imaging: a review of the current technology and clinical applications in dental practice. Eur Radiol. 2010;20 11:2637–55. https://doi.org/10.1007/s00330-010-1836-1. http://www.ncbi.nlm.nih.gov/pubmed/20544352. ISSN: 1432-1084 (Electronic) 0938-7994 (Linking).

4. Correa LR, et al. Planning of dental implant size with digital panoramic radiographs, CBCT-generated panoramic images, and CBCT cross-sectional images. Clin Oral Implants Res. 2014;25 6:690–5. https://doi.org/10.1111/clr.12126. ISSN: 1600-0501 (Electronic) 0905-7161 (Linking). http://www.ncbi.nlm.nih.gov/pubmed/23442085.
5. Chan HL, Misch K, Wang HL. Dental imaging in implant treatment planning. Implant Dent. 2010;19 4:288–98. https://doi.org/10.1097/ID.0b013e3181e59ebd. http://www.ncbi.nlm.nih.gov/pubmed/20683285. ISSN: 1538-2982 (Electronic) 1056-6163 (Linking)
6. Tyndall DA, et al. Position statement of the American academy of oral and maxillofacial radiology on selection criteria for the use of radiology in dental implantology with emphasis on cone beam computed tomography. Oral Surg Oral Med Oral Pathol Oral Radiol. 2012;113 6:817–26. https://doi.org/10.1016/j.oooo.2012.03.005. http://www.ncbi.nlm.nih.gov/pubmed/22668710. ISSN: 2212-4411 (Electronic)
7. Benavides E, et al. Use of cone beam computed tomography in implant dentistry: the international congress of oral implantologists consensus report. Implant Dent. 2012;21 2:78–86. https://doi.org/10.1097/ID.0b013e31824885b5. http://www.ncbi.nlm.nih.gov/pubmed/22382748. ISSN: 1538-2982 (Electronic) 1056-6163 (Linking).
8. Mandelaris GA, et al. American academy of periodontology best evidence consensus statement on selected oral applications for cone-beam computed tomography. J Periodontol. 2017;88 10:939–45. https://doi.org/10.1902/jop.2017.170234. http://www.ncbi.nlm.nih.gov/pubmed/28967333. ISSN: 1943-3670 (Electronic) 0022-3492 (Linking)
9. Bhaskar V, et al. Updates on ultrasound research in implant dentistry: a systematic review of potential clinical indications. Dentomaxillofac Radiol. 2018;47 6:20180076. https://doi.org/10.1259/dmfr.20180076. ISSN: 0250-832X (Print) 0250-832X (Linking). https://www.ncbi.nlm.nih.gov/pubmed/29791198.
10. Traxler M, et al. Ultrasonographic measurement of the soft-tissue of the upper jaw. Acta Radiol. 1991;32 1:3–5. http://www.ncbi.nlm.nih.gov/pubmed/2012725. ISSN: 0284-1851 (Print) 0284-1851 (Linking)
11. Culjat MO, et al. Ultrasound detection of submerged dental implants through soft tissue in a porcine model. J Prosthet Dent. 2008;99 3:218–24. https://doi.org/10.1016/S0022-3913(08)60046-3. http://www.ncbi.nlm.nih.gov/pubmed/18319093. ISSN: 0022-3913 (Print) 0022-3913 (Linking).
12. Culjat MO, et al. Ultrasound imaging of dental implants. Conf Proc IEEE Eng Med Biol Soc. 2012;2012:456–9. https://doi.org/10.1109/EMBC.2012.6345966. http://www.ncbi.nlm.nih.gov/pubmed/23365927. ISSN: 1557-170X (Print) 1557-170X (Linking)
13. De Bruyckere T, et al. Horizontal stability of connective tissue grafts at the buccal aspect of single implants: a 1-year prospective case series. J Clin Periodontol. 2015;42 9:876–82. https://doi.org/10.1111/jcpe.12448. http://www.ncbi.nlm.nih.gov/pubmed/26373422. ISSN: 1600-051X (Electronic) 0303-6979 (Linking).
14. Eghbali A, et al. Ultrasonic assessment of mucosal thickness around implants: validity reproducibility and stability of connective tissue grafts at the buccal aspect. Clin Implant Dent Relat Res. 2016;18 1:51–61.
15. Tattan M, et al. Ultrasonography for chairside evaluation of periodontal structures: a pilot study. J Periodontol. (2019). https://doi.org/10.1002/JPER.19.0342. ISSN: 1943-3670 (Electronic) 0022-3492 (Linking). https://www.ncbi.nlm.nih.gov/pubmed/31837020.
16. Traxler M, et al. Sonographic measurement versus mapping for determination of residual ridge width. J Prosthet Dent. 1992;67 3:358–61. http://www.ncbi.nlm.nih.gov/pubmed/1507101. ISSN: 0022-3913 (Print) 0022-3913 (Linking).
17. Bertram S, Emshoff R. Sonography of periimplant buccal bone defects in periodontitis patients: a pilot study. Oral Surg Oral Med Oral Pathol Oral Radiol Endod. 2008;105 1:99–103. https://doi.org/10.1016/j.tripleo.2007.01.014. https://www.ncbi.nlm.nih.gov/pubmed/17482844. ISSN: 1528-395X (Electronic) 1079-2104 (Linking).

18. Klein MO, et al. Ultrasound transmission velocity for noninvasive evaluation of jaw bone quality in vivo before dental implantation. Ultrasound Med Biol. 2008;34 12:1966–71. https://doi.org/10.1016/j.ultrasmedbio.2008.04.016. http://www.ncbi.nlm.nih.gov/pubmed/18620798. ISSN: 1879-291X (Electronic) 0301-5629 (Linking).

19. Kammerer PW, et al. Influence of a collagen membrane and recombinant platelet-derived growth factor on vertical bone augmentation in implantfixed deproteinized bovine bone–animal pilot study. Clin Oral Implants Res. 2013;24 11:1222–30. https://doi.org/10.1111/j.1600-0501.2012.02534.x. https://www.ncbi.nlm.nih.gov/pubmed/22762383. ISSN: 1600-0501 (Electronic) 0905-7161 (Linking)

20. Salmon B, Le Denmat D. Intraoral ultrasonography: development of a specific high-frequency probe and clinical pilot study. Clin Oral Investig. 2012;16 2:643–9. https://doi.org/10.1007/s00784-011-0533-z. https://www.ncbi.nlm.nih.gov/pubmed/21380502. ISSN: 1436-3771 (Electronic) 1432-6981 (Linking).

21. Degen K, et al. Assessment of cortical bone thickness using ultrasound. Clin Oral Implants Res. 2017;28 5:520–8. https://doi.org/10.1111/clr.12829. http://www.ncbi.nlm.nih.gov/pubmed/27018152. ISSN: 1600-0501 (Electronic) 0905-7161 (Linking).

22. Chan HL, et al. Non-invasive evaluation of facial crestal bone with ultrasonography. PLoS One. 2017;12 2:e0171237. https://doi.org/10.1371/journal.pone.0171237. http://www.ncbi.nlm.nih.gov/pubmed/28178323. ISSN: 1932-6203 (Electronic) 1932-6203 (Linking).

23. Lustig JP, et al. Ultrasound identification and quantitative measurement of blood supply to the anterior part of the mandible. Oral Surg Oral Med Oral Pathol Oral Radiol Endod. 2003;96 5:625–9. https://doi.org/10.1016/S107921040300516X. http://www.ncbi.nlm.nih.gov/pubmed/14600700. ISSN: 1079-2104 (Print) 1079-2104 (Linking).

24. Machtei EE, et al. Novel ultrasonic device to measure the distance from the bottom of the osteotome to various anatomic landmarks. J Periodontol. 2010;81 7:1051–5. https://doi.org/10.1902/jop2010.090621. http://www.ncbi.nlm.nih.gov/pubmed/20214439. ISSN: 1943-3670 (Electronic) 0022-3492 (Linking)

25. Rosenberg N, Craft A, Halevy-Politch J. Intraosseous monitoring and guiding by ultrasound: a feasibility study. Ultrasonics. 2014;54 2:710–9. https://doi.org/10.1016/j.ultras2013.09008. http://www.ncbi.nlm.nih.gov/pubmed/24112599. ISSN: 1874-9968 (Electronic) 0041-624X (Linking).

26. Zigdon-Giladi H, et al. Intraoperative measurement of the distance from the bottom of osteotomy to the mandibular canal using a novel ultrasonic device. Clin Implant Dent Relat Res. 2016;18 5:1034–1041. https://doi.org/10.1111/cid.12362. http://www.ncbi.nlm.nih.gov/pubmed/26134492. ISSN: 1708-8208 (Electronic) 1523-0899 (Linking).

27. Chan HL, et al. Non-invasive evaluation of facial crestal bone with ultrasonography. PLoS One 2017;12 e0171237.

28. Barootchi S, et al. Ultrasonographic characterization of lingual structures pertinent to oral, periodontal, and implant surgery. Clin Oral Implants Res. (2020). https://doi.org/10.1111/clr.13573. https://www.ncbi.nlm.nih.gov/pubmed/31925829. ISSN: 1600-0501 (Electronic) 0905-7161 (Linking).

29. Veltri M, et al. The speed of sound correlates with implant insertion torque in rabbit bone: an in vitro experiment. Clin Oral Implants Res. 2010;21 7:751–5. https://doi.org/10.1111/j1600-0501.2009.01873.x. https://www.ncbi.nlm.nih.gov/pubmed/20384706. ISSN: 1600-0501 (Electronic) 0905-7161 (Linking).

30. Kumar VV, et al. Relation between bone quality values from ultrasound transmission velocity and implant stability parameters–an ex vivo study. Clin Oral Implants Res. 2012;23 8:975–80. https://doi.org/10.1111/j.1600-0501.2011.02250.x. https://www.ncbi.nlm.nih.gov/pubmed/22092939. ISSN: 1600-0501 (Elec- tronic) 0905-7161 (Linking).

31. Ossi Z, et al. In vitro assessment of bone-implant interface using an acoustic emission transmission test. Proc Inst Mech Eng H. 2012;226 1:63–9. https://doi.org/10.1177/0954411911428696. https://www.ncbi.nlm.nih.gov/pubmed/22888586. ISSN: 0954-4119 (Print) 0954-4119 (Linking).

32. Ossi Z, et al. Transmission of acoustic emission in bones, implants and dental materials. Proc Inst Mech Eng H. 2013;227 11:1237–45. https://doi.org/10.1177/0954411913500204. https://www.ncbi.nlm.nih.gov/pubmed/23963748. ISSN: 2041-3033 (Electronic) 0954-4119 (Linking).

33. Mathieu V, et al. Numerical simulation of ultrasonic wave propagation for the evaluation of dental implant biomechanical stability. J Acoust Soc Am. 2011;129 6:4062–72. https://doi.org/10.1121/13586788. https://www.ncbi.nlm.nih.gov/pubmed/21682427. ISSN: 1520-8524 (Electronic) 0001-4966 (Linking).

34. Mathieu V, et al. Ultrasonic evaluation of dental implant biomechanical stability: an in vitro study. Ultrasound Med Biol. 2011;37 2:262–70. https://doi.org/10.1016/j.ultrasmedbio.2010.10.008. https://www.ncbi.nlm.nih.gov/pubmed/21257090. ISSN: 1879-291X (Electronic) 0301-5629 (Linking).

35. Mathieu V, et al. Biomechanical determinants of the stability of dental implants: influence of the bone-implant interface properties. J Biomech. 2014;47 1:3–13. https://doi.org/10.1016/j.jbiomech.2013.09.021. https://www.ncbi.nlm.nih.gov/pubmed/24268798. ISSN: 1873-2380 (Electronic) 0021-9290 (Linking).

36. Vayron R, et al. Assessment of in vitro dental implant primary stability using an ultrasonic method. Ultrasound Med Biol. 2014;40 12:2885–94. https://doi.org/10.1016/j.ultrasmedbio.2014.03.035. https://www.ncbi.nlm.nih.gov/pubmed/25308939. ISSN: 1879-291X (Electronic) 0301-5629 (Linking).

37. Mathieu V, et al. Biomechanical determinants of the stability of dental implants: influence of the bone-implant interface properties. J Biomech. 2014;47 1:3–13. https://doi.org/10.1016/j.jbiomech.2013.09.021. https://www.ncbi.nlm.nih.gov/pubmed/24268798. ISSN: 1873-2380 (Electronic) 0021-9290 (Linking).

38. Vayron R, et al. Finite element simulation of ultrasonic wave propagation in a dental implant for biomechanical stability assessment. Biomech Model Mechanobiol. 2015;14 5:1021–32. https://doi.org/10.1007/s10237-015-0651-7. https://www.ncbi.nlm.nih.gov/pubmed/25619479. ISSN: 1617-7940 (Elec- tronic) 1617-7940 (Linking).

39. Vayron R, et al. Assessment of the biomechanical stability of a dental implant with quantitative ultrasound: a three-dimensional finite element study. J Acoust Soc Am. 2016;139 2:773–80. https://doi.org/10.1121/1.4941452. https://www.ncbi.nlm.nih.gov/pubmed/26936559. ISSN: 1520-8524 (Electronic) 0001-4966 (Linking).

40. Kemmerer JP, et al. Assessment of high-intensity focused ultrasound treatment of rodent mammary tumors using ultrasound backscatter coefficients. J Acoust Soc Am. 2013;134 2:1559–68. https://doi.org/10.1121/1.4812877. http://www.ncbi.nlm.nih.gov/pubmed/23927196. ISSN: 1520-8524 (Electronic) 0001-4966 (Linking).

41. Fu JH, et al. The accuracy of identifying the greater palatine neurovascular bundle: a cadaver study. J Periodontol. 2011;82 7:1000–6. https://doi.org/10.1902/jop.2011.100619. https://www.ncbi.nlm.nih.gov/pubmed/21284546. ISSN: 1943-3670 (Electronic) 0022-3492 (Linking).

42. Methathrathip D, et al. Anatomy of greater palatine foramen and canal and pterygopalatine fossa in Thais: considerations for maxillary nerve block. Surg Radiol Anat. 2005;27 6, 511–6. https://doi.org/10.1007/s00276-005-0016-5. https://www.ncbi.nlm.nih.gov/pubmed/16228112. ISSN: 0930-1038 (Print) 0930-1038 (Linking).

43. Behnia H, Kheradvar A, Shahrokhi M. An anatomic study of the lingual nerve in the third molar region. J Oral Maxillofacial Surg. 2000;58 6:649–51. Discussion 652. http://sfx.lib.umich.edu:9003/sfx_local?sid=Entrez%3APubMed;id=pmid%3A10847287. ISSN: 0278-2391.

44. Pogrel MA, Goldman K, Lingual flap retraction for third molar removal. J Oral Maxillofacial Surg. 2004;62 9:1125–30. ISSN: 0278-2391. http://sfx.lib.umich.edu:9003/sfx_local?sid=Entrez%3APubMed;id=pmid%3A15346365.

45. Chan HL, et al. The significance of the lingual nerve during periodontal/implant surgery. J Periodontol. 2010;81 3:372–7. https://doi.org/10.1902/jop.2009.090506. http://www.ncbi.nlm. nih.gov/pubmed/20192863. ISSN: 1943-3670 (Electronic) 00223492 (Linking).

46. Bataineh AB. Sensory nerve impairment following mandibular third molar surgery. J Oral Maxillofac Surg. 2001;59 9:1012–7. discussion 1017. https://doi.org/S0278-2391(01)58639-5[pii]10.1053/joms.2001.25827.   http://www.ncbi.nlm.nih.gov/entrez/query.fcgi?cmd= Retrieve&db=PubMed&dopt=Citation&list_uids=11526568. ISSN: 0278-2391 (Print).

47. Gomes AC, et al. Lingual nerve damage after mandibular third molar surgery: a randomized clinical trial. J Oral Maxillofac Surg. 2005;63 10:1443–6. https://doi.org/ S0278-2391(05)01033-5[pii]10.1016/j.joms.2005.06.012.   http://www.ncbi.nlm.nih.gov/ entrez/query.fcgi?cmd=Retrieve&db=PubMed&dopt=Citation&list_uids=16182911.   ISSN: 0278-2391 (Print).

48. Gulicher D, Gerlach KL. Sensory impairment of the lingual and inferior alveolar nerves following removal of impacted mandibular third molars. Int J Oral Maxillofac Surg. 2001;30 4:306–12. https://doi.org/S0901-5027(01)90057-8[pii]10.1054/ijom.2001.0057. http://www. ncbi.nlm.nih.gov/entrez/query.fcgi?cmd=Retrieve&db=PubMed&dopt=Citation&list_uids= 11518353. ISSN: 0901-5027 (Print).

49. Hillerup S, Stoltze K. Lingual nerve injury in third molar surgery I. Observations on recovery of sensation with spontaneous healing. Int J Oral Maxillofac Surg. 2007;36 10:884–9. https:// doi.org/S0901-5027(07)00231-7[pii]10.1016/j.ijom.2007.06.004.   http://www.ncbi.nlm.nih. gov/entrez/query.fcgi?cmd=Retrieve&db=PubMed&dopt=Citation&list_uids=17766086. ISSN: 0901-5027 (Print).

50. Valmaseda-Castellon E, Berini-Aytes L, Gay-Escoda C. Lingual nerve damage after third lower molar surgical extraction. Oral Surg Oral Med Oral Pathol Oral Radiol Endod. 2000;90 5:567–73. https://doi.org/S1079-2104(00)56151-4[pii]10.1067/moe-2000. 110034. http://www.ncbi.nlm.nih.gov/entrez/query.fcgi?cmd=Retrieve&db=PubMed&dopt= Citation&list_uids=11077378. ISSN: 1079-2104 (Print).

51. Askar H, et al. Morphometric analysis of the mental foramina, accessory mental foramina, and anterior loops: a CBCT study. Acta Sci Dental Sci. 2018;2 12:126–32.

52. Bartling R, Freeman K, Kraut RA. The incidence of altered sensation of the mental nerve after mandibular implant placement. J Oral Maxillofac Surg. 1999;57 12:1408– 12. https://doi.org/10.1016/s0278-2391(99)90720-6. https://www.ncbi.nlm.nih.gov/pubmed/ 10596660. ISSN: 0278-2391 (Print) 0278-2391 (Linking).

53. Walton JN. Altered sensation associated with implants in the anterior mandible: a prospective study. J Prosthet Dent. 2000;83 4:443–9. https://doi.org/10.1016/s0022-3913(0)70039-4. https://www.ncbi.nlm.nih.gov/pubmed/10756294. ISSN: 0022-3913 (Print) 0022-3913 (Linking).

54. Wismeijer D, et al. Patients' perception of sensory disturbances of the mental nerve before and after implant surgery: a prospective study of 110 patients. Br J Oral Maxillofac Surg. 1997;35 4:254–9. https://doi.org/10.1016/s0266-4356(97)90043-7. https://www.ncbi.nlm.nih. gov/pubmed/9291263. ISSN: 0266-4356 (Print) 0266-4356 (Linking).

Ultrasonic Imaging for Evaluating Peri-Implant Diseases

8

Hsun-Liang (Albert) Chan and Oliver D. Kripfgans

8.1 Introduction

Implant therapy has become the standard of care for replacing missing teeth. It is estimated two to four million implants will be placed in the USA by 2020. While implant therapy has enjoyed a high survival rate, incidences of biological and esthetic complications are on the rise. The biological complication is mostly referring to peri-implantitis, an infectious disease affecting peri-implant hard and soft tissues. It is estimated approximately 20% implants are affected by this disease [1]. The end outcome of this disease is peri-implant bone loss and eventually implant loss. The less severe and reversible form that does not involve progressive bone loss is peri-implant mucositis. The two diseases originate and progress in soft tissues with bacterial challenge and dysbiosis before bone hemostasis disruption. In addition, nowadays, patients have a higher esthetic expectation. To achieve and sustain an esthetic outcome, a thorough soft- and hard-tissue evaluation at the treatment phase and subsequently at the maintenance phase is important. Therefore, ultrasound, being a superior imaging modality for evaluating soft tissue features, will play an important role in diagnosing peri-implantitis and evaluating tissue phenotype. This chapter will briefly discuss the current clinical methods to evaluate peri-implant structures and their limitations. Images of peri-implant tissues with various disease severity, defined by the 2017 AAP-EFP (American Academy of Periodontology/European Federation of Periodontology) World Workshop will be

H.-L. (Albert) Chan
Department of Periodontics and Oral Medicine, School of Dentistry, University of Michigan, Ann Arbor, MI, USA
e-mail: hlchan@umich.edu

O. D. Kripfgans (✉)
Department of Radiology, Medical School, University of Michigan, Ann Arbor, MI, USA
e-mail: greentom@umich.edu

© Springer Nature Switzerland AG 2021
H.-L. (Albert) Chan, O. D. Kripfgans (eds.), *Dental Ultrasound in Periodontology and Implantology*, https://doi.org/10.1007/978-3-030-51288-0_8

presented to illustrate the potential usefulness of ultrasound in diagnosing peri-implant diseases. Proper diagnosis and evaluation of peri-implant tissues will lay a foundation for decision making in treatment options and outcome assessment.

8.2   2017 AAP/EFP Classification on Peri-Implant Diseases and Conditions

In 2017 an international task force proposed a classification on peri-implant diseases and condition and formed the current foundation for studying and treating these related diseases and conditions. For details the authors can refer to the manuscripts published in 2018 [2–7]. In brief, four categories have been listed: (1) peri-implant health, (2) peri-implant mucositis, (3) peri-implantitis, and (4) soft- and hard-tissue deficiencies. The case definitions are summarized in Table 8.1. A healthy implant is surrounded by bone, with the its coronal part sealed by mucosa. This mucosa contains a core of connective tissue, comprised of mainly type 1 collagen fibers and matrix elements (85%), fibroblasts (3%), and vascular units (5%). The outer (oral) surface of the connective tissue is normally covered by keratinized epithelium. The mucosa that is in direct contact with the implant, abutment, and crown contains two components, the epithelium and the connective tissue. In health, the peri-implant mucosa height is about 3–4 mm with an epithelium that is about 2 mm long. A healthy implant should not have signs indicative of inflammation, including bleeding on gentle bleeding (BOP), erythema, swelling, suppuration. It should not have increased probing depth, mucosal recession, and pathologic bone loss. Peri-implant mucositis has signs of inflammation but a lack of bone loss beyond remodeling. On the other hand, peri-implantitis, in addition to signs of inflammation, has pathologic bone loss. Soft- and hard-tissue deficiencies, as the name indicated, have mucosal recession and/or thin mucosa and/or loss of bone in the absence of overt tissue inflammation. Therefore, diagnosis and differentiation of

Table 8.1 Summary of the four peri-implant diseases and conditions (published with permission from [8])

Clinical signs/symptoms	Case definition	Peri-implant health	Peri-implant mucositis	Peri-implantitis	Soft- and hard-tissue deficiencies
	Bleeding on gentle probing (BOP)	−	+	+	±
Inflammation	Erythema, swelling, and/or suppuration	−	+	+	−
	Increased probing depth	−	+	+	−
Tissue loss	Mucosal recession	−	−	±	±
	Bone loss beyond remodeling	−	−	+	+

these diseases and conditions center on evaluation of the soft tissue inflammatory status, tissue phenotype, and dimensions of the peri-implant hard and soft tissues.

8.3 Current Methods to Measure Peri-Implant Bone Loss and Limitations

Peri-implant bone loss is the hallmark of peri-implantitis, a prevalent disease that occurs in approximately 20% of dental implants [1]. Costly and traumatic surgical interventions impact patients' quality of life tremendously. Demands for improving quality of implant therapy have driven expansion of clinical research and patient care in this field. To provide definitive evidence, development of well-founded outcome measures and standardized diagnostic criteria are critical. Currently, peri-implant bone level measured from two-dimensional intraoral radiographs is the primary measure [9]. However, 2D radiography is incapable of providing a comprehensive evaluation of peri-implant bone level (Fig. 8.1). It only shows superimposed interproximal bone level, much less the radicular (facial and palatal/lingual) bone level and thickness. Bone thickness is another important outcome measure, especially related to esthetics and long-term peri-implant bone stability [10, 11]. This inherent limitation reduces its ability to assess disease severity and treatment outcome [9, 12, 13]. Other limitations include ionizing radiation and image distortions, etc.

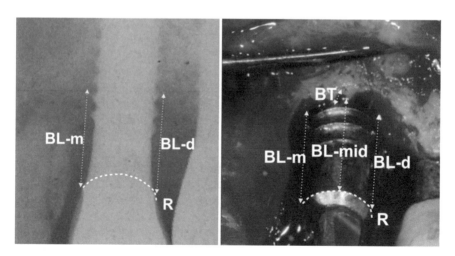

Fig. 8.1 An implant with peri-implant bone loss shown on the periapical radiograph (Right) and intraoperatively (Left). Interproximal bone level at mesial (BL-m) and distal sites (BL-d) is measured vertically from implant platform as a reference (R) to the first implant-bone contact. However, the radiographic interproximal bone level is only at its best the superimposition of the facial and palatal bone levels. Individual bone levels on the facial and palatal sides as well as bone thickness (BT), measured horizontally from the implant surface to the bone surface, are important parameters for disease characters and treatment selection and could be measured with the proposed sonography-based method

8.4   Current Methods to Estimate Tissue Phenotype and Limitations

Methods to evaluate tissue phenotype are summarized in Table 8.2. Visual evaluation is not an objective method to identify the tissue phenotype, since it was accurately identified in only about half of the cases, irrespective of the clinician's experience [14]. Probe transparency is another way to determine tissue phenotype. However, it is only accurate when the mucosal thickness is either too thin, i.e. less than 0.6 mm or more than 1.2 mm. Moderate tissue thickness cannot be differentiated with this method [15]. Bone sounding is not commonly applied because it is invasive, usually performed under local anesthesia. Injection of local anesthetic solution causes patient discomfort and is also associated with a transient local tissue volume increase. When bone is thin, penetration of the sharp instrument into bone, overestimates soft tissue thickness. Use of cone-beam computed tomography (CBCT) has also shown a high diagnostic accuracy in assessing mucosal thickness, demonstrating minimal discrepancy with clinical and radiographic measurements [16]. However, routine uses of CBCT for this purpose may not recommended [17]. Optical scanners can record tissue surfaces changes overtime, e.g. tissue thickness changes before and after a given procedure. However, it cannot measure the "absolute" soft tissue thickness. Ultrasound is an established tool to measure soft tissue thickness and therefore optimal for estimate tissue phenotype [18–22].

8.5   Rationale of Ultrasound as an Adjunctive Diagnostic Method

Unlike teeth, facial bone around implants is more susceptible for resorption [23,24], resulting in non-uniform bone loss in 34–45% of infected implants [25, 26]. Two-dimensional X-rays are not adequate to evaluate facial and lingual/palatal bone loss. CBCT might provide accurate 3D bone level values but issues like imaging artifacts arising from metal implants and radiation concerns are unsolved (Fig. 8.2) [12, 27, 28].

There have been promising research efforts to apply ultrasonography for evaluating periodontal bone level [29–31], including recent works from the authors' group [32–34]. Peri-implant bone level was evaluated by Bertram et al. [35] using ultrasound with a linear 12.5 MHz transducer. A total of 29 buccal bone defects in 25 patients who were diagnosed with peri-implantitis and scheduled for a revision surgery were recruited. The results showed that measurements made at moderate bone loss levels (3–6 mm) were the most reliable (ICC = 0.81 for reproducibility and 0.76 for accuracy). The mean absolute difference is 0.1 mm. However, the correlations in normal (<3 mm) and advanced bone loss (>6 mm) cases were moderate to poor (ICC = 0.63 to 0.73). The mean absolute difference is 0.6 mm. Recent advances in device miniaturization and image resolution improvement, coupled with other desirable properties, e.g. real-time, cost-effective, and non-ionizing make

Table 8.2 Methods to evaluate tissue phenotype

	Visual	Bone sounding	Probe transparency	CBCT	Optical scan	Ultrasound
Absolute/relative reading	Relative	Absolute	Relative	Absolute	Relative	Absolute
Reproducibility	+[a]	+++	++	+++	++++	++++
Accuracy	N/A	++++	N/A	++	N/A	++++
Cost	$[b]	$	$	$$$$	$$$	$$
Invasiveness	Minimal/none	Mild/moderate	Minor	High radiation	Minimal/none	Minimal/none
Easiness of use	Yes	Yes	Yes	Need equipment and training	Need equipment and training	Need equipment and training
General comments	First-line assessment method	Considered the "gold standard" method	Only provide relative value	Radiation might not be justifiable.	Useful only for comparing tissue dimension changes.	Chairside, instant readings
	Not able to provide absolute value as the major drawback	Invasive and not practical	Might adequate for assess tissue phenotype	Inferior soft tissue contrasts	Not feasible for providing absolute readings	
			Ethnicity, pigmentation, and site variability can influence accuracy			

[a]The number of "+" sign indicates the relative degree of reproducibility and accuracy comparisons among the modalities
[b]The number of "$" sign indicates the relative costs comparisons among the modalities

Clinical Facial   2D Radiograph   CT Cross-sectional   US Cross-sectional

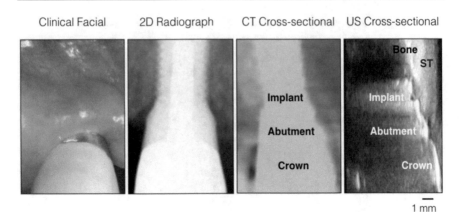

1 mm

Fig. 8.2 Comparisons of 2D radiograph, CT and ultrasound (US) images for assessing "facial" peri-implant bone of a human subject. The 2D radiograph can show superimposed interproximal bone but not facial bone. A CT cross-sectional scan example is shown; however, because of artifacts, thin facial bone could not be seen in this case. Here a representative US cross-sectional image clearly shows facial peri-implant bone surface and its spatial relation to the implant. *ST* soft tissue

ultrasonography a reality for working in the oral cavity. 3D ultrasonography can image both interproximal and radicular (facial and palatal/lingual) bone loss. This comprehensive assessment would be especially valuable for evaluating long-term bone level stability and measuring treatment efficacy because of its non-ionizing and point-of-care nature. Figure 8.3 illustrates cross-sectional ultrasound images of the mid-facial site of an implant. The facial bone level and thickness can be determined on the image that can assist in diagnosis of peri-implant diseases and conditions. The measurements can be confirmed with a transverse image stack, as shown in Fig. 8.4.

8.6 Ultrasound Case Demonstration Based on the New Classification

8.6.1 Case of Peri-Implant Health

Case Description A healthy implant should not have clinical signs of inflammation, including BOP, erythema, swelling, suppuration. It should not have probing depth increase, mucosal recession, and pathologic bone loss. Figure 8.5 exemplifies such a case. The probing depth is 3 mm without BOP. On the radiograph, the marginal bone loss is within normal range. Ultrasound images provides additional useful information, including the soft tissue height, soft tissue thickness, crestal bone thickness, etc. (see Fig. 8.5). The ultrasound soft tissue height may correlate with

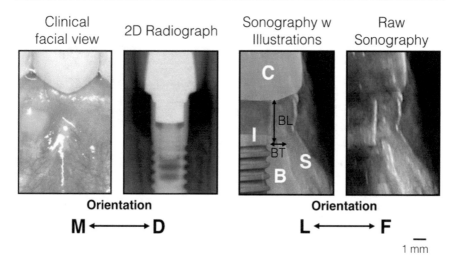

Fig. 8.3 An example of a cross-sectional ultrasound scan of an implant from a human subject. The examiners will acquire images like this example, on which the crown (C), implant (I), bone surface (B), and soft tissue (S) can be clearly identifiable. On the images, bone level (BL) and thickness (BT) will be measured and calibrated with the standard examiner

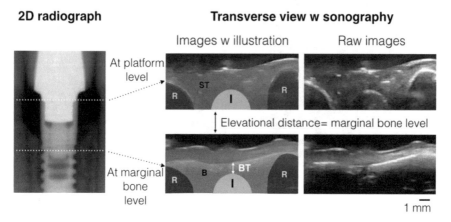

Fig. 8.4 Two ultrasound images in transverse view extracted from a volume scan. The motor drove the ultrasound probe at a constant speed in the corono-apical direction so a series of spatially oriented transverse slices could be collected. The top ultrasound image was at the level of the implant platform, whereas the bottom image was at the marginal bone level. At the marginal bone level, only the outermost part of the implant surface (I) is seen; because of attenuation, roots (R) of the adjacent teeth behind bone (B) could not be seen on ultrasound. Bone thickness (BT) can be measured on this slice. The vertical distance between these two slices can be calculated to represent the marginal bone level

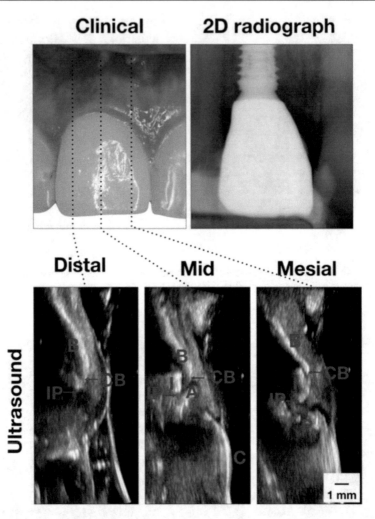

Fig. 8.5 Ultrasound images of a healthy implant, in relation to the clinical photo and 2D radiograph. *B* bone, *I* implant, *IP* implant platform, *CB* crestal bone, *P* papilla, *A* abutment, *C* crown. Published with permission from [8]

the probing depth. The soft tissue thickness and crestal bone thickness are measures of tissue phenotype.

8.6.2 Case of Peri-Implant Mucositis

Case Description Peri-implant mucositis has clinical signs of inflammation but a lack of bone loss beyond normal bone remodeling, as demonstrated in Fig. 8.6. In

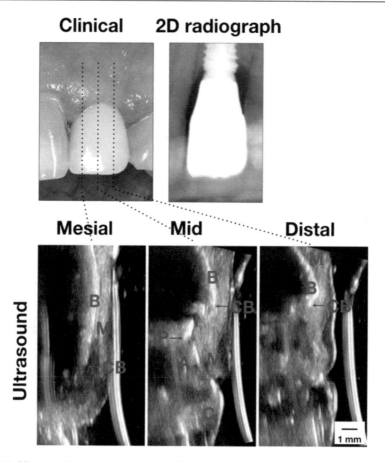

Fig. 8.6 Ultrasound images of an implant with peri-implant mucositis, in relation to the clinical photo and 2D radiograph. *B* bone, *I* implant, *IP* implant platform, *CB* crestal bone, *M* mucosa, *P* papilla, *A* abutment, *C* crown. Published with permission from [8]

this case, there is increased tissue inflammation and tissue swelling, as evidenced by visual examination and BOPs, as well as increased PD. Radiographic marginal bone loss is within normal range as a result of the initial healing process. Ultrasound images show normal soft tissue height, thickness, crestal bone level and thickness.

8.6.3 Case of Peri-Implantitis

Case Description In additional to clinical inflammation, increased bone loss is a cardinal sign of peri-implantitis. Figure 8.7 demonstrates a case defined as early stage of peri-implantitis. There is increased PD and tissue inflammation (BOPs).

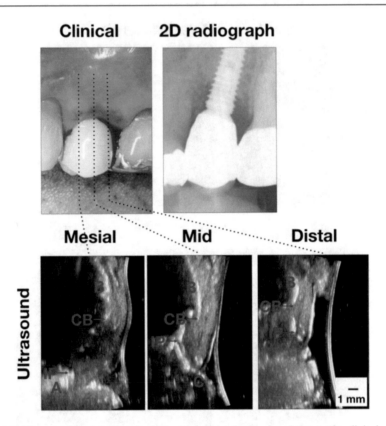

Fig. 8.7 Ultrasound images of an implant with peri-implantitis, in relation to the clinical photo and 2D radiograph. *B* bone, *I* implant, *IP* implant platform, *CB* crestal bone, *A* abutment, *C* crown. Published with permission from [8]

Radiographic marginal bone loss is more evident and beyond normal remodeling. On ultrasound images, there is increased distance between the implant platform (IP) and the crestal bone (CB), indicative of bone loss. Increased soft tissue height is also an indication of soft tissue swelling and PD increase.

8.6.4   Case of Peri-Implant Soft- and Hard-Tissue Deficiency

Case Description A case diagnosis of peri-implant soft- and hard-tissue deficiency presents as mucosal recession and/or thin mucosa and/or loss of bone in the absence of overt tissue inflammation. In a case shown in Fig. 8.8, the PD is within normal range (3 mm) without clinical inflammation. There is some radiographic marginal bone loss, as evidenced on radiographs. Ultrasound shows evidences of soft tissue deficiency, with 0.74 mm in soft tissue thickness, as well as hard-tissue deficiency,

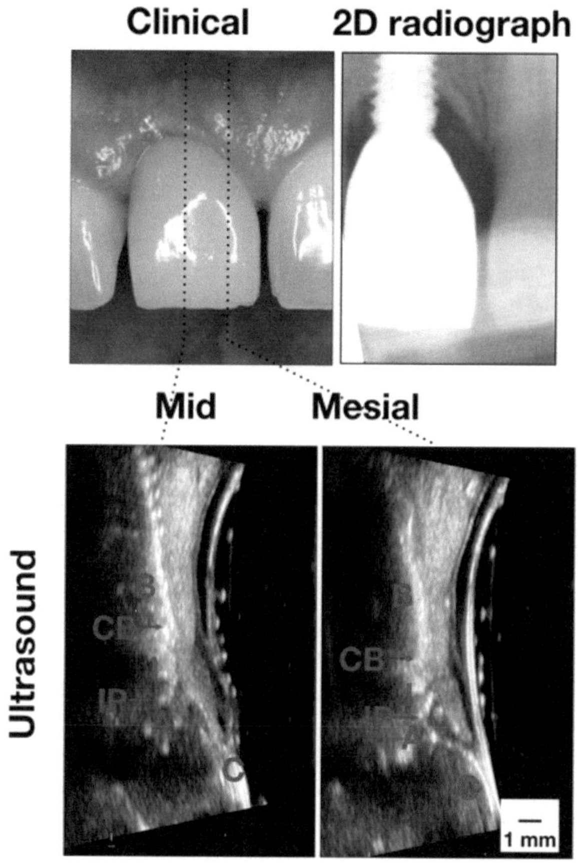

Fig. 8.8 Ultrasound images of an implant with tissue deficiency, in relation to the clinical photo and 2D radiograph. *B* bone, *I* implant, *IP* implant platform, *CB* crestal bone, *A* abutment, *C* crown. Published with permission from [8]

with close to 0 mm in crestal bone thickness on the mid-facial site. The amount of bony fenestration, i.e. implant exposure, is evident on the mid-facial site. On the ultrasound image at the mid-facial site, the implant surface with a threaded pattern is clearly seen.

In addition to anatomical images, ultrasound is able to provide various modes, including the back scatter, elasticity, color flow, power Doppler, and photoacoustic, that could be used to quantify tissue inflammation and tissue loss, which are key to evaluate aggressiveness and status of peri-implant diseases and conditions (Table 8.3). These areas are highly interesting and in active investigations. In the near future, clinicians may start to adapt to this novel technology as a tool to diagnose peri-implant diseases and conditions.

Table 8.3 Various ultrasound modes and the potential diagnostic values

Ultrasound modes	Output measures	Potential diagnostic values
B-mode	Soft-/hard-tissue anatomy	Soft tissue thickness/height Bone level/loss/thickness
Backscatter	Soft tissue content change e.g. water/collagen	Amount of destruction in soft tissues
Elasticity	Soft tissue content change e.g. water/collagen	Amount of destruction in soft tissues
Color flow	Blood velocity	Degree/features of inflammation
Power Doppler	Blood volume	Degree/features of inflammation
Photoacoustic	Oxygenated/deoxygenated Hemoglobin ratio	Degree/features of inflammation

8.7   Conclusions

Peri-implant diseases and conditions are emerging epidemic complications that do not have adequate and standard diagnostic methods currently. Conventional clinical evaluation and 2D radiographs may not grasp the whole picture of the diseases. Therefore, there is a delay in developing optimal solutions to these complications. Ultrasound can provide cross-sectional peri-implant anatomical information. It may add to the diagnostic value by offering tissue-destruction and tissue inflammation related parameters. Research ground work is being actively conducted in this field. Once validated, ultrasound can become a standard care in diagnosing peri-implant diseases and conditions in the foreseeable future.

References

1. Derks J, Tomasi C. Peri-implant health and disease. A systematic review of current epidemiology. J Clin Periodontol. 2015;42 Suppl 16:S158–71. ISSN:1600-051X (Electronic) 0303-6979 (Linking). https://doi.org/10.1111/jcpe.12334. http://www.ncbi.nlm.nih.gov/pubmed/25495683.
2. Araujo MG, Lindhe J. Peri-implant health. J Periodontol. 2018;89 Suppl 1:S249–56. ISSN:1943-3670 (Electronic) 0022-3492 (Linking). https://doi.org/10.1002/JPER.16-0424. https://www.ncbi.nlm.nih.gov/pubmed/29926949.
3. Berglundh T, et al. Peri-implant diseases and conditions: consensus report of workgroup 4 of the 2017 world workshop on the classification of periodontal and peri-implant diseases and conditions. J Periodontol. 2018;89 Suppl 1:S313–18. ISSN:1943-3670 (Electronic) 0022-3492 (Linking). https://doi.org/10.1002/JPER.17-0739. https://www.ncbi.nlm.nih.gov/pubmed/29926955.
4. Hammerle CHF, Tarnow D. The etiology of hard- and soft-tissue deficiencies at dental implants: a narrative review. J Periodontol. 2018;89 Suppl 1:S291–303. ISSN:1943-3670 (Electronic) 0022-3492 (Linking). https://doi.org/10.1002/JPER.16-0810. https://www.ncbi.nlm.nih.gov/pubmed/29926950.

5. Heitz-Mayfield LJA, Salvi GE. Peri-implant mucositis. J Periodontol. 2018;89 Suppl 1:S257–66. ISSN:1943-3670 (Electronic) 0022-3492 (Linking). https://doi.org/10.1002/JPER-16-0488. https://www.ncbi.nlm.nih.gov/pubmed/29926954.

6. Renvert S, et al. Peri-implant health, peri-implant mucositis, and peri-implantitis: case definitions and diagnostic considerations. J Periodontol. 2018;89 Suppl 1:S304–12. ISSN:1943-3670 (Electronic) 0022-3492 (Linking). https://doi.org/10.1002/JPER.17-0588. https://www.ncbi.nlm.nih.gov/pubmed/29926953.

7. Schwarz F, et al. Peri-implantitis. J Periodontol. 2018;89 Suppl 1:S267–90. ISSN:1943-3670 (Electronic) 0022-3492 (Linking). https://doi.org/10.1002/JPER.16-0350. https://www.ncbi.nlm.nih.gov/pubmed/29926957.

8. Bhaskar V, Chan H-L, MacEachern M, Kripfgans OD. Updates on ultrasound research in implant dentistry: a systematic review of potential clinical indications. Dentomaxillofac Radiol. 2018;47(6):20180076. https://doi.org/10.1259/dmfr.20180076. Epub 2018 Jun 6.

9. Sanz M, Chapple IL, Working Group 4 of the VIII European Workshop on Periodontology. Clinical research on peri-implant diseases: consensus report of Working Group 4. J Clin Periodontol. 2012;39 Suppl 12:202–6. ISSN:1600-051X (Electronic) 0303-6979 (Linking). https://doi.org/10.1111/j.1600-051X.2011.01837.x. http://www.ncbi.nlm.nih.gov/pubmed/22533957.

10. Spray JR, et al. The influence of bone thickness on facial marginal bone response: stage 1 placement through stage 2 uncovering. Ann Periodontol. 2000;5.1:119–28. ISSN:1553-0841 (Print) 1553-0841 (Linking). https://doi.org/10.1902/annals.2000.5.1.119. http://www.ncbi.nlm.nih.gov/pubmed/11885170.

11. Evans CD, Chen ST. Esthetic outcomes of immediate implant placements. Clin Oral Implants Res. 2008;19.1:73–80. ISSN:0905-7161 (Print) 0905-7161 (Linking). https://doi.org/10.1111/j.1600-0501.2007.01413x. https://www.ncbi.nlm.nih.gov/pubmed/17956569.

12. Ritter L, et al. Accuracy of peri-implant bone evaluation using cone beam CT digital intraoral radiographs and histology. Dentomaxillofac Radiol. 2014;43.6:20130088. ISSN: 0250-832X (Print) 0250-832X (Linking). https://doi.org/10.1259/dmfr.20130088. http://www.ncbi.nlm.nih.gov/pubmed/24786136.

13. Schwarz F, et al. Comparison of naturally occurring and ligature-induced peri-implantitis bone defects in humans and dogs. Clin Oral Implants Res. 2007;18.2:161–70. ISSN:0905-7161 (Print) 0905-7161 (Linking). https://doi.org/10.1111/j.1600-0501.2006.01320.x. http://www.ncbi.nlm.nih.gov/pubmed/17348880.

14. Eghbali A, et al. The gingival biotype assessed by experienced and inexperienced clinicians. J Clin Periodontol. 2009;36.11:958–63. ISSN:1600-051X (Electronic) 0303-6979 (Linking). https://doi.org/10.1111/j.1600-051X.2009.01479.x. https://www.ncbi.nlm.nih.gov/pubmed/19811580.

15. De Rouck T, et al. The gingival biotype revisited: transparency of the periodontal probe through the gingival margin as a method to discriminate thin from thick gingiva. J Clin Periodontol. 2009;36.5:428–33. ISSN:0303-6979.

16. Fu JH, et al. Tissue biotype and its relation to the underlying bone morphology. J Periodontol. 2010;81.4:569–74. ISSN:1943-3670 (Electronic) 0022-3492 (Linking). https://doi.org/10.1902/jop.2009.090591. https://www.ncbi.nlm.nih.gov/pubmed/20367099.

17. Benavides E, et al. Use of cone beam computed tomography in implant dentistry: the international congress of oral implantologists consensus report. Implant Dent. 2012;21.2:78–86. ISSN:1056-6163.

18. Eger T, Muller HP, Heinecke A. Ultrasonic determination of gingival thickness. Subject variation and influence of tooth type and clinical features. J Clin Periodontol. 1996;23.9:839–45. ISSN:0303-6979 (Print) 0303-6979 (Linking). http://www.ncbi.nlm.nih.gov/pubmed/8891935.

19. Kloukos D, et al. Gingival thickness assessment at the mandibular incisors with four methods: a cross-sectional study. J Periodontol. 2018;89.11:1300–09. ISSN:1943-3670 (Electronic) 0022-3492 (Linking). https://doi.org/10.1002/JPER-180125. https://www.ncbi.nlm.nih.gov/pubmed/30043972.

20. Muller HP, Barrieshi-Nusair KM, Kononen E. Repeatability of ultrasonic determination of gingival thickness. Clin Oral Investig. 2007;11.4:439–42. ISSN:1432-6981 (Print) 1432-6981 (Linking). https://doi.org/10.1007/s00784-007-0125-0. http://www.ncbi.nlm.nih.gov/pubmed/17522899

21. Muller HP, Kononen E. Variance components of gingival thickness. J Periodontal Res. 2005;40.3:239–44. ISSN:0022-3484 (Print) 0022-3484 (Linking). https://doi.org/10.1111/j1600-0765.2005.00798.x. http://www.ncbi.nlm.nih.gov/pubmed/15853970.

22. Zweers J, et al. Characteristics of periodontal biotype, its dimensions, associations and prevalence: a systematic review. J Clin Periodontol. 2014;41.10:958–71. ISSN:1600-051X (Electronic) 0303-6979 (Linking). https://doi.org/10.1111/jcpe.12275. https://www.ncbi.nlm.nih.gov/pubmed/24836578.

23. Kehl M, Swierkot K, Mengel R. Three-dimensional measurement of bone loss at implants in patients with periodontal disease. J Periodontol. 2011;82.5:689–99. ISSN:1943-3670 (Electronic) 0022-3492 (Linking). https://doi.org/10.1902/jop.2010.100318. https://www.ncbi.nlm.nih.gov/pubmed/21080785.

24. Parlar A, et al. Effects of decontamination and implant surface characteristics on re-osseointegration following treatment of peri-implantitis. Clin Oral Implants Res. 2009;20.4:391–9. ISSN:1600-0501 (Electronic) 0905-7161 (Linking). https://doi.org/10.1111/j.1600-0501.2008.01655.x. https://www.ncbi.nlm.nih.gov/pubmed/19298293

25. Schwarz F, Claus C, Becker K. Correlation between horizontal mucosal thickness and probing depths at healthy and diseased implant sites. Clin Oral Implants Res. 2017;28.9:1158–63. ISSN:1600-0501 (Electronic) 0905-7161 (Linking). https://doi.org/10.1111/clr.12932. http://www.ncbi.nlm.nih.gov/pubmed/27458093.

26. Serino G, Turri A, Lang NP. Probing at implants with peri-implantitis and its relation to clinical peri-implant bone loss. Clin Oral Implants Res. 2013;24.1:91–5. ISSN:1600-0501 (Electronic) 0905-7161 (Linking). https://doi.org/10.1111/j.1600-0501.2012.02470.x. http://www.ncbi.nlm.nih.gov/pubmed/22462625.

27. Benic GI, et al. Dimensions of buccal bone and mucosa at immediately placed implants after 7 years: a clinical and cone beam computed tomography study. Clin Oral Implants Res. 2012;23.5:560–6. ISSN:0905-7161.

28. Fienitz T, et al. Accuracy of cone beam computed tomography in assessing peri-implant bone defect regeneration: a histologically controlled study in dogs. Clin Oral Implants Res. 2012;23.7:882–7. ISSN:1600-0501 (Electronic) 0905-7161 (Linking). https://doi.org/10.1111/j.1600-0501.2011.02232.x. http://www.ncbi.nlm.nih.gov/pubmed/21707753.

29. Marotti J, et al. Recent advances of ultrasound imaging in dentistry–a review of the literature. Oral Surg Oral Med Oral Pathol Oral Radiol. 2013;115.6:819–32. ISSN:2212-4411 (Electronic). https://doi.org/10.1016/j.oooo.2013.03.012. http://www.ncbi.nlm.nih.gov/pubmed/23706922.

30. Tsiolis FI, Needleman IG, Griffiths GS. Periodontal ultrasonography. J Clin Periodontol. 2003;30.10:849–54. ISSN:0303-6979 (Print) 0303-6979 (Linking). http://www.ncbi.nlm.nih.gov/pubmed/14710764.

31. Nguyen KT, et al. High-resolution ultrasonic imaging of dento-periodontal tissues using a multi-element phased array system. Ann Biomed Eng. 2016;44.10:2874–86. ISSN:1573-9686 (Electronic) 0090-6964 (Linking). https://doi.org/10.1007/s10439-016-1634-2. http://www.ncbi.nlm.nih.gov/pubmed/27160674.

32. Chan HL, et al. Non-invasive evaluation of facial crestal bone with ultrasonography. PLoS One. 2017;12.2:e0171237. ISSN:1932-6203 (Electronic) 1932-6203 (Linking). https://doi.org/10.1371/journal.pone.0171237. http://www.ncbi.nlm.nih.gov/pubmed/28178323.

33. Chan HL, et al. Ultrasonography for noninvasive and real-time evaluation of peri-implant tissue dimensions. J Clin Periodontol. 2018;45.8:986–95. ISSN:1600-051X (Electronic) 0303-6979 (Linking). https://doi.org/10.1111/j.cpe.12918. https://www.ncbi.nlm.nih.gov/pubmed/29757464.

34. Chan HL, et al. Non-ionizing real-time ultrasonography in implant and oral surgery: a feasibility study. Clin Oral Implants Res. 2017;28.3:341–347. ISSN:1600-0501 (Electronic) 0905-7161 (Linking). https://doi.org/10.1111/clr.12805. http://www.ncbi.nlm.nih.gov/pubmed/26992276.
35. Bertram S, Emshoff R. Sonography of periimplant buccal bone defects in periodontitis patients: a pilot study. Oral Surg Oral Med Oral Pathol Oral Radiol Endod. 2008;105.1:99–103. ISSN:1528-395X (Electronic) 1079-2104 (Linking). https://doi.org/10.1016/j.tripleo.2007.01.014. http://www.ncbi.nlm.nih.gov/pubmed/17482844.

Ultrasonography for Wound Healing Evaluation of Implant-Related Surgeries

9

Hsun-Liang (Albert) Chan and Oliver D. Kripfgans

9.1 Introduction

Wound healing is a complex and dynamic process of replacing devitalized and missing cellular structures and tissue layers [1]. The wound healing process can be divided into three phases: inflammatory, proliferation, and remodeling. The inflammatory stage also includes a hemostasis phase [2]. The healing outcome can be either regeneration or repair, depending on whether the lost structures and function are fully or partially restored. In the context of surgical dentistry, there are broadly two categories of procedures: resective and regenerative procedures. As the name implies, a resective procedure is to remove part of diseased oral soft or hard tissue to facilitate the reversal of a disease to healthy status. The healing of most resective cases is inconsequential, as long as patients healing capacity is not compromised. On the other hand, a regenerative procedure is to apply the tissue engineering concept by adding scaffold, cells, and/or signaling molecules to improve or replace biological tissue [3]. This type of procedures requires meticulous surgical handling and post-op care, or the complication rate is high. Common complications are wound exposure, sustained inflammation, and infection, resulting in partial or total loss of the grafting materials and incomplete regeneration. Patient morbidity, time effort, and costs are all considerable to remedy these complications. A rule of thumb is to identify early the occurrence of complications and intervene so adverse consequences can be reduced. Early signs of complications mostly show

H.-L. (Albert) Chan
Department of Periodontics and Oral Medicine, School of Dentistry, University of Michigan, Ann Arbor, MI, USA
e-mail: hlchan@umich.edu

O. D. Kripfgans (✉)
Department of Radiology, Medical School, University of Michigan, Ann Arbor, MI, USA
e-mail: greentom@umich.edu

© Springer Nature Switzerland AG 2021
H.-L. (Albert) Chan, O. D. Kripfgans (eds.), *Dental Ultrasound in Periodontology and Implantology*, https://doi.org/10.1007/978-3-030-51288-0_9

altered soft tissue characteristics, i.e. increased blood flow and water content and reduced collagen amount. Therefore, ultrasound can be very beneficial to evaluate healing of these regenerative procedures, aside from its inherent advantages, e.g. real-time, non-radiation, etc. In this chapter, we will demonstrate ultrasound images of wound healing after the most commonly performed surgical procedures related to implant therapy, including socket augmentation, guided bone regeneration, implant placement, and soft tissue grafting procedures.

9.2   Current Methods to Assess Wound Healing

Vision and palpation are currently the primary methods to examine healing [4]. They are quick and simple to perform. Obvious changes in soft tissue appearance, hue, and size are often indicative of unfavorable healing. For procedures requiring primary intention healing, the flap edges should stay approximated during the entire healing period. At approximately 2 weeks after a regenerative surgery, the soft tissue should reappear in its normal pink color and firm consistency because inflammation should have already subsided. In cases of wound exposure without infection, regenerative materials, e.g. bone grafts and membrane, may be visible at the open wound, along with tissue erythema, edema, and clear exudate. If infection exists, purulence, typically in yellow color, is a very common finding that drains through the wound opening, a fistula, or sinus tract. Apparent signs of inflammation and infection just described above can be confirmed by visual means and palpation. However, visual evaluation may not be sensitive to subtle changes indicative of incipient wound healing disturbance that may later become obvious and detrimental, causing more tissue loss if not controlled. Visual examination is also subjective to examiners' interpretation. Last, visual inspection cannot directly evaluate bone quantity and quality simply because overlying soft tissue obscures the bone.

Bone is primarily evaluated by 2D/3D radiographs. A normally healed ridge after a bone augmentation procedure is comprised of a layer of cortical bone on the surface of the edentulous ridge, cancellous bone, and a marrow space with a minimal amount of residual bone grafts [5]. Because of the addition of bone grafts, not only bone quantity but also quality are changed [6]. Residual bone graft materials may influence implant success. Failed healing includes irregularly shaped crestal bone, soft tissue invagination, and decreased mineralization. Intraoral radiographs can indicate the degree of mineralization and available bone height efficiently; however, the major limitation is that they only provide superimposed image; therefore, the ridge width cannot be revealed. This method is also limited in soft tissue contrast. Three-dimensional radiographs, i.e. cone-beam computed tomography (CBCT), are very useful to evaluate available bone width and height; however, inferior image quality due to artifacts from adjacent metal structures, high cost, and increased radiation dose have to be considered. Table 9.1 summarizes the current methods for wound healing evaluation and the potential roles ultrasound may have.

Table 9.1 Current methods to evaluate healing of socket augmentation, guided bone regeneration, implant surgery, and soft tissue grafting and potential usefulness of ultrasound

Surgical procedures	Current evaluation methods	Ultrasound method
Socket augmentation	Visual examination, palpation 2D and 3D radiographs, Direct open access	• Soft tissue thickness measures • Quantitative soft tissue inflammation evaluation • Bone width and quality estimation • Timing of implant surgery determination
Guided bone regeneration		• Soft tissue thickness measures • Quantitative soft tissue inflammation evaluation • Bone width and quality estimation • Detection of micrometer-sized wound exposure • Fixation screw identification • Timing of implant surgery determination
Implant placement		• Soft tissue thickness measures • Quantitative soft tissue inflammation evaluation • Bone width and quality estimation • Implant marginal bone level and thickness
Soft tissue grafting		• Soft tissue thickness, height, and quality measures • Quantitative soft tissue inflammation evaluation

9.3   Ultrasound as a Novel Tool to Assess Wound Healing

In light of the limitations of clinical examination and radiographic imaging, ultrasound can be used as a first-line device to assess wound healing because it provides cross-sectional images in real-time without radiation. More specifically, ultrasound can evaluate soft tissue thickness and quality, blood velocity and volume in soft tissue, crestal bone surface, and crestal bone width (Table 9.1). Soft tissue thickness is useful to determine tissue phenotype [7]. Tissue thickness is correlated with marginal bone remodeling around implants [8]. Thin phenotype may require an additional soft tissue graft procedure to improve esthetics and implant longevity [9]. Blood velocity and volume are good indicators of tissue inflammation; elevated color flow and power Doppler signals are normal within the first 2 weeks. However, increased signals beyond that time frame may indicate uncontrolled inflammation process and require further investigation. It can also detect micrometer-sized wound exposure because the image resolution of a high-frequency probe, e.g. 25 MHz is less than 100 μm.

Although not being able to image intraosseous structures, ultrasound can delineate crestal bone surface well [10, 11]. Ultrasound crestal bone surface can reveal the degree of surface bone maturation and crestal bone width (see Table 9.1). A strong and continuous hyperechoic line is suggestive of complete healing, as compared to irregular, less strong hyperechoic line, suggesting soft tissue invagination and incomplete crestal bone healing.

By observing the extent of bone surface maturation with ultrasound, optimal timing for implant surgery may be objectively determined. A crestal bone width of 2–3 mm in additional to the planned implant diameter is required for an optimal implant surgery. A small bony deficiency may require additional bone grafting at the same visit as implant surgery; however, a large deficiency may require a separate bone grafting procedure before an implant can be placed [12]. Finally, ultrasound can locate fixation screws/tacks that are commonly used to secure an occlusive membrane, making minimal flap reflection possible during screws removal so as to minimize patient morbidity. In the following sections, ultrasound images will be demonstrated specific to healing of socket augmentation, guided bone regeneration, implant surgery, and soft tissue grafting surgery.

9.4   Socket Augmentation Healing

9.4.1   Procedure Description

After tooth extraction, the alveolar ridge inevitably undergoes dimensional decrease, especially the width dimension, compared to the height. To reduce the amount of bone resorption, bone grafting materials, e.g. allografts and xenografts are commonly placed in the socket. Coronally to the grafts, a collagen plug or a non-resorbable/resorbable membrane is placed, depending on the presence of missing

Fig. 9.1 Procedures of socket augmentation. After the hopeless is extracted and the socket is thoroughly debrided, bone particulate graft is placed into the socket. In uncomplicated socket, a collagen plug is placed to seal the socket and non-resorbable sutures are used to stabilize the wound

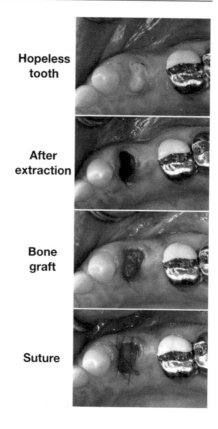

Hopeless tooth

After extraction

Bone graft

Suture

bone walls surrounding the socket. The wound may be left as second intention healing or less commonly a primary wound closure is attempted. Figure 9.1 demonstrates the clinical procedures. The literature has shown efficacy of this type of treatment. After such a bone grafting procedure, the healing is most commonly assessed at 2 weeks for any early signs of healing failure and for suture removal. If the healing is uneventful, an arbitrary time frame of 4–6 months, the socket, now an edentulous ridge, is evaluated again in preparation for an implant surgery.

9.4.2   Ultrasound Case Demonstration

Ultrasound can be used to evaluate the crestal bone quality after socket augmentation. Figure 9.2 contrasts the two scenarios: (1) the crestal bone was intact (normal healing) and (2) incomplete crestal bone formation (soft tissue invagination). In cases with incomplete socket healing, soft tissue invagination into alveolar bone, intermingled with residual bone particles is a common finding. Soft tissue invagination can be imaged with ultrasound and shows hyperechoic appearance in the socket.

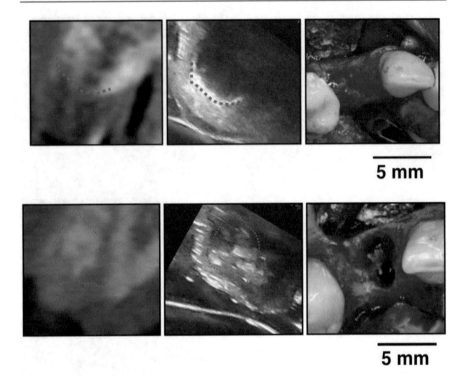

5 mm

5 mm

Fig. 9.2 Top: Normal healing with enclosure of the crestal cortical plate. A bright (hyperechoic) line (red dotted line) is shown on the ultrasound (US) image, indicative of intact bone surface. The image is consistent with the CBCT image and clinical photo. Bottom: Impaired healing with soft tissue invagination, encircled by the red dotted line, in the bone and failure of crestal cortical bone formation on the US and CBCT images. The clinical photo confirms this finding after removal of the soft, non-integrated soft tissues and bone particles

Ultrasound may image the socket immediately before and after socket augmentation is performed to serve as baselines for evaluation of the efficiency of socket augmentation (Fig. 9.3).

9.5   Guided Bone Regeneration

9.5.1   Procedure Description

Guided bone regeneration (GBR) is a surgical procedure that applies a membrane, that is either resorbable or non-resorbable, and commonly bone grafts to augment alveolar ridge [13]. After a full-thickness flap reflection, bone grafts of surgeon's choice are placed on the denuded bone. A membrane is then used to cover bone grafts. The membrane may be fixed to the underlying native bone with sutures, tacks, or fixation screws. After that, the flap is released for primary wound closure. The

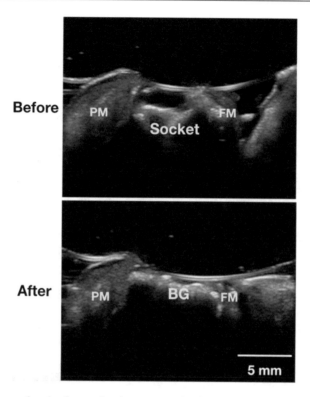

Fig. 9.3 Ultrasound occlusal scan of socket augmentation before and immediately after the bone graft is Placed. *PM* palatal mucosa; *FM* facial mucosa

GBR procedure is summarized in Fig. 9.4. Like socket augmentation, the surgical site is commonly evaluated at 2 weeks to assess early healing and approximately at 4–6 months if uneventful in preparation for implant surgery.

9.5.2 Ultrasound Case Demonstration

Wound healing after GBR procedures can be evaluated by ultrasound. Figure 9.5 shows ultrasound images of a GBR case with a membrane exposure. Ultrasound B-mode images can show the tissue thickness overlying the membrane, bone surface not covered by a non-resorbable membrane, and the membrane. Color flow images show blood velocity and blood vessel density. In cases of inflammation/infection, blood vessel intensity is expected to increase. Research to validate ultrasound for the estimation of the degree of inflammation is needed. Figures 9.6, 9.7, and 9.8 demonstrate healing after the membrane was removed. Crestal bone width and morphology can be evaluated on B-mode images. There is a significant reduction in blood vessel intensity, as shown on color flow images, compared to Fig. 9.5, suggesting resolution of inflammation.

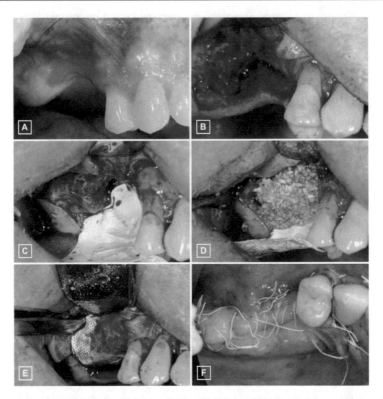

Fig. 9.4 Demonstration of a guided bone regeneration procedure. (**a**) Presence of a ridge defect in need of a GBR procedure before implant placement. (**b**) After a full-thickness flap reflection, the bony defect is evident. (**c**) A non-resorbable membrane is fixed to the palatal bone. (**d**) Bone particulates are placed onto the defect. (**e**) The membrane is folded to the buccal side and fixed. Another resorbable membrane is placed on top of the non-resorbable membrane. This additional membrane is not necessary for every case. (**f**) Primary wound closure is achieved with sutures

9.6   Healing After Implant Surgery

9.6.1   Procedure Description

An implant surgery typically involves a full-thickness flap elevation, osteotomy, and insertion of an implant fixture. After an implant is placed, the flaps are approximated with sutures. In certain cases when the ridge width is abundant, a flapless approach is applied for possible accelerated soft tissue healing. Flap implant surgery has become a standard, predictable procedure. Once integrated with the surrounding bone, which takes approximately 3 months, the implant is ready to be restored. The three most critical factors for surgical success are (1) adequate quantity and quality of hard and soft tissues, (2) optimal implant positioning, and (3) achievement of implant primary stability. Nevertheless, postoperative complications may occur, especially

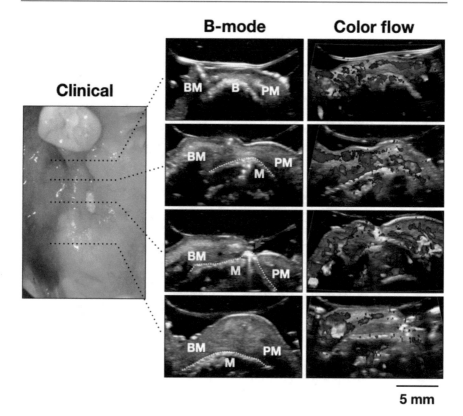

Fig. 9.5 Ultrasound B-mode and color flow images of impaired GBR wound healing due to exposure of the non-resorbable membrane. Images were taken from the occlusal side. *M* membrane; *BM* buccal mucosa; *PM* palatal mucosa. Due to wound exposure and possible bacterial invasion, blood flow as seen on color flow images increases, an indicator of tissue inflammation

when bone graft is placed simultaneously. The most common complication is soft tissue dehiscence/wound opening at the crestal region, which may result in tissue inflammation and infection. The final consequence is loss of crestal bone around the implant. Once the rough implant surface is exposed, pathologic bacteria may populate and proliferate, inducing further bone loss, a disease termed "peri-implantitis" [14]. Additionally, hard and soft tissue undergo remodeling after the surgery. Physiological remodeling is on a smaller scale, associated with acceptable crestal bone loss. However, pathological remodeling can cause excessive bone loss and subsequent soft tissue recession, compromising long-term implant function and esthetics [15]. Bone loss as a result of physiological remodeling may last for approximately a year after placement of a final restoration; pathological remodeling occurs when there is a presence of adverse influences (Table 9.2). Therefore, a careful evaluation of peri-implant structures is crucial during initial healing and subsequently after implants are in function.

| Site | B-mode | Color flow |

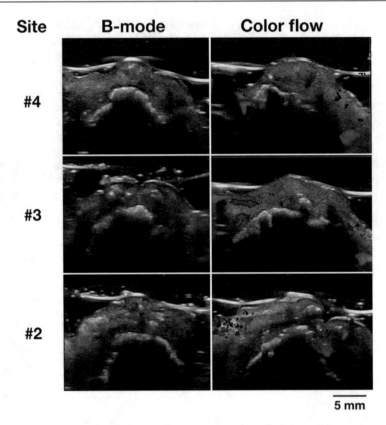

5 mm

Fig. 9.6 Ultrasound occlusal images of the same case at 1 week after membrane was removed. On the B-mode, there are some residual particles (hyperechoic) in soft tissue. Color flow images show much less blood flow, compared to Fig. 9.5

9.6.2   Ultrasound Case Demonstration

Ultrasound can be used to identify the implant location, the soft tissue thickness, marginal bone level, and marginal bone thickness before the second stage. This information can be useful to assist surgeons in determining the most appropriate second stage surgical approach. If the bone quantity is adequate, a minimally invasive approach, e.g. tissue punch, can be adopted. If the facial plate is too thin, another GBR procedure might be indicated to prevent future biological and esthetical complications. Figures 9.9 and 9.10 show an implant with normal healing and Fig. 9.11 shows an implant with impaired healing. With impaired healing, there is prominent marginal bone loss with the presence of elevated blood flow and possible hypoechoic soft tissue appearance. This hypoechoic feature might be due to loss of collagen content and fluid accumulation in the extracellular matrix.

Site   B-mode   Color flow

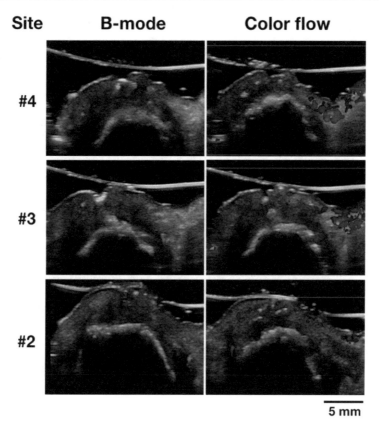

5 mm

Fig. 9.7 Ultrasound occlusal images of the same case at 1 month after the membrane was removed. On the B-mode images, residual particles are less visible in the soft tissues. Color flow images show normal blood flow, compared to Fig. 9.5, indicative of resolution of inflammation

9.7   Soft Tissue Graft Surgery Around Implants

9.7.1   Procedure Description

Facial mucosal recession, an arising complication, can affect implant function and esthetics. The etiology is not fully known; however, the recession is strongly associated with thin tissue phenotype, inadequate bone thickness, malpositioned implants, and inappropriately designed restorations [9]. Currently such a defect is treated with a soft tissue graft. In Fig. 9.12, after flap reflection, a soft tissue graft, harvested from the hard palate, is placed to cover the exposed implant. Alternatively, an allogenic graft may be used. Then the flap is released coronally to cover the graft for providing vascularization and sutured in place. By adding a graft, the therapeutic goal is to increase soft tissue thickness; the coronally advanced flap is to cover the exposed implant/implant abutment. The initial healing is typically evaluated at 2

| Site | B-mode | Color flow |

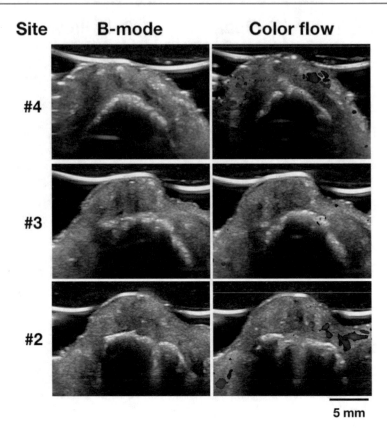

5 mm

Fig. 9.8 Ultrasound occlusal images of the same case at 2 months after the membrane was removed. On the B-mode images, soft tissue thickness and ridge width can be measured in preparation for the implant placement surgery. The edentulous ridge at tooth #2 location shows discontinuous crestal bone surface and a hyperechoic structure into the bone, indicating some soft tissue invagination into bone in this area. Color flow images show normal blood flow

weeks; however, an earlier visit may be needed. After 1-month, the new mucosal margin level should stay stable. In this case, up to 1 month, the facial mucosa is still slightly erythematic but much reduced in intensity, compared to 1-week follow-up. On the tissue donor site, granulation tissue is dominant at 1- and 2-week follow-ups. At one month, most of the re-epithelialization seems complete. At 3 months, the donor site appears almost normal, except for slight erythema. Figure 9.13 presents the course of healing over 3 months.

9.7.2 Ultrasonography Case Demonstration

Ultrasound can evaluate available tissue volume at the donor site, soft tissue thickness, and mucosal level changes over time after the soft tissue graft procedure,

Table 9.2 Comparisons of physiological and pathological crestal bone loss around implants

Crestal bone loss	Physiological	Pathological
Causes	• Controlled surgical trauma • Normal occlusion • Foreign body (implant) reaction • Normal skeletal remodeling • Others	• Uncontrolled surgical trauma • Excessive occlusion • Inadequate bone quality/quantity • Improper implant positioning • Compromised/impaired wound healing • Pathogen-induced • Others
Duration	Mostly noticeable bone loss ends at 1-year after function	When presence of a cause and can last if the cause is not controlled
Scale of bone loss	Crestal bone stops at either smooth–rough surface border or the first thread	Cumulative and beyond physiological remodeling

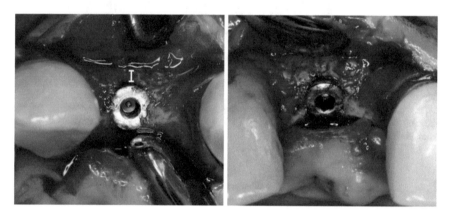

Fig. 9.9 A clinical case with implant #7 undergoing second stage exposure surgery. On the right, a layer of facial bone is present, as indicated by the white bar

and blood flow in various time points. Figure 9.14 demonstrates longitudinal B-mode and color flow images of the same case shown in Figs. 9.12 and 9.13.

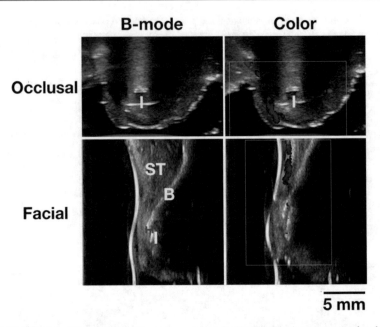

Fig. 9.10 Ultrasound illustration of the same case seen in Fig. 9.9. The images were taken before flap releasing. On the occlusal view, the cover screw has a strong sound reflection and hence hyperechoic. On the facial view, the facial bone thickness can be measured and corresponds to the dimension seen in the clinical photo in Fig. 9.9. Color flow images show normal blood flow *I* implant, *B* bone, *ST* soft tissue

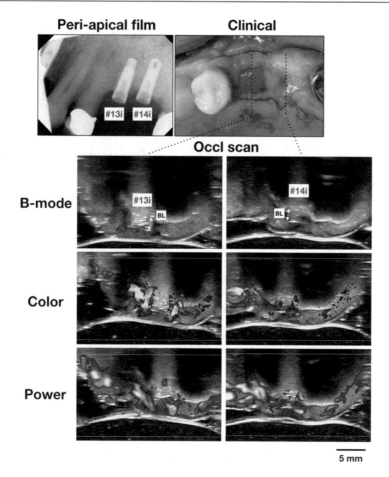

Fig. 9.11 A clinical case with compromised implant healing. The B-mode occlusal scans show intensity changes in soft tissue around the implants, indicating loss of collagen and matrix structures due to inflammation. Bone loss (BL) is evident in this view direction, corresponding to the amount of bone loss on the 2D radiograph. Overt blood flow is seen on color (middle) and power Doppler (bottom) images, indicative of tissue inflammation

Fig. 9.12 Procedures of soft tissue graft on implant #9. The initial photo is evident of mucosal recession (black arrow). A connective tissue is harvested from the palate (donor site) and this soft tissue graft (ST graft) is transferred to the donor site. The overlying flap is released to cover the graft and secured with sutures. Courtesy of Dr. Lorenzo Tavelli, faculty at the University of Michigan

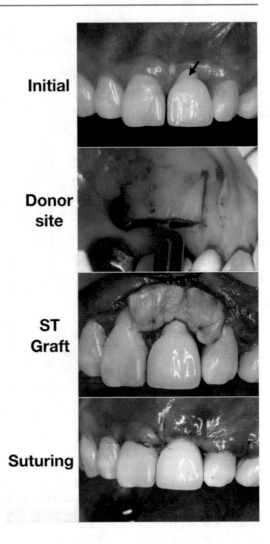

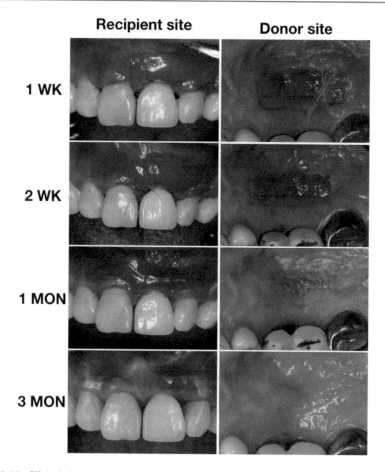

Fig. 9.13 Clinical photos of the recipient and donor sites at various time points. Even at 1 month, there is still some inflammation present at the recipient and donor sites, indicated by edematous and erythematous tissue appearance. At 3 months, the tissues look normal in color and the recession is largely corrected. Courtesy of Dr. Lorenzo Tavelli, faculty at the University of Michigan

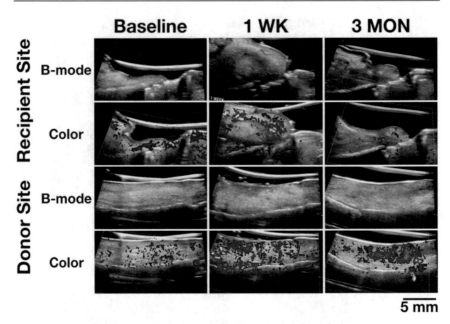

Fig. 9.14 At the recipient site, B-mode shows at 1 week the soft tissue thickness increases significantly due to the additional graft, swelling, and inflammation. At 3 months, the tissue is more condensed yet already thicker than at the baseline, indicative of a successful procedure. In addition, the mucosal margin is more coronally placed at 3 months. The color flow images show increase of blood flow at 1 week and normal blood flow at 3 months. At the donor site, the tissue intensity changes in B-mode images, suggesting remodeling of the soft tissues. In the color flow images, the blood flow increases significantly at 1 week and even at 3 months, suggesting at 3 months the revascularization and healing is still occurring

9.7.3   Conclusions

Current clinical and radiographic examinations are the primary methods to evaluate wound healing of implant-related surgical procedures. Although they can identify apparent healing impairment, they may not be sensitive enough to detect early signs of complications. In addition, visual exams are limited by only soft tissue surface screening. Intraoral radiographs cannot provide cross-sectional images nor tissue activity. This chapter demonstrated the potential use of ultrasound to evaluate healings of socket augmentation, guided bone regeneration, implant surgery, and soft tissue augmentation. Being cross-sectional and functional imaging, it can acquire essential clinical information, e.g. soft tissue thickness measures, quantitative evaluation of soft tissue inflammation, ridge width and quality, and marginal bone level and bone thickness around implants. These pieces of information, along with clinical and radiographic findings, allow for clinicians to grasp a full picture of the healing event that is necessary for making clinical decisions and provide recommendations to the patients. Although at its rudimentary stage, ultrasonography has showed its potential as a useful imaging modality to evaluate tissue healing. Subject variability may influence ultrasound blood flow and velocity measures and has to be taken into consideration. Other ultrasound parameters that are worth investigating for evaluating wound healing are, among others, elasticity and backscatter imaging.

References

1. Hammerle CH, Giannobile WV, Working Group 1 of the European Workshop on Periodontology. Biology of soft tissue wound healing and regeneration–consensus report of Group 1 of the 10th European Workshop on Periodontology. J Clin Periodontol. 2014;41 Suppl 15:S1–5. ISSN:1600-051X (Electronic) 0303-6979 (Linking). https://doi.org/10.1111/jcpe. 12221. https://www.ncbi.nlm.nih.gov/pubmed/24640995.
2. Wang HL, et al. Periodontal regeneration. J Periodontol. 2005;76.9:1601–22. ISSN:0022-3492 (Print) 0022-3492 (Linking). https://doi.org/10.1902/jop.2005.76.9.1601. https://www.ncbi.nlm.nih.gov/pubmed/16171453.
3. Pilipchuk SP, et al. Tissue engineering for bone regeneration and osseointegration in the oral cavity. Dent Mater. 2015;31.4:317–38. ISSN:1879-0097 (Electronic) 0109-5641 (Linking). https://doi.org/10.1016/j.dental.2015.01.06. https://www.ncbi.nlm.nih.gov/pubmed/25701146.
4. Polimeni G, Xiropaidis AV, Wikesjo UM. Biology and principles of periodontal wound healing/regeneration. Periodontol 2000. 2006;41:30–47. ISSN:0906-6713 (Print) 0906-6713 (Linking). https://doi.org/10.1111/j.1600.0757.2006.00157.x. https://www.ncbi.nlm.nih.gov/pubmed/16686925.
5. Pagni G, et al. Postextraction alveolar ridge preservation: biological basis and treatments. Int J Dent. 2012;2012:151030. ISSN:1687-8736 (Electronic) 1687-8728 (Linking). https://doi.org/10.1155/2012/151030. https://www.ncbi.nlm.nih.gov/pubmed/22737169.
6. Chan HL, et al. Alterations in bone quality after socket preservation with grafting materials: a systematic review. Int J Oral Maxillofac Implants. 2013;28.3:710–20. ISSN:1942-4434 (Electronic) 0882-2786 (Linking). https://doi.org/10.11607/jomi.2913. http://www.ncbi.nlm. nih.gov/pubmed/23748301.
7. Fu JH, et al. Tissue biotype and its relation to the underlying bone morphology. J Periodontol. 2010;81.4:569–74. ISSN:1943-3670 (Electronic) 0022-3492 (Linking). https://doi.org/10. 1902/jop.2009.090591. https://www.ncbi.nlm.nih.gov/pubmed/20367099.
8. Linkevicius T, et al. The influence of soft tissue thickness on crestal bone changes around implants: a 1-year prospective controlled clinical trial. Int J Oral Maxillofac Implants. 2009;24.4:712–9. ISSN:0882-2786 (Print) 0882-2786 (Linking). http://www.ncbi.nlm.nih. gov/pubmed/19885413.
9. Hammerle CHF, Tarnow D. The etiology of hard- and soft-tissue deficiencies at dental implants: a narrative review. J Periodontol. 2018;89 Suppl 1:S291–303. ISSN:1943-3670 (Electronic) 0022-3492 (Linking). https://doi.org/10.1002/JPER-160810. https://www.ncbi. nlm.nih.gov/pubmed/29926950.
10. Chan HL, et al. Non-invasive evaluation of facial crestal bone with ultrasonography. PLoS One. 2017;12.2:e0171237. ISSN:1932-6203 (Electronic) 1932-6203 (Linking). https://doi.org/ 10.1371/journal.pone.0171237. http://www.ncbi.nlm.nih.gov/pubmed/28178323.
11. Chan HL, et al. Ultrasonography for noninvasive and real-time evaluation of peri-implant tissue dimensions. J Clin Periodontol. 2018;45.8:986–95. ISSN:1600-051X (Electronic) 0303-6979 (Linking). https://doi.org/10.1111/jcpe.12918. https://www.ncbi.nlm.nih.gov/pubmed/29757464.
12. Fu JH, Wang HL. Horizontal bone augmentation: the decision tree. Int J Periodontics Restorative Dent. 2011;31.4:429–36. ISSN:1945-3388 (Electronic) 0198-7569 (Linking). https://www.ncbi.nlm.nih.gov/pubmed/21837309.

13. Wang HL, Boyapati L. "PASS" principles for predictable bone regeneration. Implant Dent. 2006;15.1:8–17. ISSN:1056-6163 (Print) 1056-6163 (Linking). https://doi.org/10.1097/01.id. 0000204762. 39826.0f. https://www.ncbi.nlm.nih.gov/pubmed/.16569956.
14. Schwarz F, et al. Peri-implantitis. J Periodontol. 2018;89 Suppl 1:S267–S290. ISSN:1943-3670 (Electronic) 0022-3492 (Linking). https://doi.org/10.1002/JPER.16.0350. https://www.ncbi.nlm.nih.gov/pubmed/29926957.
15. Oh TJ, et al. The causes of early implant bone loss: myth or science? J Periodontol. 2002;73.3:322–33. ISSN:0022-3492 (Print) 0022-3492 (Linking). https://doi.org/10.1902/jop. 2002.73.3.322. https://www.ncbi.nlm.nih.gov/pubmed/11922263.

Ultrasonic Evaluation of Dental Implant Stability

10

Yoann Hériveaux, Vu-Hieu Nguyen, Romain Vayron, and Guillaume Haïat

10.1   Introduction

Dental implants are now routinely used in clinical practice [1] to replace missing teeth in fully or partially edentulous patients, allowing considerable progress in dental, oral, and maxillofacial surgery. However, failures of implant integration still occur and may lead to aseptic loosening, which is one of the major causes of surgical failure [2]. These failures remain difficult to anticipate and may require additional hazardous painful and expensive surgical interventions for the patient. Assessing dental implant stability, which is determined by the quantity and biomechanical quality of bone tissue around the implant [3], is therefore determinant for the surgical success [4]. Two different kinds of implant stability have to be considered. The primary stability occurs during the implant insertion within bone tissue, and is related to bone quality at the implant site. Implant stability should be sufficiently high to avoid micromotion at the bone–implant interface (BII) without being too high to avoid bone necrosis that may occur if the bone tissue is overloaded [5]. Secondary stability is obtained after healing, as the initial stability gets reinforced by newly formed bone tissue growing at the bone–implant interface [6]. Despite the

Y. Hériveaux · G. Haïat (✉)
CNRS, Laboratoire Modélisation et Simulation Multi-Échelle, MSME UMR 8208 CNRS, Créteil Cedex, France
e-mail: guillaume.haiat@cnrs.fr

V.-H. Nguyen
Université Paris-Est, Laboratoire Modélisation et Simulation Multi Echelle, MSME UMR 8208 CNRS, Créteil Cedex, France
e-mail: vu-hieu.nguyen@u-pec.fr

R. Vayron
Université Polytechnique des Hauts de France, Laboratoire d'Automatique, de Mécanique et d'Informatique Industrielles et Humaines, LAMIH UMR 8201 CNRS, Valenciennes, France
e-mail: romain.vayron@uphf.fr

© Springer Nature Switzerland AG 2021
H.-L. (Albert) Chan, O. D. Kripfgans (eds.), *Dental Ultrasound in Periodontology and Implantology*, https://doi.org/10.1007/978-3-030-51288-0_10

routine use of dental implants, there is still an important lack of standardization of the surgical procedures. In particular, the time between the implant insertion and loading with the prosthesis is often determined empirically and may vary from 0 to 6 months [7]. A patient-specific compromise should be found between an early implant loading, which may further stimulate osseointegration phenomena, and a late implant loading, which prevents the degradation of the consolidating BII [8]. Meanwhile, shortening the time of implant loading has become a priority in recent implant developments to (1) minimize the time of social disfigurement and (2) avoid gum loss. Therefore, accurate measurements of the stability of dental implants are of interest because they could improve the surgical strategy by adapting the choice of the healing period to each patient [4]. Various approaches have been suggested to investigate the stability of dental implants. X-rays or Magnetic Resonance Imaging based techniques [9, 10] are not adapted due to the distortion effects generated by the presence of titanium. Impact methods as, for example, the Periotest (Medizintechnik Gulden, Bensheim, Germany) [11, 12] have also been developed (initially to assess the periodontal ligament properties), but present a low reproducibility due to their sensitivity to striking height and handpiece angulation [13]. Resonance frequency analysis (RFA) [14–16] is the most commonly used biomechanical technique to investigate the stability of dental implants. However, the RFA cannot be used to directly identify the BII characteristics [17], and the orientation and fixation of the transducers were found to have important effects on the Implant Stability Quotient (ISQ) [18]. Ultrasound represent an interesting alternative method and the use of quantitative ultrasound (QUS), which was first suggested in [19], constitutes an attractive alternative to assess dental implant stability as it is non-invasive, non-ionizing, and relatively cheap. Other studies showed the potential of non-linear ultrasound techniques to retrieve information on implants stability [20–22]. Furthermore, ultrasound being mechanical waves, it is adapted to capture the biomechanical properties of living tissues.

This chapter reviews various types of work including in silico, in vitro, and in vivo studies dealing with QUS approaches to assess dental implant stability. First, the evolution of periprosthetic bone properties during healing and its influence on the ultrasonic response of the BII will be described. Second, the validation of a QUS device will be considered in vitro, then numerically, and eventually in vivo. Finally, perspectives of clinical applications will be detailed.

10.2 Quantitative Ultrasound Evaluation of the Bone–Implant Interface

10.2.1 Evolution of Periprosthetic Bone Properties During Healing

Implant stability is highly dependent on the biomechanical properties of bone tissue at a distance lower than around 200 μm from the implant surface [23, 24]. Different experimental approaches may be used to retrieve information on newly formed bone properties at the scale of a few micrometers around the implant. Histology is the

Table 10.1 Mean values and standard deviation of the apparent Young's modulus and hardness measured by nanoindentation and of the ultrasound velocity measured with micro-Brillouin scattering in newly formed (NB) and mature (MB) bone tissue of New Zealand White Rabbits

Healing time	7 weeks		13 weeks	
	NB	MB	NB	MB
Young's Modulus (GPa)	15.85 ($\pm$1.55)	20.46 ($\pm$2.75)	17.82 ($\pm$2.10)	20.69 ($\pm$2.41)
Hardness (GPa)	0.660 ($\pm$0.101)	0.696 ($\pm$0.150)[a]	0.668 ($\pm$0.074)	0.696 ($\pm$0.150)[a]
Ultrasound velocity (m.s^{-1})	4966 ($\pm$145)	5305 ($\pm$36)	5030 ($\pm$80)	5360 ($\pm$10)
Mass density	0.878 ρ_{7w}[b]	ρ_{7w}[b]	0.978 ρ_{13w}[b]	ρ_{13w}[b]

Data in means $\pm$ standard deviation in parentheses [29, 30]
[a]Values of hardness for mature bone were not differentiated for the samples with healing times of 7 and 13 weeks
[b]Only a relative variation of the bone mass density was obtained

standard technique used to assess the degree of osseointegration of an implant [25–27]. Histological analyses allow clinicians (1) to distinguish pre-existing mature from newly formed bone tissue, (2) to measure the evolution of the bone-implant contact ratio (BIC) as a function of healing time, and (3) to obtain a qualitative estimation of the increase of mineralization of newly formed bone tissue. However, histology does not provide quantitative information on the biomechanical properties of newly formed bone tissue. Nanoindentation and micro-Brillouin scattering have been employed to retrieve quantitative information on bone properties around an implant. Nanoindentation is widely used to measure the apparent Young's modulus and the hardness of different materials at the microscopic scale [28]. Micro-Brillouin scattering technique uses the photo acoustic interaction between a laser beam and a sample to measure the speed of sound of bone with a resolution of a few micrometers. Table 10.1 summarizes the biomechanical properties of newly formed bone tissue obtained by coupling histology with nanoindentation [27, 29, 30] and micro-Brillouin scattering [30, 31]. Newly formed bone tissue has lower Young's modulus, hardness, and ultrasonic velocities compared to mature bone tissue, which is due to a lower mineral content. Since the two measurements were realized at the same scale, coupling nanoindentation with micro-Brillouin analysis also allowed to derive the relative variation of mass density between newly formed and mature bone tissues.

10.2.2 Influence of Healing Time on the Ultrasonic Response of the Bone–Implant Interface

Mathieu et al. [32] investigated the effect of bone healing on the ultrasound response of the BII in the case of coin-shaped implants placed on rabbit tibiae, in cortical bone tissue. The ultrasound response of the BII was measured in vitro at 15 MHz after 7 and 13 weeks of healing time. The BIC was measured by histomorphometry and the degree of mineralization of bone was estimated qualitatively by histological staining. A significant decrease of the amplitude of the echo of the BII as a function of healing time was obtained, which was explained by (1) the increase of the BIC ratio as a function of healing time from 27 to 69% and (2) the increase of mineralization of newly formed bone tissue, which modifies its Young's modulus and its ultrasound velocity (see Table 10.1). This study demonstrated the sensitivity of QUS to osseointegration phenomena, opening up new path in dental implantology. These results were confirmed in silico [33] in a study investigating the impact of osseointegration and of the implant roughness on the ultrasonic response of a BII. Finite element analyses were used to model the implant ultrasonic response and to determine its sensitivity to variations of a thin layer of soft tissues (representing fibrous tissues) introduced between the bone and the implant. Osseointegration was simulated by progressively reducing the thickness of the soft tissue layer, which leads to a decrease of the echo reflected by the BII.

10.3 Estimation of Dental Implant Stability using a Quantitative Ultrasound Device In Vitro

The use of QUS to assess dental implant biomechanical stability was first suggested in [19], which measured the variations of the 1 MHz response of a screw inserted in an aluminum block. Based on this pioneer work, dental implants have been used as an ultrasound wave guide in order to assess their stability, using a QUS device that was validated in vitro [34–37] and in vivo [38,39]. The principle of this QUS device is to place an ultrasonic transducer with a central frequency of 10 MHz in contact with the top surface of a dental implant inserted in bone, as represented in Fig. 10.1. The ultrasonic probe is linked to an analyzer, and a transient recorder monitors the

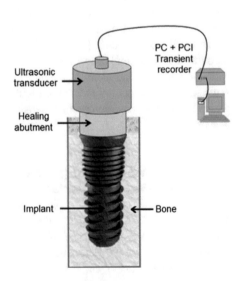

Fig. 10.1 Ultrasonic device including the implant, the transducer and the adapted dedicated electronics. Figure adapted from [35]

radiofrequency (rf) signal from the analyzer with a sampling frequency equal to 100 MHz. An indicator I is then derived from the rf signals by computing its Hilbert envelope to get a simple score representing the average amplitude of the measured signal. The precise definition of I may depend on the specific study so that the values obtained for different studies could not be compared. Note that a multifractal analysis was also performed to retrieve information from the inner structure of the rf signal [40]. The amplitude of the rf signals depends on the biomechanical properties of the media in the vicinity of the BII. The acoustical impedance gap is lower when the implant is surrounded by bone than by fluids (blood, water or air), and the energy leakage of the ultrasonic wave out of the implant is therefore more important. Moreover, evolutions of the bone mechanical properties described in Sect. 10.2.1 also influence the ultrasonic propagation at the BII [29, 33]. Consequently, I is sensitive to the mechanical properties of the BII, and its evolution is representative of the dental implant stability.

10.3.1 Preliminary Study with Titanium Cylinders

An in vitro experimental preliminary study was first carried out with prototype titanium cylinder-shaped implants in Mathieu et al. [34]. The aim of this study was to propose an in vitro methodology to identify the amount of bone surrounding titanium cylinders, paving the way for the assessment of implant stability by QUS techniques. Identical implants were inserted into rabbit distal femurs with four different geometric configurations represented in Fig. 10.2, each configuration corresponding to a given amount of bone in contact with the implants. All implants were placed in defects created in bone tissue with the same depth (6 μm). However,

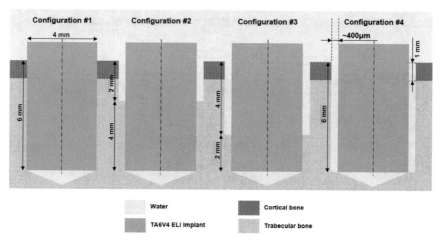

Fig. 10.2 Schematic illustrations of the four drilling configurations used to mimic different configurations of primary stability. Figure adapted from [34]

the diameter of the defect changed (from 4 to 4.8 mm) at a different depth depending on the configuration. All samples were then analyzed using the QUS device. The obtained rf signals exhibited an approximately periodic repetition of echoes recorded on the upper surface of the implant. Moreover, the amplitudes of the echoes decreased faster as a function of time when the amount of bone in contact with the implant increases, and the value of the indicator I was correlated to the amount of bone in contact with the implant.

10.3.2 Studies in Biomaterials

A second in vitro study [35] was performed using real dental implants in the tricalcium silicate-based cement (TSBC) Biodentine [41, 42], which is used as bone substitute biomaterials for dental implant surgery in the case of edentulous patients with poor bone quality. Synthetic biomaterials present the possibility of avoiding invasive surgery procedures of autogenous bone grafts while preventing the higher risks of rejection and infection of allografts [43]. In particular, TSBCs could be used as bone substitutes for dental implantology because of (1) their adapted mechanical properties [44, 45], (2) their biocompatibility [46], (3) their bioactive properties [41, 42], (4) their adhesive properties with calcified tissues [47], and (5) the relatively low duration necessary to prepare the mixture before application (9–12 min) [44]. For these reasons, [35] studied the evolution of the ultrasonic response of an implant embedded in TSBC and subjected to fatigue stresses. Six titanium dental implants were embedded in Biodentine™ (Septodont, Saint-Maur-des Fossés, France). Cyclic lateral stresses were then applied to the implants during 24 h via a custom-made mechanical device, and the stability of the implant was regularly evaluated with the QUS device. Figure 10.3 shows the variation of the mean values of I as a function of fatigue time and the associated linear regression for 2 different implants, as well as the results obtained without mechanical stresses

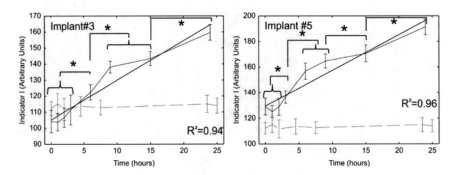

Fig. 10.3 Variation of the QUS indicator I as function of fatigue duration for two implants. The stars indicate that the corresponding fatigue times give significantly different results according to Tukey–Kramer analysis. The gray dashed lines correspond to results obtained without mechanical stresses applied to the implant. Figure adapted from [35]

applied to the implant. One-way analysis of variance (ANOVA) showed a significant effect of fatigue time on the mean value of I for all samples.

Different values of I may be obtained for different implants at time $t = t_0$, (i.e. without mechanical solicitation, see Fig. 10.3), which may be due to (1) variations of implant positioning in Biodentine (e.g. depth of insertion) and (2) possible air bubbles present at the Biodentine-implant interface. However, without mechanical solicitation, I remains constant as a function of time. When subjected to cyclic stresses, a significant increase of I was obtained as a function of fatigue time for all implants, which is due to the progressive debonding of the Biodentine-implant interface, leading to a higher acoustic energy recorded at the upper surface of the implant.

10.3.3 Studies in Bone-Mimic Materials

The use of bone-mimic phantoms made of polyurethane foams allows working under standardized and reproducible conditions. Therefore, it has recently been used to compare the performance of the QUS and RFA methods [37]. Bone test blocks composed of rigid polyurethane foam (Orthobones; 3B Scientific, Hamburg, Germany) with different values of bone density and of cortical thickness (1 and 2 mm) were used to perform this study. Cortical bone was modeled by the material type #40 PCF with a mass density equal to $0.55\,g/cm^3$. Three types of trabecular mimicking phantoms were considered (#10, #20, and #30 PCF) with mass density values, respectively, equal to 0.16, 0.32, and $0.48\,g/cm^3$. Conical cavities were created in the blocks with surgical drills, and implants were then screwed into these cavities. Four different parameters affecting the implant stability were considered in the study, namely (1) the trabecular bone density, (2) the cortical bone thickness, (3) the final drill diameter, and (4) the implant insertion depth. The RFA response of the implant was measured in ISQ units (on a scale from 1 to 100) using the Osstell device (Osstell, Gothenburg, Sweden). The ultrasonic response of the implant was measured thanks to the indicator I, corresponding to the average amplitude of the signal between 10 and $120\,\mu s$. Figure 10.4 shows the variation of the values of the ISQ and of I as a function of the different input parameters.

The results shown in Fig. 10.4 indicate that the values of ISQ (respectively, I) increase (respectively, decrease) as a function of trabecular density, cortical thickness, and the screwing of the implant. However, ANOVA and Tukey–Kramer tests indicate significant difference for the values of I obtained for all the tested trabecular densities and cortical thickness, which was not the case for the ISQ values (see Fig. 10.4a, b). When the final drill diameter varies, values of I were significantly different for all considered configurations except for two (see Fig. 10.4c), while the ISQ values were similar for all final drill diameters lower than 3.2 mm and higher than 3.3 mm. Moreover, Table 10.2 shows that the errors committed with the RFA technique on the estimation of the different parameters was between 4 and 8 times higher compared to that made with the QUS device. QUS has a better sensitivity

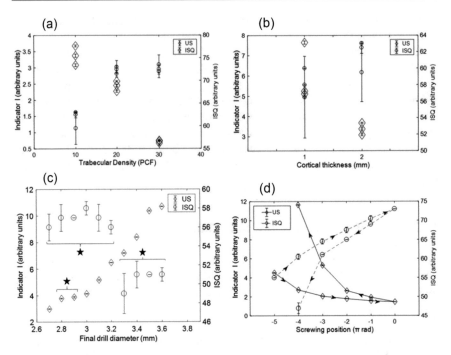

Fig. 10.4 Variations of the values of the ISQ and of the indicator I for implants inserted in bone-mimicking phantoms with different values of (**a**) trabecular density (#10, #20, and #30 PCF), (**b**) cortical thickness (1 or 2 mm), (**c**) final drill diameter, and (**d**) screwing of the implant. Three implants are considered per test block for (**a**) and (**b**). The stars indicate the results that are statistically similar for (**c**). The error bars correspond to the reproducibility of each measurement. Figure adapted from [37]

Table 10.2 Error realized in the estimation of each parameter in [37]

Indicator	Trabecular density (PCF)	Cortical thickness (mm)	Insertion depth (mm)
ISQ	2.73	0.31	0.16
I	0.6	0.04	0.04

to changes of the parameters related to the implant stability and thus a higher potentiality to assess correctly the dental implant stability than the RFA technique.

10.3.4 Studies in Bone Tissue

An in vitro validation of the QUS device has been carried out with implants inserted in bone tissue [36] to establish the dependence of I on the amount of bone in contact with the implant. Ten identical implants were fully inserted in cylindrical cavities (3.5 mm) diameter and 13 mm deep created in the proximal part of bovine humeri. After recording the ultrasonic response of the implant, it was unscrewed by 2π rad

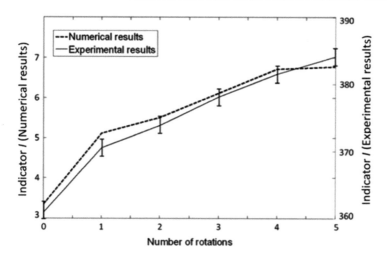

Fig. 10.5 Variation of the simulated and experimental values of I as a function of the number of unscrewing rotations of the dental implant in bone tissue. Figure adapted from [48]

in order to reduce the surface area of the implant in contact with bone tissue. The procedure of unscrewing the implant and recording its ultrasonic response was then repeated until the implant was detached from bone tissue. Figure 10.5 compares results obtained experimentally in [36] with numerical data [48] and shows that the value of the indicator I significantly increases as a function of the number of rotations when the implant is unscrewed. Therefore, despite the more complex wave propagation occurring within the implant than in the preliminary study with titanium cylinders [34], the ultrasonic response is shown to be still sensitive to the implant environment.

10.4 Simulation of Ultrasonic Wave Propagation in Dental Implants

The development of acoustical modeling and of the associated numerical simulation is mandatory in order to understand the interaction between an ultrasonic wave and the bone-implant system because it allows to improve the performances of the device. Moreover, using acoustical modeling is the only solution in order to discriminate the effects of the different bone parameters (such as bone structure, geometry, and material properties) on the ultrasonic response of the implant, which is impossible to achieve in vivo because all parameters vary in parallel. In the studies described below, the ultrasonic source was modeled by a broadband longitudinal velocity pulse centered at 10 MHz in the direction normal to the implant surface. Note that all media were assumed to have homogeneous, elastic, and isotropic mechanical properties, and that the values of ultrasound velocity and of density of all media were taken from [18, 49–51].

10.4.1 2D Model

A 2D numerical study of the ultrasonic propagation in cylinder-shaped titanium implants positioned in bone tissue was first performed in [52] using SIMSONIC, a 2D finite-difference time-domain (FDTD) algorithm. The geometry considered in this study was identical as the one described in Sect. 10.3.1 (see Fig. 10.2). A good qualitative agreement with experimental results was obtained. However, for numerical simulations, a faster decay of the amplitude of the ultrasonic response was observed, and contributions due to mode conversions were lower, which may be related to the 2D approximation made on the study. Therefore, 3D modeling is necessary to derive a more precise description of the interaction between the ultrasonic wave and the bone-implant system.

10.4.2 3D Model

Vayron et al. [53] considered the same configuration as the one considered in [52] (see Fig. 10.2) but using a 3D axisymmetric finite element model and COMSOL Multiphysics (Stockholm, Sweden). Figure 10.6 shows a comparison between the relative evolution of the ultrasonic indicator I obtained experimentally [34], and numerically with the 2D FDTD and with the 3D finite element models. The indicator I is shown to increase when bone quantity around the implant increases for all models. However, there is some discrepancy between data obtained numerically and experimentally, which may be explained by possible experimental errors on the geometry of the configuration as well as on material properties. Nonetheless, 3D data are closer to experimental data than 2D data, which is due to a more realistic description of the problem.

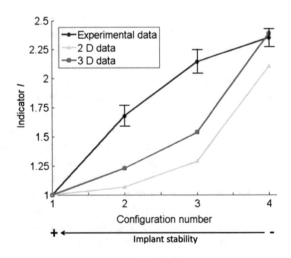

Fig. 10.6 Variation of the normalized value of the ultrasonic indicator as a function of the configuration number corresponding to the amount of bone in contact with the implant (see Fig. 10.2) for results obtained experimentally, with 2D FDTD simulations and with the 3D finite element model. Figure adapted from [53]

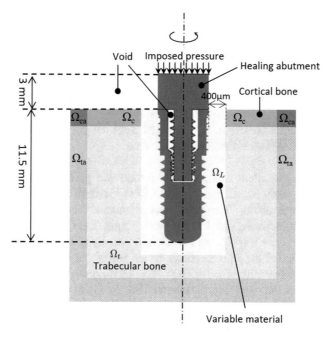

Fig. 10.7 Cross-section view of the 3D axisymmetric geometrical configuration used in [48]. Ω_L corresponds to the region where the material properties are varied. Ω_i, Ω_c, and Ω_t, respectively, denote the implant, the cortical bone, and the trabecular bone. Ω_{ca} and Ω_{ta}, respectively, correspond to absorbing layers associated to trabecular bone and cortical bone. The white parts inside the implant are filled with void. Figure adapted from [48]

The evolution of the indicator I as a function of healing time was also simulated by progressively modifying the mechanical properties of bone tissue around the dental implant considering experimental values measured in Table 10.1. The indicator I was shown to significantly decrease as a function of healing time and therefore to be sensitive to bone quality. In order to derive a more realistic description of the implant structure, another 3D axisymmetric study was performed in [48] considering actual geometries of dental implants, as shown in Fig. 10.7. The effects of changes of three different parameters on the ultrasonic response of the implant were assessed, namely (1) introducing fibrous tissue in part Ω_L (see Fig. 10.7) and progressively reducing the depth of this fibrous layer, (2) unscrewing the implant, and (3) modifying the peri-implant bone mechanical properties from ± 20%.

Figure 10.5 shows that I increases as a function of the number of rotation when unscrewing the implant, and a good agreement with experimental results [36] was obtained. Increasing longitudinal wave velocity and mass density of bone tissue around the implant also leads to a decrease of the values of I. These results may be explained by the decrease of the gap of material properties between bone tissue and the implant, which leads to a lower gap of acoustic impedance between bone and the implant and therefore to a higher transmission coefficient at the bone–implant interface. Heriveaux et al. [33] further studied this point with a 2D numerical model and conclusions were in agreement with [48]. As a conclusion, in all the aforementioned numerical simulations, the indicator I was shown to decrease as a function of the implant stability.

10.5   In Vivo Estimation of Implant Stability Using the Quantitative Ultrasound Device

An initial in vivo validation of the QUS device was performed in [38] using a rabbit model. Twenty-one dental implants were inserted in the femur of eleven New Zealand white rabbits. Two (respectively, three and six) rabbits were sacrificed after 2 weeks (respectively, 6 and 11) of healing time. The QUS device was used to measure the ultrasonic response of the implant directly after implantation and just before the sacrifice of the animals. Each measurement was reproduced 10 times to assess their reproducibility. The BIC was also determined by histological analyses. Figure 10.8 shows that the rf signals obtained on the day of the implantation have a higher amplitude than signals obtained after 11 weeks of healing time. A significant decrease of the ultrasonic indicator was obtained between the initial and the final measurements for all but one (respectively, for all) implants after 6 (respectively, 11) weeks of healing time, whereas no global tendency could be assessed after 2 weeks of healing time. Moreover, the indicator I had significantly different values for samples obtained after 2, 6, and 13 weeks of healing, which validates the use of QUS to assess dental implant stability.

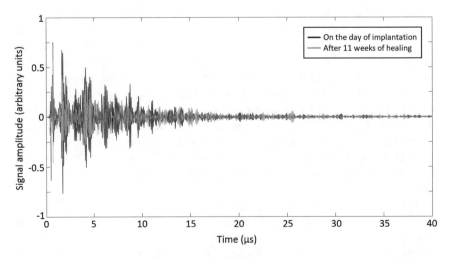

Fig. 10.8 Time gated rf signals obtained on the day of the implantation (black line) and after 11 weeks of healing time (gray line). Figure adapted from [38]

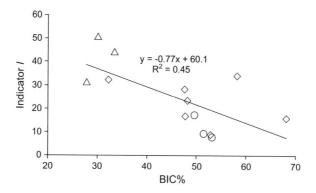

Fig. 10.9 Variation of the indicator I as function of the BIC ratio. The triangles (respectively, the circles and the squares) represent the samples with 2 (respectively, 6 and 11) weeks of healing time. Figure adapted from [38]

Figure 10.9 shows the variation of the indicator I as function of the BIC ratio for 13 implants. A significant but limited correlation was obtained between I and the BIC, which may be explained by (1) the low number of analyzed samples, (2) the measurement of the BIC ratio in a given plane rather than in 3D, and (3) the dependence of the implant ultrasonic response on the mechanical properties of bone tissue in contact with the implant, which are not described by the BIC ratio.

Recently, a second in vivo study was performed with sheep by [39] in order to compare the performance of the RFA (Osstell was used) and of QUS techniques to retrieve dental implant stability. Compared to [38], the study considered (1) a larger number of samples, (2) a bigger animal model inducing bone properties closer to those of human tissue, (3) the comparison with the RFA technique, and (4) a controlled torque of insertion (3.5 N cm) when screwing the ultrasonic probe on the implant, which allowed a better reproducibility compared to the manual positioning performed in the former study. Eighty-one dental implants were inserted in the iliac crests of eleven sheep. QUS and RFA measurements were performed after healing times of 5, 7, and 15 weeks. The RFA response was measured in ISQ as described in Sect. 10.3.3. The ultrasonic indicator I that was used in previous studies was modified in order to obtain an ultrasonic indicator UI$= 100 - 10\times$ I having values from 1 to 100 and increasing when bone quality and quantity increases around the implant.

Figure 10.10 shows the variations of UI and of ISQ as a function of healing time for 2 given implants. ISQ measurements were performed following two perpendicular directions, denoted 0 and 90°. ANOVA showed that UI significantly increased from 0 to 5 healing weeks and from 0 to 7 healing weeks for 97% of implants. However, variations of UI between 5 and 15 healing weeks were implant dependent and UI decreased as a function of healing time for several implants. This result may be explained by the fact that implants were not loaded mechanically in the iliac crest, which is likely to lead to bone tissue resorption around the implants [54]. Results obtained by the RFA technique were shown not to be dependent on

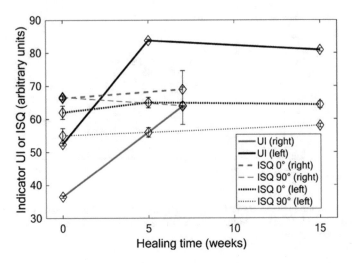

Fig. 10.10 Results obtained for implant #2 right and left of the sheep #3 for the different healing times for UI, ISQ 0° and ISQ 90° values. Error bars show the reproducibility of the measurements. Figure adapted from [39]

Table 10.3 Comparison of the error realized in the estimation of the healing time using the QUS and RFA measurements in both directions (0 and 90°)

Healing times (weeks)	UI	ISQ 0°	ISQ 90°
0–5	0.56 ± 2.04	4.59 ± 3.21	4.93 ± 4.56
5–15	1.28 ± 1.03	9.24 ± 11.9	13.93 ± 16.7
0–7	4.45 ± 5.33	0.90 ± 1.38	9.67 ± 13.2

The mean and standard deviation values are shown for all implants and each time interval

the healing time, with significant variations of the ISQ values for only 18% of the implants. Moreover, Table 10.3 shows that the error on the estimation of the healing time when analyzing the results obtained with QUS was around 10 times lower than that made when using RFA, which may be explained by a better reproducibility of measurements. The conclusion of the study is that QUS allow to determine the evolution of dental implant stability with a better accuracy than RFA.

10.6 Perspectives

The studies summarized in this chapter have shown the potential of QUS techniques to retrieve information on the BII and pave the way for the development of an ultrasonic device that could be used clinically to estimate dental implant stability. Comparisons with the RFA technique highlight the better sensitivity and precision of QUS. However, it remains difficult to precisely define implant stability [4, 55]. Moreover, clinical studies are now needed in order to define a target value for the ultrasonic indicator above which an implant is considered to be stable enough to be loaded. Such QUS device could be used in clinical practice i) at the time of implant surgery (in order to assess dental implant primary stability), which may lead to an estimation of the loading time and at the time of implant loading (in order to assess dental implant secondary stability), which may help the surgeon determine whether the implant can actually be loaded or more time is needed to secure the process.

References

1. Albrektsson T, et al. Osseointegrated oral implants. A Swedish multicenter study of 8139 consecutively inserted Nobelpharma implants. J Periodontol. 1988;59 5:287–96. https://doi.org/10.1902/jop.1988.59.5.287. ISSN: 0022-3492 (Print) 0022-3492.
2. Pilliar RM, Lee JM, Maniatopoulos C. Observations on the effect of movement on bone ingrowth into porous-surfaced implants. Clin Orthop Relat Res. 1986;208:108–13. https://www.ncbi.nlm.nih.gov/pubmed/3720113. ISSN: 0009-921X (Print) 0009-921X (Linking).
3. Franchi M, et al. Influence of different implant surfaces on peri-implant osteogenesis: histomorphometric analysis in sheep. J Periodontol. 2007;78 5:879–888. ISSN: 1943-3670.
4. Mathieu V, et al. Biomechanical determinants of the stability of dental implants: influence of the bone–implant interface properties. J Biomech. 2014;47 1:3–13. ISSN: 0021-9290.
5. Grandi T, et al. Clinical outcome and bone healing of implants placed with high insertion torque: 12-month results from a multicenter controlled cohort study. Int J Oral Maxillofac Surg. 2013;42 4:516–520. ISSN: 0901-5027.
6. Abrahamsson I, et al. Early bone formation adjacent to rough and turned endosseous implant surfaces: an experimental study in the dog. Clin Oral Implants Res. 2004;15 4:381–392. ISSN: 0905-7161.
7. Raghavendra S, Wood MC, Taylor TD. Early wound healing around endosseous implants: a review of the literature. Int J Oral Maxillofac Implants. 2005;20 3:425–31. https://www.ncbi.nlm.nih.gov/pubmed/15973954. ISSN: 0882-2786 (Print) 0882-2786 (Linking).
8. Serra G, et al. Sequential bone healing of immediately loaded mini- implants. Am J Orthod Dentofacial Orthop. 2008;134 1:44–52. ISSN: 0889-5406.
9. Shalabi MM, et al. Evaluation of bone response to titanium-coated polymethyl methacrylate resin (PMMA) implants by X-ray tomography. J Mater Sci Mater Med. 2007;18 10:2033–2039. ISSN: 0957-4530.
10. Gill A, Shellock FG. Assessment of MRI issues at 3-Tesla for metallic surgical implants: findings applied to 61 additional skin closure staples and vessel ligation clips. J Cardiovasc Magn Reson. 2012;14 1:3. ISSN: 1532-429X.
11. Schulte W. Periotest-a new measurement process for periodontal function. Zahnarztl Mitt. 1983;73:1229–1240.
12. Van Scotter DE, Wilson CJ. The Periotest method for determining implant success. J Oral Implantol. 1991;17 4:410–413. ISSN: 0160-6972.
13. Meredith N, et al. Relationship between contact time measurements and PTV values when using the Periotest to measure implant stability. Int J Prosthodont. 1998;11 3. ISSN: 0893-2174
14. Meredith N, Alleyne D, Cawley P. Quantitative determination of the stability of the implant-tissue interface sing resonance frequency analysis. Clin Oral Implants Res. 1996;7 3:261–267. ISSN: 0905-7161.
15. Georgiou AP, Cunningham JL. Accurate diagnosis of hip prosthesis loosening using a vibrational technique. Clin Biomech. 2001;16 4:315–323. ISSN: 0268-0033.
16. Pastrav LC et al. In vivo evaluation of a vibration analysis technique for the per-operative monitoring of the fixation of hip prostheses. J Orthop Surg Res. 2009;4:10. https://doi.org/10.1186/1749-799X-4-10. https://www.ncbi.nlm.nih.gov/pubmed/19358703. ISSN: 1749-799X (Electronic) 1749-799X (Linking).
17. Aparicio C, Lang NP, Rangert B. Validity and clinical significance of biomechanical testing of implant/bone interface. Clinical Oral Implants Res. 2006;17 S2:2–7. ISSN: 0905-7161.

18. Pattijn V, et al. Resonance frequency analysis of implants in the guinea pig model: influence of boundary conditions and orientation of the transducer. Med Eng Phys. 2007;29 2:182–90. https://doi.org/10.1016/j.medengphy.2006.0201. https://www.ncbi.nlm.nih.gov/pubmed/16597507. ISSN: 1350-4533 (Print) 1350-4533 (Linking).

19. De Almeida M, Maciel C, Pereira J. Proposal for an ultrasonic tool to monitor the osseointegration of dental implants. Sensors. 2007;7 7: 1224–1237.

20. Riviere J, et al. Nonlinear ultrasound: potential of the cross-correlation method for osseointegration monitoring. J Acoust Soc Am. 2012;132 3:EL202–7. https://doi.org/10.1121/1.4742138. https://www.ncbi.nlm.nih.gov/pubmed/22979833. ISSN: 1520-8524 (Electronic) 0001-4966 (Linking).

21. Riviere J, et al. Time reversed elastic nonlinearity diagnostic applied to mock osseointegration monitoring applying two experimental models. J Acoust Soc Am. 2012;131 3:1922–7. https://doi.org/10.1121/1.3683251. https://www.ncbi.nlm.nih.gov/pubmed/22423689. ISSN: 1520-8524 (Electronic)0001-4966 (Linking).

22. Riviere J, et al. Nonlinear acoustic resonances to probe a threaded interface. J Appl Phys. 2010;107 12:124901. ISSN: 0021-8979.

23. Huja S, et al. Microdamage adjacent to endosseous implants. Bone. 1999;25:217–22. https://doi.org/10.1016/S87563282(99)001519.

24. Luo G, et al. The effect of surface roughness on the stress adaptation of trabecular architecture around a cylindrical implant. J Biomech. 1999;32 3:275–84. ISSN: 0021-9290.

25. Nkenke E, et al. Implant stability and histomorphometry: a correlation study in human cadavers using stepped cylinder implants. Clin Oral Implants Res.2003;14 5:601–9. https://doi.org/10.1034/j.1600.0501.2003.00937.x. https://www.ncbi.nlm.nih.gov/pubmed/12969364. ISSN: 0905-7161 (Print) 0905-7161 (Linking).

26. Scarano A, et al. Correlation between implant stability quotient and bone-implant contact: a retrospective histological and histomorphometrical study of seven titanium implants retrieved from humans. Clin Implant Dent. Relat. Res. 2006;8 4:218–22. ISSN: 1523-0899.

27. Vayron R, et al. Variation of biomechanical properties of newly formed bone tissue determined by nanoindentation as a function of healing time. Comput Methods Biomech Biomed Eng. 2011;14 sup1:139–40. ISSN: 1025-5842.

28. Zysset PK, et al. Elastic modulus and hardness of cortical and trabecular bone lamellae measured by nanoindentation in the human femur. J Biomech. 1999;32 10:1005–12. https://doi.org/10.1016/S0021.9290(99).00111.6. http://www.sciencedirect.com/science/article/pii/S0021929099001116. ISSN: 0021-9290.

29. Vayron R, et al. Nanoindentation measurements of biomechanical properties in mature and newly formed bone tissue surrounding an implant. J Biomech Eng. 2012;134 2:021007. ISSN: 0148-0731.

30. Vayron R, et al. Assessment of in vitro dental implant primary stability using an ultrasonic method. Ultrasound Med Biol. 2014;40 12:2885–94. ISSN: 0301-5629.

31. Mathieu V, et al. Micro-Brillouin scattering measurements in mature and newly formed bone tissue surrounding an implant. J Biomech Eng. 2011;133 2:021006. ISSN: 0148-0731.

32. Mathieu V, et al. Influence of healing time on the ultrasonic response of the bone-implant interface. Ultrasound Med Biol. 2012;38 4:611–8. https://doi.org/10.1016/j.ultrasmedbio.2011.12.014. ISSN: 0301-5629.

33. Heriveaux Y, Nguyen VH, Haiat G. Reflection of an ultrasonic wave on the bone-implant interface: a numerical study of the effect of the multiscale roughness. J Acoust Soc Am. 2018;144 1:488. https://doi.org/10.1121/1.5046524. ISSN: 0001-4966.

34. Mathieu V, et al. Ultrasonic evaluation of dental implant biomechanical stability: an in vitro study. Ultrasound Med Biol. 2011;37 2:262–70. ISSN: 0301-5629.

35. Vayron R, et al. Variation of the ultrasonic response of a dental implant embedded in tricalcium silicate-based cement under cyclic loading. J Biomech. 2013;46 6:1162–8. ISSN: 0021-9290.

36. Vayron R, et al. Assessment of in vitro dental implant primary stability using an ultrasonic method. Ultrasound Med Biol. 2014;40 12:2885–94. https://doi.org/10.1016/j.ultrasmedbio.2014.03.035. http://wwwsciencedirectcom/science/article/pii/S0301562914004104. ISSN: 0301-5629.

37. Vayron R, et al. Evaluation of dental implant stability in bone phantoms: comparison between a quantitative ultrasound technique and resonance frequency analysis. Clin Implant Dent Relat Res. 2018;20 4:470–8. ISSN: 1523-0899.

38. Vayron R, et al. Evolution of bone biomechanical properties at the micrometer scale around titanium implant as a function of healing time. Phys Med Biol. 2014;59 6:1389. ISSN: 0031-9155.

39. Vayron R, et al. Comparison of resonance frequency analysis and of quantitative ultrasound to assess dental implant osseointegration. Sensors. 2018;18 5:1397.

40. Scala I, et al. Ultrasonic characterization and multiscale analysis for the evaluation of dental implant stability: A sensitivity study. Biomed Signal Proces. 2018;42:3744. https://doi.org/10.1016/j.bspc.2017.12.007.

41. Koubi S, et al. Quantitative evaluation by glucose diffusion of microleakage in aged calcium silicate-based open-sandwich restorations. Int J Dentistry. 2012;2012:105863. ISSN: 1687-8728.

42. Koubi G, et al. Clinical evaluation of the performance and safety of a new dentine substitute, Biodentine, in the restoration of posterior teeth—a prospective study. ClinOral Investig. 2013;17 1:243–9. ISSN: 1432-6981.

43. Jones KS. Assays on the influence of biomaterials on allogeneic rejection in tissue engineering. Tissue Eng B Rev. 2008;14 4:407–17. ISSN: 1937-3368.

44. Golberg M, et al. Biocompatibility or cytotoxic effects of dental composites, Chapter VI: Emerging trends in (bio)material researches. Oxfordshire: Coxmoor;2009.

45. Sawyer, AN et al. Effects of calcium silicate-based materials on the flexural properties of dentin. J Endod. 2012;38 5:680–3. https://doi.org/10.1016/j.joen.2011.12.036. https://www.ncbi.nlm.nih.gov/pubmed/22515902. ISSN: 1878-3554 (Electronic) 0099-2399 (Linking).

46. Leiendecker, AP, et al. Effects of calcium silicate–based materials on collagen matrix integrity of mineralized dentin. J Endodontics. 2012;38 6:829–33. ISSN: 0099-2399.

47. Kenny SM, Buggy M. Bone cements and fillers: a review. J Mater. Sci Mater. Med. 2003;14 11:923–38. ISSN: 0957-4530.

48. Vayron R, et al. Assessment of the biomechanical stability of a dental implant with quantitative ultrasound: a three-dimensional finite element study. J Acoust Soc Am. 2016;139 2:773–80. ISSN: 0001-4966.

49. Njeh CF, et al. An in vitro investigation of the dependence on sample thickness of the speed of sound along the specimen. Med Eng Phys. 1999;21 9:651–9. https://doi.org/10.1016/s1350-4533(99)00090-9. https://www.ncbi.nlm.nih.gov/pubmed/10699567. ISSN: 1350-4533 (Print) 1350-4533 (Linking).

50. Pattijn V, et al. The resonance frequencies and mode shapes of dental implants: rigid body behaviour versus bending behaviour a numerical approach. J Biomech. 2006;39 5:939–47. https://doi.org/10.1016/j.jbiomech.2005.01.035. https://www.ncbi.nlm.nih.gov/pubmed/16488232. ISSN: 0021-9290 (Print) 0021-9290 (Linking).

51. Padilla, F, et al. Variation of ultrasonic parameters with microstructure and material properties of trabecular bone: a 3D model simulation. J Bone Miner Res. 2007;22:665–74. https://doi.org/10.1359/jbmr.070209.

52. Mathieu V, et al. Numerical simulation of ultrasonic wave propagation for the evaluation of dental implant biomechanical stability. J Acoust Soc Am. 2011;129 6:4062–72. ISSN: 0001-4966.

53. Vayron R, et al. Finite element simulation of ultrasonic wave propagation in a dental implant for biomechanical stability assessment. Biomech Model Mechanobiol. 2015;14 5:1021–32. ISSN: 1617-7959.

54. Li Z, Muller R, Ruffoni D. Bone remodeling and mechanobiology around implants: insights from small animal imaging. J Orthop Res. 2018;36 2:584–93. https://doi.org/10.1002/jor.23758. ISSN: 0736-0266.

55. Haiat G, Wang H-L, Brunski J. Effects of biomechanical properties of the bone–implant interface on dental implant stability: from in silico approaches to the patient's mouth. Ann Rev Biomed Eng. 2014;16:187–213. ISSN: 1523-9829.

Photoacoustic Ultrasound for Enhanced Contrast in Dental and Periodontal Imaging

11

Colman Moore and Jesse V. Jokerst

11.1 Introduction

Ultrasound is a long-standing tool in medical diagnosis. Its benefits include affordability, high spatiotemporal resolution, sensitivity, and safety—it is ideally suited for imaging soft tissue and bone surfaces simultaneously. Despite these advantages, it is surprisingly uncommon in clinical dentistry. Nevertheless, a variety of reports have been published on oral applications of ultrasound; for an overview of the field to date, we recommend previously published reviews on this topic as well as the other chapters in this textbook [1–8]. Briefly, the scope of ultrasound applications includes visualization of dental and gingival anatomy, the detection of caries, dental fractures and cracks, gingival thickness measurements, periapical lesions, maxillofacial fractures, periodontal bony defects, muscle thickness, temporomandibular disorders, and implant dentistry [9].

Ultrasound imaging systems use piezoelectric transducers to transmit high frequency (1–50 MHz) pulses through target tissue and detect the reflected waves. Because sound waves are mechanical vibrations, the speed of sound through a particular medium depends on the acoustic impedance of the material. At interfaces between tissue types with distinct acoustic impedances, a fraction of the ultrasonic pulse is backscattered, while the other part is transmitted. The magnitude of the

C. Moore
Department of NanoEngineering, University of California San Diego, La Jolla, CA, USA
e-mail: cam081@ucsd.edu

J. V. Jokerst (✉)
Department of NanoEngineering, University of California San Diego, La Jolla, CA, USA

Materials Science and Engineering Program, University of California San Diego, La Jolla, CA, USA
Department of Radiology, University of California San Diego, La Jolla, CA, USA
e-mail: jjokerst@ucsd.edu

© Springer Nature Switzerland AG 2021
H.-L. (Albert) Chan, O. D. Kripfgans (eds.), *Dental Ultrasound in Periodontology and Implantology*, https://doi.org/10.1007/978-3-030-51288-0_11

reflected pulse (echo) scales with the impedance mismatch at the boundary. Therefore, the intensity of the returning echo and the time it takes to reach the transducer
are the two main components used to reconstruct images. However, one of the main
drawbacks of ultrasound is its limited contrast. The modality can resolve anatomical
features but cannot probe molecular components of disease (nucleic acids, proteins,
enzymes, etc.). Recent progress has been made in activatable ultrasound contrast
agents, but these still can only boost the grayscale intensity in a given region; they
cannot produce spectrally unique signal. Fortunately, photoacoustic ultrasound has
emerged as a fast-growing and promising technique for augmenting conventional
ultrasound with the spectral contrast of optical imaging.

Photoacoustic ultrasound harnesses the photoacoustic effect—a phenomenon
first observed by Alexander Graham Bell that occurs when the energy from light
is absorbed by a material and released as an acoustic vibration. For imaging,
a near-infrared (NIR) light source is used to pulse photons (1–100 ns) onto an
absorbing target or tissue. NIR light is used because it can propagate through
tissue better than blue or green wavelengths. The tissue being irradiated by the
NIR absorbs the light and experiences brief (nanosecond) thermoelastic expansion.
This expansion generates broadband acoustic waves that can be detected with
conventional ultrasound transducers. Importantly, there is no bulk heating of the
tissue. This is because the incident laser pulse is shorter than the thermal and stress
relaxation times of the target; thus, the system becomes mechanically and thermally
confined and the fractional volume expansion of the target can be neglected
[10]. Therefore, the initial pressure rise (i.e. the generated photoacoustic wave) is
proportional to the optical fluence and absorption coefficient of the material. The
resulting photoacoustic wave propagates in three dimensions and is detected by
either a single element ultrasound transducer or an array of transducer elements.
From here, if the fluence is assumed to be locally homogenous, an image can be
reconstructed based primarily upon differences in the absorption coefficient of tissue
components effectively mapping the pressure wave distribution.

A variety of hardware configurations are commonly used in research
applications: These primarily include photoacoustic tomography, photoacoustic
microscopy, and photoacoustic endoscopy [11]. The body possesses a number of
endogenous absorbers but exogenous contrast agents can also be used. The main
sources of endogenous contrast are NIR-absorbing molecules such as oxygenated
and deoxygenated hemoglobin, melanin, lipids, and water [12]. These targets have
often been used to image hemodynamics [13], blood oxygen saturation [14, 15],
and cancers [16, 17]. However, a wide variety of exogenous contrast agents—often
small molecules or nanoparticles—have also been developed to boost contrast and
probe specific biomarkers or disease states [18]. From a materials perspective, the
current landscape of these agents primarily consists of organic small molecules
[19], inorganic nanomaterials [20, 21], and organic nanoparticles [22, 23].

The preclinical applications of photoacoustic imaging for oral health have been
growing in the past decade. Early work on this topic was focused on optical and
photoacoustic spectroscopic measurements of oral tissue. The induced temperature
distributions of photoacoustic excitation and the absorbing/scattering behavior of
incident light have also been characterized. Following this, investigations have pro-

ceeded on dental pulp characterization as well as enamel/dentin imaging for early detection of caries and cracks. Recently, the field has expanded into characterization of the periodontium via non-invasive imaging of the periodontal pocket. Here, we review the developments in oral photoacoustics to date and offer perspectives on future progress in this burgeoning field.

11.2 Optical and Photoacoustic Characterization of Oral Tissues

Early investigations into dental applications of photoacoustics largely focused on the determination of optical and photoacoustic properties of oral tissue within the optical window. In medical imaging, the optical window refers to a range of wavelengths between 650–900 nm in which tissue absorbance and scattering are reduced relative to other wavelengths [24]. Optical imaging techniques typically operate in this range to maximize resolution, contrast, and penetration depths. The optical properties of tissue that govern these parameters, primarily absorption and scattering, vary across tissue types; therefore, the investigation of these properties preceded imaging applications. Furthermore, they are relevant to both photoacoustic imaging and optical coherence tomography—another modality has seen recent growth in oral diagnostic research.

Initial work focused on understanding the absorption and scattering properties of NIR light in healthy and carious/demineralized enamel [25–27]. For many years, dental caries have been diagnosed with visual, tactile, and radiographic exams; however, a significant level of variation exists across examiners. Healthy enamel is primarily composed of hydroxyapatite $(Ca_{10}(PO_4)_6(OH)_2)$ and is highly transparent to NIR light (Fig. 11.1a). During demineralization and decay, individual mineral crystals dissolve which causes micropores to form in carious lesions [28].

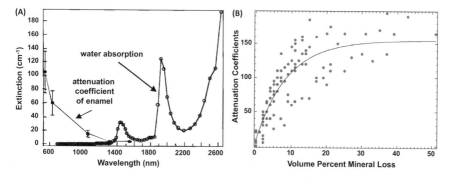

Fig. 11.1 Optical properties of enamel. (**a**) Plot of the attenuation coefficient of dental enamel versus the absorption profile of water in the NIR. (**b**) The attenuation coefficient has an exponential relationship ($r^2 = 0.74$) to the extent of mineral loss in enamel caries lesions. Adapted with permission from the Society of Photo-Optical Instrumentation Engineers [25]

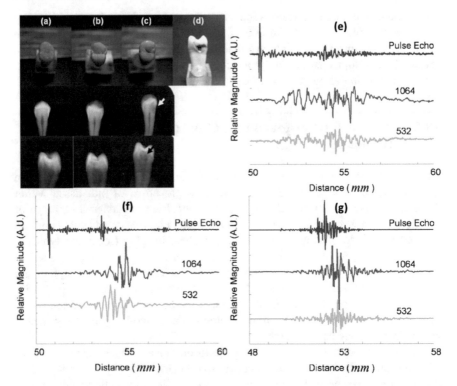

Fig. 11.2 Characterization of upper premolar health status through visual, radiographic, and photoacoustic indicators. The top row of photographs shows occlusal views of (**a**) healthy tooth, (**b**) incipient caries, (**c**) advanced caries, and (**d**) advanced from a proximal view, revealing penetration through the dentin. The lower radiographs show buccolingual views (second row) and proximal views (third row) of the same teeth—they exhibit low contrast from the caries. Pulse-echo and photoacoustic A-line signals are shown at 1064 nm and 532 nm for (**e**) healthy tooth, (**f**) incipient caries, and (**g**) advanced caries. Adapted with permission from the Society of Photo-Optical Instrumentation Engineers [34]

These pores strongly scatter visible and NIR light (Fig. 11.2b) [29]. Darling et al. found that the porosity of these lesions increased the scattering coefficient one to two orders of magnitude above healthy enamel. Indeed, the interactions of NIR light with enamel are dominated by scattering rather than absorption making absorption properties difficult to measure using optical methods [30]. Nevertheless, because photoacoustic intensity is proportional to optical absorption, photoacoustic ultrasound can measure relative absorption coefficients as well as true values if the light fluence is known quantitatively [31].

One of the earliest studies of photoacoustics for dentistry used a pulsed Nd:YAG (neodymium-doped yttrium aluminum garnet) laser to study the absorption and ablation properties of 1064 nm light on dentin and enamel [30]. The authors found that enamel absorbs poorly at 1064 nm so the photoacoustic signal is low. However, it increases with caries due to the presence of melanin from pigmented anaerobic bacteria and their metabolites. In addition, the pulsed laser could be used for ablation of caries lesions, which could be monitored due to the higher photoacoustic signal from ablation (rapid expansion of vaporized organic material) compared to non-pigmented tissue. The acoustic properties of teeth following laser irradiation have also been studied to elucidate the acoustic differences between healthy and decayed teeth. El-Sharkawy et al. used an interferometric detection scheme for measuring surface acoustic waves, which propagate parallel to surfaces of irradiated teeth [32, 33]. The system could differentiate healthy and decayed teeth by calculating the longitudinal speed of sound, optical penetration depth, and Gruneisen coefficient for each sample—this photoacoustic spectroscopy scheme suggests the potential of automated caries diagnosis if used with pattern recognition algorithms. In 2006, Kim et al. extended the concept of detecting early-stage caries using photoacoustics [34]. They used a Nd:YAG laser (15-ns pulse width at 100 mJ, 10 Hz, 1064/532 nm) and an unfocused single element transducer (12 MHz) to analyze extracted human molars split into three groups (healthy, incipient caries, and advanced caries) as determined visually and radiographically. Here, incipient caries only affected the enamel, while advanced caries penetrated to the dentin. They found that the photoacoustic signal at 1064 nm was significantly stronger from regions of teeth with incipient caries than normal regions. This signal was further elevated for teeth with advanced caries. There was elevated signal between regions of teeth with incipient caries and normal teeth at 532 nm; importantly, the signal did not increase for advanced caries. This work was an important proof-of-concept but full photoacoustic imaging was not possible because the data acquisition was limited to one-dimension, i.e., only spectroscopic data.

11.3   Dentin and Enamel Imaging for Caries and Crack Detection

The photoacoustic technique was extended for imaging of dental caries in 2D and 3D in 2010 by Li et al. [35, 36]. They used a Q-Switched Nd:YAG laser (8-ns pulse width at 6 mJ, 2 Hz, 1064 nm) with a needle hydrophone aligned with an optical fiber for acoustic transduction. To acquire images, the probe was raster scanned using step motors. They also performed temperature and pressure field simulations in teeth to validate the safety of laser excitation. The 2D finite element modeling results suggested that the maximum local temperature change would be below 1 °C (where ≥ 5 °C is required for pulpal necrosis). In addition, the modeled pressure change in the dentin was <0.7 MPa, much less than its fatigue limit of 20 MPa. The authors could image both an extracted healthy tooth and one with caries (Fig. 11.3).

Photoacoustic tomography has been further investigated for early detection of dental lesions [37, 38]. Cheng et al. used a similar imaging system (8-ns pulse width, 10 Hz, 11 mJ/cm^2, 532 nm with 4.39 MHz ultrasound center frequency) to study extracted teeth with white spot enamel caries and artificially induced cracks. They used both typical B-mode photoacoustic tomography (contrast is proportional to the relative optical absorption in tissue) and "S-mode" tomography (where contrast is

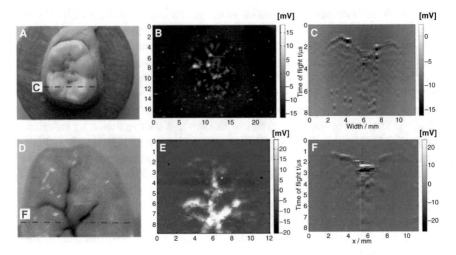

Fig. 11.3 Photoacoustic tomography of healthy versus carious teeth. (**a**) Occlusal photograph of a healthy extracted tooth. (**b**) Top-down (C-scan) photoacoustic image of the healthy tooth. (**c**) B-scan photoacoustic cross-section of a healthy tooth taken at the red line shown in Panel **a**. (**d**) Occlusal photograph of an extracted tooth with caries. (**e**) Top-down (C-scan) photoacoustic image of the diseased tooth. (**f**) B-scan photoacoustic cross-section of the diseased tooth at the red line shown in Panel **d**. Adapted with permission from the Institute of Physics [36]

determined by the spectral slope of the photoacoustic signal). This S-mode exploits the spectral profile of the photoacoustic echo rather than just its time-domain properties; it has shown potential for better differentiation of tissue types based on physical properties (such as the Young's modulus) than conventional photoacoustic imaging [39]. These authors found that the conventional B-mode technique was useful for imaging the structure of teeth including the enamel, dentin, and pulp. However, their images could not distinguish early enamel lesions. This limitation was primarily attributed to insufficient changes in optical absorption. Nevertheless, S-mode imaging could correlate differences in photoacoustic spectral slope to differences in stiffness between enamel and dentin as well as early enamel lesions. Rao et al. improved the resolution and contrast of these techniques with photoacoustic microscopy [40]. Photoacoustic microscopy is a form of photoacoustic imaging that can drastically improve resolution by using lenses to focus the excitation light analogous to traditional optical microscopy. There are two primary forms, and they are classified by the property that limits resolution: optical-resolution photoacoustic microscopy (OR-PAM) and acoustic-resolution photoacoustic microscopy (AR-PAM). In OR-PAM, the optical excitation and acoustic detection (single element ultrasound transducer) are co-focused to create dual foci that increase sensitivity. OR-PAM can generally achieve 0.5–3.0 μm resolutions with imaging depths of 1.2 mm. In AR-PAM, a cone of light is used for dark-field excitation of tissue and offers ~45 μm resolutions with 5 mm imaging depths. Both of these modalities have been used to image extracted teeth. The authors found that the darkened

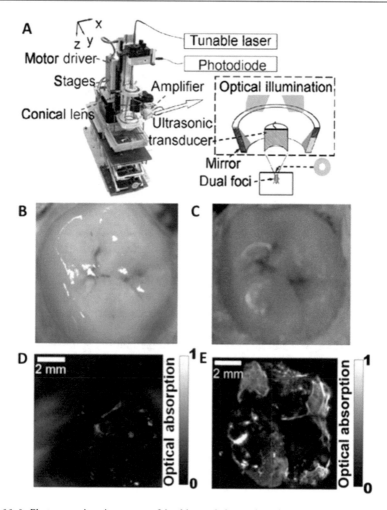

Fig. 11.4 Photoacoustic microscopy of healthy and decayed teeth. (**a**) Schematic of the AR-PAM hardware. (**b**) Occlusal photograph of a healthy extracted tooth and (**c**) a decaying extracted tooth. (**d**) AR-PAM image of the healthy tooth and (**e**) the decaying tooth. These images show significantly elevated optical absorption in the decayed tooth due to the pigmentation associated with dental lesions. Adapted with permission from the Society of Photo-Optical Instrumentation Engineers [40]

color characteristic of dental decay was correlated with increased photoacoustic intensity. Furthermore, healthy vs. decayed teeth showed significantly different intensities under AR-PAM (Fig. 11.4); of course, longitudinal tracking would be required to reliably quantify the progression of dental decay. One challenge noted by Periyasamy et al. is that photoacoustic signal from metal fillings can dominate the signal generated by the tooth itself introducing undesirable background when looking for dental lesions [41].

Hughes et al. also utilized photoacoustic microscopy in an all-optical configuration for early-stage detection of dental caries [42]. They showed that the optically generated ultrasonic signal in one-dimension alone could differentiate pre-caries lesions from healthy enamel; in addition, the sample could be scanned to acquire depth-resolved images revealing the extent of the sub-surface lesion (confirmed with histology). The authors noted that error in the measurement of enamel lesion thickness was about 3%, which they attributed to variation in the speed of sound caused by the lesions themselves. A larger error (30%) was present when measurements were made closer to the enamel dentine junction possibly due to the higher depth. Perhaps the largest limitation of photoacoustic microscopy is that it is not suited for in vivo imaging. To this end, a handheld PAM probe was recently reported, but it has not yet been demonstrated for dental applications [43].

11.4   Imaging Dental Pulp, Implants, and Periodontal Features

Accurate assessment of the pulp status is critical for the diagnosis of a number of conditions such as reversible/irreversible pulpitis, acute/chronic abscess, and necrosis. However, the objective measurement and characterization of pulp vitality remain a significant challenge in dental practice. The clinical gold standard is to perform sensitivity tests: these primarily refer to thermal testing (assessment of the response to hot and cold stimuli) and electric pulp testing, which is used to assess the status of pulpal nerve fibers. Unfortunately, these techniques are painful for the patient and do not necessarily reflect the status of the vascular supply. An ideal diagnostic tool would supply an objective, reproducible, non-painful, and accurate method for quantifying the vascular supply of a tooth. Some optical techniques such as pulse oximetry and laser Doppler flowmetry have been applied to probing pulpal blood oxygen saturation; however, these are primarily limited by the high scattering and absorption coefficients of the surrounding hard dental tissues. Yamada et al. conducted an early feasibility study on photoacoustic imaging of dental pulp in 2016 [44]. They investigated both 532 nm and 1064 nm wavelengths (100 Hz repetition rate, 1.2 ns pulsewidth, 1 mJ pulse energy, 4.6 MHz central frequency) for imaging extracted teeth. First, they imaged teeth split in half. In the first case, the root canal was filled with water and in the second case it was filled with 3% hemoglobin solution. At 532 nm, the water and the hemoglobin-filled samples could not be distinguished, primarily due to the strong scattering by the enamel and dentin. However, at 1064 nm, high frequency vibrations could be detected in the photoacoustic waveform of the hemoglobin-filled tooth that were not present in the water-filled tooth. Furthermore, the intensity of the high frequency signals had a linear correlation to the hemoglobin concentration. Unfortunately, the differences in frequency spectra between hemoglobin and water-filled whole teeth were much less significant than in split teeth. Photoacoustic imaging for diagnosis of pulp vitality is an attractive concept but is still largely unexplored. The intense reflection, scattering, and absorption of dentin and enamel will pose the largest challenge going forward. Another interesting application is in implant dentistry. Ultrasound has recently been growing as a promising tool for evaluating implant status across multiple stages of treatment, and we recommend a recent review for a systematic discussion of this topic [1]. One of its limitations, however, is the lack of molecular contrast, which can be desirable for diagnosis and quantification of peri-implantitis. Peri-implantitis is an umbrella term for "destructive inflammatory processes around osseointegrated implants" that contribute to pocket deepening and crestal/alveolar bone loss [45, 46]. Lee et al. conducted initial work on this topic with photoacoustic imaging using porcine jaws ex vivo [47, 48]. They used a 532/1064 nm Q-switched Nd:YAG laser with a tunable (680–950 nm) OPO laser at 17.7 mJ/cm^2 for excitation with both an AR-PAM system (5 MHz central frequency) and a commercial US system (3–12 MHz central frequency) for detection. They then imaged a titanium implant with abutment and fixture both under chicken breast of varying thickness (10–20 mm) and after implantation at the site of the molar in an extracted porcine jawbone (Fig. 11.5). The authors found that the structure of the jawbone and internal position of the implant could be easily visualized with both systems. Of course, the entire bone structure could not be resolved as in radiographic techniques because the optical illumination and ultrasonic emission cannot penetrate through bone like X-rays. Nevertheless, they could determine the angle and length of the position under the jawbone in addition to the depth of the layer of soft tissue above it.

Finally, resolving the periodontal anatomy, especially the pocket depth, is of significant interest to clinical practice. Periodontal disease is currently and has historically been diagnosed by a combination of factors: pocket (probing) depth, attachment loss, mobility, bone loss, and degree of inflammation. The periodontal probe is often used for physically measuring the extent of apical epithelial attachment relative to the gingival margin. However, it is a highly variable technique that is time consuming and uncomfortable for patients; furthermore, the threads of dental implants often impede the physical probe measurements [49]. A facile imaging technique could potentially address these issues and improve the poor clinical rate of pocket depth charting [50, 51]. Optical coherence tomography is one option that has recently been explored for imaging the gingiva and periodontal structures in high resolution [52, 53]. This technique can resolve tissue microstructures and capillary vasculature with impressive detail, but unfortunately is limited to penetration depths of 2 mm due to optical tissue scattering. Though photoacoustic ultrasound cannot significantly improve the penetration depth through hard tissues, it can penetrate through centimeters of soft tissue (e.g. gingiva) because even diffuse photons can generate acoustic waves.

Our group has recently leveraged this ability for imaging the periodontal pocket in both swine jaws ex vivo [54] and the human mouth in vivo [55]. This work used a commercial, tomographic photoacoustic ultrasound system (16–40 MHz central frequency, 680–970 nm, 5-ns pulse width at 20 Hz) along with a food-grade contrast agent derived from cuttlefish ink. The spatial resolution of this system was roughly 300 μm in the photoacoustic mode and 100 μm in the ultrasound-only mode. The contrast agent contained melanin nanoparticles with broad absorption in the NIR and was used to irrigate the gingival sulcus using a micropipette tip or oral gavage, thereby enabling visualization of the pocket with photoacoustics. This contrast

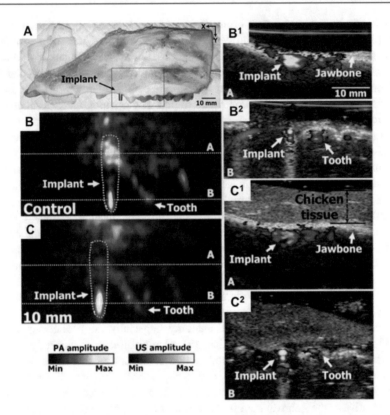

Fig. 11.5 Ex vivo imaging of a dental implant in a porcine jawbone using a clinical photo-acoustic/ultrasound tomography system. (a) Photograph of the porcine jawbone with implant. (b) Photoacoustic maximum amplitude projection of the titanium implant in the jawbone where (b1) and (b2) correspond to cross-sections of the dashed region in (a). (c) Photoacoustic maximum amplitude projection of the implant at the same location, under 10 mm of chicken breast tissue. (c1) and (c2) correspond to the dashed region in (c). Adapted with permission from The Optical Society [48]

media was chosen for its broad NIR absorbance, food-grade biocompatibility, and simple formulation. The technique was first conducted on 39 porcine teeth in extracted swine jaws, both with natural and artificially deepened pockets, and was validated with the conventional Williams probe (bias values $<\pm0.25$ mm, $<11\%$ variance) (Fig. 11.6). Shallow (1.65 mm), intermediate (2.04 mm), deep (4.45 mm), and artificially deep pockets (4.60 mm) were successfully measured. The ultrasound mode was also leveraged to measure 45 gingival thicknesses and compared to measurement with a needle. These measurements were only 0.07 mm larger than invasive examination. This bias could potentially be accounted for by the pressure generated by the needle during physical measurement. The contrast agent was also easily removed following rinsing with water (applied via a 5-mL syringe without needle) and normal tooth brushing.

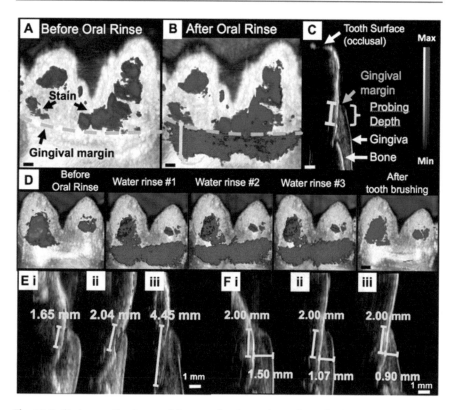

Fig. 11.6 Photoacoustic ultrasound images of swine molars using a food-grade contrast agent. (**a**) A mandibular molar prior to the administration of contrast agent using 680-nm excitation. Ultrasound signal is in grayscale while photoacoustic is in color; the blue signal is from tartar/calculus on the enamel. The green line shows the gingival margin. (**b**) The same tooth following irrigation of the pocket with contrast agent, shown in red. Differentiation between stain and contrast agent is possible by using both 680 and 800 nm excitation, due to their different absorption peaks. The red region reveals the pocket geometry and the probing depth for an arbitrary plane is shown with a yellow bar. (**c**) A sagittal plane from the 3D scan in (**b**) reveals the probing depth for that particular plane. The occlusal tooth surface, gingival margin, probing depth, gingiva, and bone are easily distinguished. Panel (**d**) shows the stability of labeling and the removal of the label with a toothbrush. The contrast agent remained in the pocket for multiple water rinses but was easily removed with brushing. (**e**) Representative sagittal images of a range of probing depths including 1.65 mm, 2.04 mm, and 4.45 mm. (**f**) Representative gingival thickness measurements taken 2.00 mm from the gingival margin with thicknesses of 1.50 mm, 1.07 mm, and 0.90 mm from different swine [54]

Subsequently, this application was extended to a case study in a healthy adult subject (Fig. 11.7). The relative standard deviation of five replicate measurements for a mandibular incisor was 10%. The depths measured by imaging agreed with conventional probing. Of note, all measurements were ≤2 mm because the imaging site was healthy incisors. One of the benefits of this approach was that the whole pocket could be mapped as opposed to single positions (e.g. mesiobuccal, central

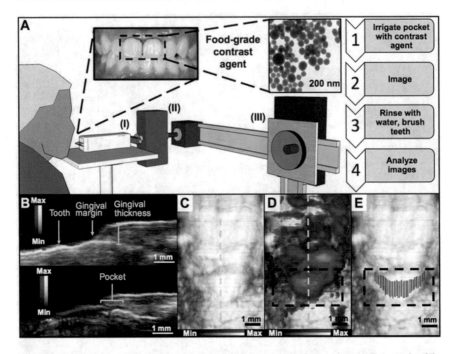

Fig. 11.7 Human data of photoacoustic ultrasound for pocket depth mapping. (a) Schematic of the imaging setup and workflow. The subject was scanned in an upright position by a photoacoustic ultrasound transducer (i) attached to a stepper motor (ii) and sliding frame (iii) for 3D imaging and positioning, respectively. Ultrasound gel was used for coupling. (b) A cross-section in the sagittal plane of a mandibular incisor at a central buccal position (yellow dashed line in c, d) showing the gingival margin before (top) and after (bottom) irrigation with contrast agent. The pocket depth was measured from the gingival margin to the edge of photoacoustic signal. The same incisor is shown in the frontal plane before (c) and after (d) irrigation. (e) The shape of the pocket could be reconstructed by measuring the pocket depth for each sagittal plane in the frontal image (∼0.076 mm spacing) and overlaying these measurements onto the ultrasound-only image to remove nonspecific signal from the tooth and gingival surfaces [55]

buccal, and distobuccal) at a time. Additionally, the contrast agent was easily removed by rinsing with water and brushing the teeth as in the ex vivo porcine model. Current efforts are focused on streamlining the post-processing steps and miniaturizing the imaging hardware for improved access to distal teeth.

11.5   Outlook and Practical Considerations

One of the main advantages of ultrasound for dentistry is its ability to image the gingiva, which is mostly transparent to the common dental imaging modalities such as X-ray and cone beam computed tomography. In addition, it can resolve the surfaces and contours of hard tissues (e.g. tooth, bone) and integrate these with the depth-resolved data from the gingiva. It follows, however, that the major limitations are its relative inability to image through tooth/bone and its limited grayscale contrast. Photoacoustic imaging can help overcome these limitations by shifting the contrast mechanism to the absorption of light rather than differences in refractive index, and extending penetration depths from the ballistic to the diffusive regime. Nevertheless, research to date suggests that photoacoustic analysis of teeth alone will probably be restricted to their surfaces (enamel and cementum).

Currently, a handful of practical challenges face the translation of photoacoustics to dentistry but we believe these are largely solvable. One example is the form factor of existing photoacoustic hardware. Most research-grade systems are meant for general purpose applications and utilize relatively large transducers that can only access the anterior teeth. Furthermore, the laser is housed separately. However, new hardware can be envisioned for the specific purpose of imaging within the oral cavity. These designs could potentially take the form of a mouthpiece transducer with coupled optical excitation or a handheld "hockey-stick" transducer for reaching the posterior teeth [56]. Another consideration for eventual clinical adoption is the price: Ultrasound is an inexpensive technique but the laser associated with photoacoustic imaging raises the cost significantly. It is possible, however, for systems to harness LED excitation sources that drastically reduce both the cost and overall footprint [57].

When taking 3D scans with a linear array transducer, it is necessary for the head of the subject to remain still. Otherwise, artifacts from minor movements will distort the final image. To combat this, a clinical setup would likely use a head immobilizer similar to those used for dental radiographs. Post-processing algorithms can also be employed to minimize these effects. Furthermore, since ultrasound waves do not propagate through air, the choice of coupling agent between oral surfaces and the transducer requires some consideration. Ultrasound gel is functional but requires re-sterilization of the transducer between patients in a clinical setting. Single-use materials for dry coupling may be useful in this context.

Photoacoustic imaging is a young technology but is developing at a rapid pace due to its optical contrast, good spatial resolution, and real-time imaging. Dental-specific investigations are still in their very early stages, but they show potential for caries detection, analysis of tooth surface integrity (crack detection), implant imaging, and characterization of the periodontium. With the growing availability of commercial photoacoustic systems, and the prevalence of custom preclinical systems, it is likely that photoacoustic imaging will continue to complement the developments in ultrasound techniques for dental applications.

References

1. Bhaskar V, et al. Updates on ultrasound research in implant dentistry: a systematic review of potential clinical indications. Dentomaxillofac Radiol. 2018;47(6):20180076. ISSN:0250-832X.

2. David CM, Tiwari R. Ultrasound in maxillofacial imaging: a review. J Med Rad Pathol Surg. 2015;1(4):17–23. ISSN:2395-2075.

3. Evirgen Ş, Kamburoğlu K. Review on the applications of ultrasonography in dentomaxillofacial region. World J Radiol. 2016;8(1):50.

4. Hall A, Girkin JM. A review of potential new diagnostic modalities for caries lesions. J Dental Res. 2004;83 Suppl 1:89–94. ISSN:0022-0345.

5. Kocasarac HD, Angelopoulos C. Ultrasound in dentistry: toward a future of radiation-free imaging. Dent Clin N Am. 2018;62(3):481–89. ISSN:0011-8532.

6. Musu D, et al. Ultrasonography in the diagnosis of bone lesions of the jaws: a systematic review. Oral Surg Oral Med Oral Pathol Oral Radiol. 2016;122(1):e19–e29. ISSN:2212-4403.

7. Sharma S, et al. Ultrasound as a diagnostic boon in Dentistry a review. Int J Sci Stud. 2014;2:2.

8. Singh GP, Dogra S, Kumari E. Ultrasonography: maxillofacial applications. Ann Dent Spec 2014;2(3):104–7.

9. Marotti J, et al. Recent advances of ultrasound imaging in dentistry – a review of the literature. Oral Surg Oral Med Oral Pathol Oral Radiol. 2013;115(6):819–32. ISSN:2212-4403. https://doi.org/10.1016/j.oooo.2013.03.012. http://www.sciencedirect.com/science/article/pii/S2212440313001727%20https://ac.els.cdn.com/S2212440313001727/.1.s2.0-S2212440313001727-main.pdf?_tid=7f0abd15-9b8b-4118-8d81-69e9a69c3eda&acdnat=1550271867_b0e72fb1058ebf78347938676ee6c2fb.

10. Zhou Y, Yao J, Wang LV. Tutorial on photoacoustic tomography. J Biomed Opt. 2016;21(6):1–14, 14. https://doi.org/10.1117/1.JBO.21.6.061007.

11. Wang LV, Hu S. Photoacoustic tomography: in vivo imaging from organelles to organs. Science. 2012;335(6075):1458–62. ISSN:0036-8075.

12. Xu M, Wang LV. Photoacoustic imaging in biomedicine. Rev Sci Instrum. 2006;77(4):041101. ISSN:0034-6748.

13. Rich LJ, Seshadri M. Photoacoustic imaging of vascular hemodynamics: validation with blood oxygenation level-dependent MR imaging. Radiology 2014;275(1):110–18. ISSN:0033-8419.

14. Hariri A, et al. In vivo photoacoustic imaging of chorioretinal oxygen gradients. J Biomed Opt 2018;23(3):036005. ISSN:1083-3668.

15. Zhang HF, et al. Imaging of hemoglobin oxygen saturation variations in single vessels in vivo using photoacoustic microscopy. Appl Phys Lett. 2007;90(5):053901. ISSN:0003-6951.

16. Mallidi S, Luke GP, Emelianov S. Photoacoustic imaging in cancer detection, diagnosis, and treatment guidance. Trends Biotechnol. 2011;29(5):213–21. ISSN:0167-7799.

17. Mehrmohammadi M, et al. Photoacoustic imaging for cancer detection and staging. Curr Mol Imaging. 2013;2(1):89–105. ISSN:2211-5552.

18. Moore C, Jokerst JV. Strategies for image-guided therapy surgery and drug delivery using photoacoustic imaging. Theranostics 2019;9(6):1550–71. ISSN:1838-7640. https://doi.org/10.715/thno.32362. https://www.ncbi.nlm.nih.gov/pubmed/31037123%20https://www.ncbi.nlm.nih.gov/pmc/articles/PMC6485201/.

19. Borg RE, Rochford J. Molecular photoacoustic contrast agents: design principles & applications. Photochem Photobiol. 2018;94(6):1175–1209. ISSN:0031-8655. https://doi.org/10.1111/php.12967. https://onlinelibrary.wiley.com/doi/abs/10.1111/php.12967.

20. Lemaster JE, Jokerst JV. What is new in nanoparticle-based photoacoustic imaging? Wiley Interdiscip Rev Nanomed Nanobiotechnol. 2017;9(1). ISSN:1939-0041 1939-5116. https://doi.org/10.1002/wnan.1404. https://www.ncbi.nlm.nih.gov/pubmed/27038222%20https://www.ncbi.nlm.nih.gov/pmc/articles/PMC5045757/.

21. Swierczewska M, Lee S, Chen X. Inorganic nanoparticles for multimodal molecular imaging. Mol Imaging. 2011;10(1). https://doi.org/10.2310/7290.2011.00001. https://journals.sagepub.com/doi/abs/10.2310/7290.2011.00001.

22. Jiang Y, Pu K. Multimodal biophotonics of semiconducting polymer nanoparticles. Acc Chem Res 2018;51(8):1840–49. ISSN:0001-4842. https://doi.org/10.1021/acs.accounts.8b00242.

23. Jiang Y, Pu K. Advanced photoacoustic imaging applications of near-infrared absorbing organic nanoparticles. Small. 2017;13(30):1700710. ISSN:1613-6810. https://doi.org/10.1002/smll.201700710. https://onlinelibrary.wiley.com/doi/abs/10.1002/smll.201700710.

24. Weissleder R. A clearer vision for in vivo imaging. Nat Biotechnol. 2001;19:316. https://doi. org/10.1038/86684.
25. Darling CL, Huynh G, Fried D. Light scattering properties of natural and artificially demineralized dental enamel at 1310 nm. J Biomed Opt 2006;11(3):034023. ISSN:1083-3668.
26. Fried D, et al. Nature of light scattering in dental enamel and dentin at visible and near-infrared wavelengths. Appl Opt 1995;34(7):1278–85. ISSN:2155-3165.
27. Spitzer D, Ten Bosch JJ. The absorption and scattering of light in bovine and human dental enamel. Calcif Tiss Res 1975;17(2):129–37. ISSN:0008-0594.
28. Neel EAA, et al. Demineralization-remineralization dynamics in teeth and bone. Int J Nanomed 2016;11:4743–63. ISSN:1178-2013; 1176-9114. https://doi.org/10.2147/IJN. S107624. https://www.ncbi.nlm.nih.gov/pubmed/27695330%20https://www.ncbi.nlm.nih. gov/pmc/PMC5034904/.
29. Fried D, et al. Early caries imaging and monitoring with near-infrared light. Dental Clin N Am 2005;49(4):771–93. ISSN:0011-8532. https://doiorg/10.1016/j.cden.2005.05.008. http://www. sciencedirect.com/science/article/pii/S0011853205000352.
30. Harris DM, Fried D. Pulsed Nd:YAG laser selective ablation of surface enamel caries: I. Photoacoustic response and FTIR spectroscopy. In: BiOS 2000 the international symposium on biomedical optics. SPIE. Vol. 3910; 2000. https://doi.org/10.1117/12.380823.
31. Rajian JR, Carson PL, Wang X. Quantitative photoacoustic measurement of tissue optical absorption spectrum aided by an optical contrast agent. Opt Express 2009;17(6):4879–89. https://doi.org/10.1364/OE.17.004879. http://www.opticsexpress.org/abstract.cfm?URI= oe-17-6-4879.
32. El-Sharkawy YH, El Sherif AF. Photoacoustic diagnosis of human teeth using interferometric detection scheme. Opt Laser Technol 2012;44(5):1501–06. ISSN:0030-3992.
33. El-Sharkawy YH, et al. Diagnostic of human teeth using photoacoustic response. In: Lasers in dentistry XII. Vol. 6137. San Francisco: International Society for Optics and Photonics; 2006. p. 613701.
34. Kim K, et al. Early detection of dental caries using photoacoustics. In: Photons plus ultrasound: imaging and sensing 2006: the seventh conference on biomedical thermoacoustics, optoacoustics, and acousto-optics. Vol. 6086. San Francisco: International Society for Optics and Photonics; 2006. p. 60860G.
35. Li T, Dewhurst RJ. Photoacoustic non-destructive evaluation and imaging of caries in dental samples. In: AIP conference proceedings. Vol. 1211. New York: AIP; 2010. p. 1574–81. ISBN:0735407487.
36. Li T, Dewhurst RJ. Photoacoustic imaging in both soft and hard biological tissue. In: Journal of physics: conference series. Vol. 214. Bristol: IOP Publishing; 1999. p. 012028. ISBN:1742-6596.
37. Cheng R, et al. Noninvasive assessment of early dental lesion using a dual-contrast photoacoustic tomography. Sci Rep 2016;6:21798. https://www.nature.com/articles/srep21798# supplementary-information. https://doi.org/10.1038/srep21798%20https://www.ncbi.nlm.nih. gov/pmc/articles/PMC4763185/pdf/srep21798.pdf.
38. Koyama T, Kakino S, Matsuura Y. Photoacoustic imaging of hidden dental caries by using a fiber-based probing system. In: Biomedical imaging and sensing conference. Vol. 10251. Bellingham: International Society for Optics and Photonics; 2017. p. 1025119.
39. Wang S, et al. Theoretical and experimental study of spectral characteristics of the photoacoustic signal from stochastically distributed particles. IEEE Trans Ultrason Ferroelectr Freq Control 2015;62(7):1245–55. ISSN:0885-3010. https://doi.org/10.1109/TUFFC.2014.006806.
40. Rao B, et al. Photoacoustic microscopy of human teeth. In: Lasers in dentistry XVII. Vol. 7884. San Francisco: International Society for Optics and Photonics; 2011. p. 78840U.
41. Periyasamy V, Rangaraj M, Pramanik M. Photoacoustic imaging of teeth for dentine imaging and enamel characterization. In: Lasers in dentistry XXIV. Vol. 10473. San Francisco: International Society for Optics and Photonics; 2018. p. 1047309.

42. Hughes DA, et al. Imaging and detection of early stage dental caries with an all-optical photoacoustic microscope. In: Journal of Physics: Conference Series. Vol. 581. Bristol: IOP Publishing; 2015. p. 012002. ISBN:1742-6596.
43. Electronic Article. 2017/10// 2017. https://doi.org/10.1038/s41598-017-132243.
44. Yamada A, Kakino S, Matsuura Y. Detection of photoacoustic signals from blood in dental pulp. Opt Photon J 2016;6(09):229.
45. Mombelli A, Müller N, Cionca N. The epidemiology of peri-implantitis. Clin Oral Implants Res 2012;23(s6):67–76. ISSN:0905-7161. https://doi.org/10.1111/j.1600-0501.2012.02541.x. https://onlinelibrary.wiley.com/doi/abs/10.1111/j.16000-501.2012.02541.x.
46. Naveau A, et al. Etiology and measurement of peri-implant crestal bone loss (CBL). J Clin Med 2019;8(2):166. ISSN:2077-0383. https://www.mdpi.com/2077-0383/8/2/166.
47. Lee D, Park S, Kim C. Dual-modal photoacoustic and ultrasound imaging of dental implants. In: SPIE BiOS. SPIE. Vol. 10494; 2018. p. 5.
48. Lee D, et al. Photoacoustic imaging of dental implants in a porcine jawbone ex vivo. Opt Lett 2017:42(9):1760–63. ISSN:1539-4794.
49. Schou S, et al. Probing around implants and teeth with healthy or inflamed peri-implant mucosa/gingiva: a histologic comparison in cynomolgus monkeys (Macaca fascicularis). Clin Oral Implants Res 2002;13(2):113–26. ISSN:0905-7161.
50. McFall WT, et al. Presence of periodontal data in patient records of general practitioners. J Periodontol 1988;59(7):445–49. ISSN:1943-3670.
51. Cole A, McMichael A. Audit of dental practice record-keeping: a PCT-coordinated clinical audit by Worcestershire dentists. Prim Dent Care 2009;16(3):85–93. ISSN:1355-7610.
52. Fernandes LO, et al. In vivo assessment of periodontal structures and measurement of gingival sulcus with optical coherence tomography: a pilot study. J Biophoton 2017;10(6–7):862–69. ISSN:1864-063X. https://onlinelibrary.wiley.com/doi/pdf/10.1002/jbio.201600082.
53. Le NM, et al. A noninvasive imaging and measurement using optical coherence tomography angiography for the assessment of gingiva: an in vivo study. J Biophoton 2018;11(12):e201800242. ISSN:1864-063X. https://doi.org/10.1002/jbio.201800242. https://onlinelibrary.wiley.com/doi/abs/10.1002/jbio.201800242.
54. Lin CY, et al. Photoacoustic imaging for noninvasive periodontal probing depth measurements. J Dent Res 2018;97(1):23–30. ISSN:0022-0345. https://www.ncbi.nlm.nih.gov/pmc/articles/PMC5755810/pdf/10.1177_0022034517729820.pdf.
55. Moore C, et al. Photoacoustic imaging for monitoring periodontal health: a first human study. Photoacoustics 2018;12:67–74. ISSN:2213-5979. https://www.ncbi.nlm.nih.gov/pmc/articles/PMC6226559/pdf/main.pdf.
56. Pirotte T, Veyckemans F. Ultrasound-guided subclavian vein cannulation in infants and children: a novel approach. Br J Anaesth 2007;98(4):509–14. ISSN:1471-6771.
57. Hariri A, et al. The characterization of an economic and portable LED-based photoacoustic imaging system to facilitate molecular imaging. Photoacoustics 2018;9:10–20. ISSN:2213-5979.

Volumetric Ultrasound and Related Dental Applications

12

Oliver D. Kripfgans and Hsun-Liang (Albert) Chan

12.1 Review of 3D Ultrasound Technology

Three-dimensional ultrasonic imaging is well established and many manufacturers are offering 3D and 4D imaging on their platforms (see Table 12.1). The latter is live 3D imaging and allows the visualization of 3D structures in real-time or in gated mode, such as cardiac gating, which is beneficial for cardiovascular applications. Computed tomography (CT), cone-beam CT (CBCT), and MRI (magnetic resonance imaging) are natural 3D imaging modalities. They are accepted as diagnostic tools and operate with a standardized patient orientation for each procedure. Ultrasound differs not only in its physical principle of imaging, i.e. mechanical versus atomic/electronic, but also from a procedural concept. Ultrasound has a very narrow field of view and is always directed to the immediate location of the body part of interest. Images are taken in real-time and the probe is positioned under this real-time guidance by the sonographer or other healthcare personnel. CT, CBCT, and MRI on the other hand use a few scout scans and then obtain a 3D volume for post-scan slicing of the image volume. In addition, CT, CBCT, and MRI slice thicknesses can be selected such that an almost isotropic voxel resolution results, which then lends itself for 3D reslicing after the scan. Ultrasound on the other hand has poor out of plane beam resolution such that the lateral–elevational slice plane has a poor resolution in comparison to the axial–lateral plane. This is especially true for 1D (transducer) arrays. There are predominantly two methods for

O. D. Kripfgans (✉)
Department of Radiology, Medical School, University of Michigan, Ann Arbor, MI, USA
e-mail: greentom@umich.edu

H.-L. (Albert) Chan
Department of Periodontics and Oral Medicine, School of Dentistry, University of Michigan, Ann Arbor, MI, USA
e-mail: hlchan@umich.edu

© Springer Nature Switzerland AG 2021
H.-L. (Albert) Chan, O. D. Kripfgans (eds.), *Dental Ultrasound in Periodontology and Implantology*, https://doi.org/10.1007/978-3-030-51288-0_12

Table 12.1 Review of commercial clinical ultrasound scanners with 3D capabilities

Company	3D methods	Probes	Applications
Alpinion	Mechanical	SVC1-6H VE3-10H	Abdomen, OB/GYN, emergency medicine (EM) OB/GYN, urology web reference (http://www.alpinion.com/web/download/low/E-CUBE15%20Platinum%20OBGYN%20Catalog.pdf, 2020)
BK	2×	8824	Intraoperative biplane, intraoperative
	2D static	I12C5b	Intraoperative biplane, intraoperative, musculoskeletal, peripheral vascular web reference (https://www.bkmedical.com/transducers/?product=flex-focus)
Biosound Esaote	Not specified	BC441 and SB2C41	Abdominal, OB/GYN, contrast agents procedures, 3D biopsy variable-band bi-scan volumetric convex array web reference (https://www.esaote.com/en-US/ultrasound/probes/, 2020)
Butterfly Network	2D array (CMUT)	No 3D modes	General imaging, only 2D however web reference (https://www.butterflynetwork.com/iq, 2020)
Canon	Mechanical	4D 9CV2	Wideband, OB, radiology
	2D array	i6SVX2	Abdominal, OB examinations, real-time 3D biopsy guidance, 4D SMI and CEUS, TEE
	2D array	i7SVX2	3D cardiac (pediatric heart) web reference (https://us.medical.canon/products/ultrasound/aplio-i-series/technology/#i6SVX2)
Chison	Mechanical	V4C40L	Volume scans web reference (http://www.chison.com/Images/UpFile/2019826103753611.pdf, 2020)
Edan	Mechanical	C5-2MD	OB, abdomen, gynecology web reference (http://www.edan.com/html/EN/products/ultrasound/CDUltrasound/201601/292173.html, 2020)
GE	Mechanical	RNA5-9-D H48651MY	Abdomen, small parts, cardiology, obstetrics, pediatrics
	Mechanical	RSP6-16-D H48651MR	Small parts, breast, peripheral vascular, pediatrics, musculoskeletal
	Mechanical	RIC6-12D H48651NA	Obstetrics, gynecology, urology
	Mechanical	RAB4-8-D H48651MP	Abdomen, obstetrics, gynecology, pediatric, urology
	2D matrix array	RM14L H48681AR	Small parts, breast, peripheral vascular, pediatrics, musculoskeletal
	2D matrix array	RM6C H48671ZG	Abdomen, obstetrics, gynecology, pediatrics, urology

(continued)

Table 12.1 (continued)

Company	3D methods	Probes	Applications
	Mechanical	Invenia ABUS 2.0	Breast web reference (https://www.gehealthcare.co.uk/-/media/c34db4de9e774c5e99f41f42b6251f18.pdf?la=en-gb&rev=b2bb13b216064d199fe454e8d8dbe48a&hash=2FC3A215E7BD7476DC20946ECF8723AD, 2020) web reference (https://www.gehealthcare.com/products/ultrasound/abus-breast-imaging/invenia-abus, 2020)
Hitachi Aloka	Mechanical	VC41V	3D/4D endocavity, endocavity volume
		Not named	Biplane imaging, 3D live imaging, 3D and 4D cardiac evaluation and analysis web reference (http://www.hitachi-aloka.com/products/lisendo-880/cardiovascular, 2020)
Konica Minolta	–	No 3D transducers	web reference (https://www.konicaminolta.com/medicalusa/product/sonimage-hs1/, 2020)
Mindray	Mechanical	DE10-3U	OB/GYN, urology, volume CEUS
		D8-4U	Adult abdomen, OB/GYN, volume CEUS web reference (https://www2.mindraynorthamerica.com/Resona7-transducer-family-pdf, 2020)
Philips	Mechanical	V6-2	General purpose abdominal, obstetrical, and gynecological volumetric applications. Supports interventional applications
	Mechanical	3D9-3v	Endovaginal obstetrics and gynecology
	Mechanical	VL13-5	High resolution superficial applications including small parts, breast, and vascular imaging
	Mechanical		
	2D matrix array	V9-2	OB/GYN
	2D matrix array	X6-1	Abdominal, obstetrics, fetal, gynecology, vascular
	2D matrix array	XL14-3	Vascular, MSK
	2D matrix array	X7-2t	Adult TEE applications web reference (https://www.usa.philips.com/healthcare/solutions/ultrasound/ultrasound-transducer, 2020) web reference (https://www.usa.philips.com/healthcare/product/HC989605409251/xl14-3-xmatrix-transducer/specifications)
Samsung	Mechanical	CV1-8AD	Abdomen, obstetrics, gynecology
	Mechanical	VE4-8	Abdomen, obstetrics, gynecology
	Mechanical	V5-9	Abdomen, obstetrics, gynecology
	Mechanical	3D4-9	Abdomen, obstetrics, gynecology

(continued)

Table 12.1 (continued)

Company	3D methods	Probes	Applications
	Mechanical	LV3-14A	Musculoskeletal, small parts, vascular web reference (https://www.samsunghealthcare.com/en/products/UltrasoundSystem/RS85/Radiology/transducers)
Siemens Acuson	Mechanical	EV9F3 EV9F4	Early OB, OB/GYN
	2D matrix array	4Z1c	Transthoracic adult echo, volume stress echo, contrast agent studies
	2D matrix array	Z6Ms	Transesophageal echo
	Mechanical	S2000 ABVS	Breast web reference (https://static.healthcare.siemens.com/siemens_hwem-hwem_ssxa_websites-context-root/wcm/idc/groups/public/@global/@imaging/@ultrasound/documents/download/mdaz/mzc1/~edisp/acuson_x700_womens_imaging_transducer_flyer-01433431.pdf)
SIUI	Mechanical	Not named	Real-time and static stereoscopic fetal imaging
	Mechanical	IBUS BE3	Breast web reference (http://www.siui.com/ax0/a/caichao/20190419/277.html)
Sono Scape	Mechanical	Not named	Volumetric abdominal probe web reference (http://www.sonoscape.com/html/2018/exceed_0921/86.html)
Sonosite	–	No 3D transducers	web reference (https://www.sonosite.com/products/transducers, 2020)
Super Sonic Imagine	Mechanical	SLV16-5 12-3	Breast, general OB-GYN, genitourinary, general web reference (https://www.supersonicimagine.com/Aixplorer-R/TRANSDUCERS, 2020)
Terason	–	No 3D transducers	web reference (https://www.terason.com/usmart-3300/, 2020)
Visual Sonics	Mechanical	No specific transducer	MS and MX series transducers web reference (https://www.visualsonics.com/, 2020)
Whale Imaging	–	No 3D transducers	web reference (https://whaleimaging.com/products/p-series-benefits/probes/, 2020)

Given are the company name, the method of 3D provided in their product description, the associated probe label as well as clinical target applications. Reviewed from companies' official websites on August 20th, 2019. Dashes ("–") indicate information missing from the websites. Highlighted companies offer products with 2D matrix arrays. Note: The 3D methods are listed as "Mechanical" if not stated by the manufacturer as 2D matrix array

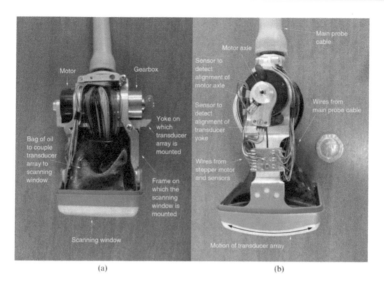

Fig. 12.1 Example of a mechanically steered commercial transducer (RSP6-12) from GE Healthcare. (**a**) Axial–lateral view of the interior body of the transducer. The main probe cable enters the housing from the top and passes the motor and gearbox to then enter a bag filled with oil in which it is connected to the transducer elements. Oil is used to couple the transducer array to the scanning window, seen on the bottom of both panels. An axial–elevational view of the same transducer is shown on the right side in panel (**b**) [1]

3D ultrasonic imaging. The first one is based on mechanically moving a 2D imaging transducer (1D array) in the elevational direction to form a 3D image. Some systems might support this motion to be free-hand. However, most systems provide modified 1D transducers, for 2D imaging, that employ a motorized mechanical sweep of the transducer in the elevational direction to obtain a lateral, axial, elevational image volume. Figures 12.1 and 12.2 provide examples of these two methods. Mechanically sweeping a transducer in the elevational direction is a direct extension of the axial–lateral scan plane. It comes in several implementations:

- Angular sweep of (curvi-)linear array transducer for abdominal and vascular applications, for example (see vendors listed in Table 12.1).
- Angular sweep of phased array transducer for cardiac or neonatal applications, for example (see vendors listed in Table 12.1).
- Linear sweep of linear array transducer for breast applications, for example (see GE, Siemens, and SIUI in Table 12.1).

Angular sweep transducers can achieve a very large field of view (e.g. >140° elevationally for neonatal applications) and currently form the majority of 3D imaging ultrasound transducers. However, they suffer from a decrease in elevational resolution as axial distance increases. The angular beam density is constant, but the linear spacing increases by $d \times \sin(\alpha)$ for d being the axial distance from

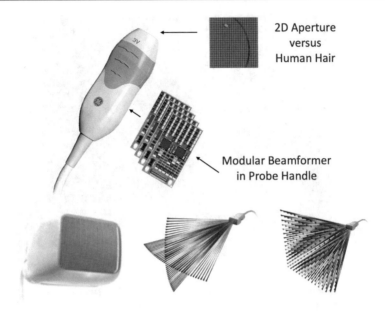

Fig. 12.2 Example illustrations of 2D array matrix transducers. Top: 3V from GE Healthcare (adapted from [1]), bottom: xMatrix (X6-1, X5-1, or XL14-3) from Philips Healthcare web reference (https://www.usa.philips.com/healthcare/resources/feature-detail/xmatrix). A 2D aperture allows the system to produce an ultrasound beam that is electronically focused in the lateral and in the elevational directions as well as steerable in both of these directions. Thus 2D matrix array transducer can produce 3D image volumes without the need for mechanically moving the transducer. Left: Illustration of transducer housing. Middle: Schematic of beams fanning a 3D volume. Right: Schematic of beams fanning 2 orthogonal image planes in 3D, predominantly one in the axial–lateral slice and the other in the axial–elevational slice

the elevational pivot point and α being the angular step size. The left and middle panels of Fig. 12.3 illustrate this change in resolution. Curvilinear and phased array transducers also suffer from a loss of lateral image resolution for increasing distance for the same reason, which is an immediate trade-off to an increase in the field of view. While linear sweeping transducers (right panel of Fig. 12.3) form a smaller field of view, they yield constant image resolution, independent of image depth. Associated applications are those that require a great level of spatial detail even at depth, such as breast ultrasound.

Ideally a two-dimensional transducer aperture would be employed to obtain 3D ultrasound images. These are called matrix arrays and are able to rapidly steer the acoustic beam in the lateral and elevational directions using electronic phasing in the same fashion as one-dimensional transducers can steer the beam in the lateral direction for phased arrays or virtual phased arrays. However, matrix arrays are technologically difficult as they require an equal number of acoustic transmit–receive elements in the lateral and elevational directions. Without these, the resulting field of view is significantly limited. Matrix arrays started within the field of cardiology, where real-time volumetric images are crucial to depict the

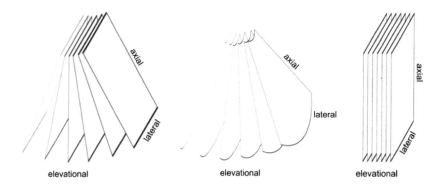

Fig. 12.3 Example illustrations of elevational transducer plane steering of a mechanically swept array transducer. Left: Angular steering of a linear array transducer. Middle: Angular steering of a phased array transducer. Right: Linear sweep of a linear array transducer

function of heart valves and other cardiac structures. Even though early transducers already had thousands of transmit–receive elements (1000–2000), the resulting images had poor spatial resolution due to the inherent low frequency of cardiac imaging, the required high temporal resolution of cardiac imaging, and small apertures. Phased arrays typically possess 96 or more transmit–receive elements, all of which are used for beamforming. Linear arrays, while being composed of 128 or more elements, usually use variable sized subapertures for constant f-number beamforming. However, linear arrays can only steer up to approximately 20°. Thus, a matrix phased array should ideally be composed of at least $96^2 = 9216$ transmit–receive elements. It is obvious that managing to integrate drive circuits for almost 10,000 elements below a surface of approximately 3 by 3 cm is challenging. One has to keep in mind the required dynamic range of nominally at least 120 dB of a state-of-the-art clinical ultrasound scanner, which corresponds to transmitting electric pulses between 10 and 100 V, and being sensitive to receive signals of the order of 10–100 μV for up to 6 MHz for pediatric cardiac applications. A 2019 online assessment of commercially available matrix arrays yields a matrix array with as many as 65,000 elements at up to 14 MHz operating frequency. This number of elements corresponds to a true 128×128 aperture with equal lateral and elevational resolution. Specifically a lateral resolution of $\Delta x = \lambda \times f\#$, where λ is the wavelength in tissue, i.e. 1.54 mm for 1 MHz operating frequency and 0.11 mm for 14 MHz operating frequency. Typical f-numbers, i.e. f#, for linear array imaging are of the order of 3–5. Thus the lateral and elevational resolution of a 2D matrix array is of the order of 330–550 μm, which compares favorably to 200–500 μm spatial resolution of cone-beam CT. The axial resolution at 14 MHz operating frequency is with 165 μm (assuming a 1.5-cycle transmit–receive pulse) even higher.

12.2 Geometry Considerations

A large variety of clinical 3D ultrasound transducers exist. Most of them are based on mechanically swept arrays and thus have large housings to cover the array, motor, gearbox, and cabling (see Fig. 12.1). The smallest devices using mechanically swept arrays are those for endocavitary use, due to the spatial constraints of the particular clinical application. However, they are small only in two dimensions, namely in the lateral and elevational directions (typically less than 2 cm). The axial dimension of this class of 3D transducers is on the order of 20–30 cm. Overall, none of these devices lend themselves for dental imaging except for the buccal side of the frontal incisors or canines. And even those will be difficult to image given the physical dimensions of mechanically swept arrays. Matrix arrays offer smaller geometries due to the replacement of mechanical components (motor, gearbox, etc.) with electronic components (larger aperture, local beamforming circuits). Despite these reductions in the spatial requirements, matrix arrays are still too large for routine dental applications. While this is true in general, there is one exception. Transesophageal echo, abbreviated as TEE, also requires small form factors. Currently at least one commercially available TEE device exists that allows for 3D imaging and is based on matrix arrays. The Philips X7-2t is composed of 2500 elements and operates at 2–7 MHz. Its aperture is the size of a US quarter coin, i.e. 24 mm, and it is oriented sideways, i.e. the aperture is perpendicular to the transducer cable. This geometry would allow the user to place the transducer deep inside the oral cavity and image gum tissue and jaw bone, root, and crown surfaces. However, the lower operating frequencies also lower the achievable spatial resolution, which in this case at most 660–1100 μm laterally and 330 μm axially. Several key factors have to be addressed to obtain a clinically relevant 3D imaging transducer. Namely physical size, spatial resolution, and form factor. Physical size is constrained by the need to reach deep into the oral cavity to image 2nd molars from the buccal and the lingual side. For such applications, a device of the order of the toothbrush would be ideal. Second, spatial resolution; CBCT is currently providing a detailed resolution of approximately 200–500 μm, which is realistically achievable, even for matrix array transducers. The last key factor, i.e. form factor, relates to the orientation of the aperture with respect to the transducer housing and the cable. The above comparison to a toothbrush also holds for this key factor. As the bristles of the brush are oriented perpendicular to the handle, the transducer aperture needs to also be oriented perpendicular to the transducer cable.

12.3 Volume Imaging Considerations

Ultrasonic imaging is a real-time scanning modality with immediate feedback to the user, similar to fluoroscopy. However, this is potentially misleading as only 2D images are obtained. Mechanically swept array transducers typically take several seconds to sweep a volume and thus lose the real-time character of ultrasonic scanning. While it is possible to achieve real-time volume scanning even on mechanically sweeping transducers, it is only possible when reducing scan line density in the lateral and elevational directions, which significantly reduces the resulting image quality, which might be suitable for some applications. The underlying reason for slow ultrasonic scanning is the slow speed of sound, which is nominally 1540 m/s compared to the speed of light which is 3×10^8 m/s. Taking the example of a mechanically swept linear array with nominally 100 lateral scan lines, 100 elevational frames, and a scan depth of 4 cm, one computes $100 \times 100 \times 40$ mm $\times 2/1.54$ mm/µs, i.e. 519 ms to obtain one image volume. While this time might seem fast, i.e. 2 Hz volume rate due to 519 ms per volume, it would present itself for a user monitoring the image(s) as laggy. Typical real-time 2D images are at least 10 Hz, more likely 20 Hz, keeping in mind that the human eye can detect changes up to 70 Hz. Real-time visualization of 3D image volumes is difficult. Only 3D surfaces or 2D cross-sections can be visualized. Thus either the former or the latter would be shown to a user. In cardiology and obstetrics segmentation can be used to obtain 3D surfaces. Either the low echogenicity of the blood (cardiac imaging) or of the amniotic fluid (OB imaging) is used to perform real-time segmentation and visualize a 3D surface. Figure 12.4 illustrates both of these cases. The left panel shows a cardiac 4D image with removal (segmentation) of image voxels of small acoustic backscatter, i.e. voxels with little intensity. In particular, the right side of the left panel shows the 3D surface visualization and the left side shows two cross-sectional images (2D grayscale, i.e. B-mode). This allows the user to maneuver the ultrasound transducer in the right position with respect to the desired anatomical view. By means of the cross-sectional image the user can also see the underlying tissues. The right panel of Fig. 12.4 shows a 3D obstetrics imaging example, a yawning fetus. Segmentation was done here also by removing low intensity voxels. All diagnostic ultrasound imaging procedures are based on 2D images. Three-dimensional visualization for ultrasound is diagnostically not required. However, retrospective visualization beyond a given 2D image plane might be helpful. Yet, the real-time character of ultrasound creates the certain difference between CT and MRI imaging procedures, where retrospective visualization is the standard method as real-time images are (a) not available, (b) scanning does not rely on acoustic windows, i.e. there is unblocked view from any direction, (c) the image resolution can be close to isotropic, which allows for retrospective visualization in oblique planes. In contrast to that, ultrasound benefits from real-time placement of the transducer to ensure adequate acoustic access (acoustic window) and to align the desired anatomical structures in the axial–lateral scan plane, where the resolution is the highest.

12.4 Dental Applications of Volumetric Imaging

Dental imaging spans across several modalities and levels of dimensions, including but not limited to one-dimensional pocket-depth assessment, two-dimensional plain-film, panoramic or optical, three-dimensional cone-beam CT (CBCT). Soft-

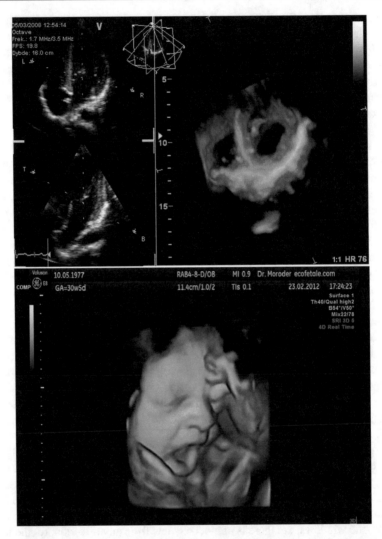

Fig. 12.4 Examples of 3D surface visualization based on tissue segmentation between high intensity tissue and low intensity fluids, such as blood in cardiac imaging (top) or amniotic fluid on obstetric imaging (bottom). Source: https://upload.wikimedia.org/wikipedia/commons/6/61/Apikal4D.gif (2020) Kjetil Lenes [CC BY-SA 3.0] (https://creativecommons.org/licenses/by-sa/3.0). Source: This Photo was taken by Wolfgang Moroder (web page: https://commons.wikimedia.org/wiki/File:Fetal_yawning_4D_ultrasound_ecografia_4D_Dr._Wolfgang_Moroder.theora.ogv, 2020)

tissue imaging is currently limited to low contrast X-ray methods, namely CBCT and superficial optical imaging including visual assessment of the care provider. Ultrasound naturally provides cross-sectional images of high soft-tissue contrast and thus extends the currently available diagnostic information. Volumetric ultrasonic scanning would allow the clinician to coregister images between, for example, CBCT and ultrasound. Contrary to that the position and orientation of single images without the possibility of coregistration might leave spatial uncertainties. The significance of these uncertainties depends on the individual patient imaging cases.

Three-dimensional ultrasonic imaging in dentistry can yield anatomically referenced information. Figure 12.5 shows the example of a 3D ultrasound scanned implant. A coronal section is shown in the left panel, as the interior of 3D solid tissue cannot be visualized except by means of cut-sections. The section was placed in the anterior–posterior direction such that both adjacent teeth and the central implant crown are demarcated. In this view the facial bone level can be seen relative to the spatial position of the adjacent teeth and the implant crown. The absolute value and any subsequent change in the bone level can thus be quantified. The middle panel illustrates the anterior–posterior position of the coronal plane as a vertical yellow line. Analogous, the cross-sectional plane position is also shown in the coronal plane as a vertical yellow line. Bone width and level relative to the implant can be quantified in this cross-sectional view and the absolute position of the view is determined by the coronal slice. The 3D volume data can also be superimposed with CBCT data as available to further its diagnostic value. The right panel shows the corresponding photographic view of the same anatomical location with a virtual view of the placed implant. The red and yellow lines indicate the relative positions between the ultrasonic and optical images.

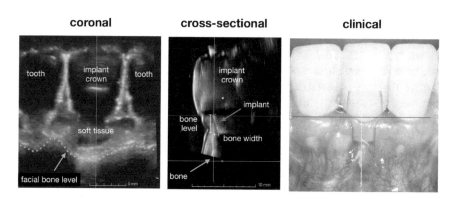

Fig. 12.5 Example of an ultrasonic 3D implant scan. The yellow vertical and red horizontal lines correspond to each other in all three panels. Left: Coronal cut-plane at an anterior–posterior position where the implant crown and adjacent teeth are fully demarcated. The resulting facial bone level is labeled by the green dotted line. Middle: Midfacial, cross-sectional, view of the implant. Here bone level and width can be directly measured. The red and yellow slice plane markers define the absolute position of the 2D cut-sections within the complete 3D image data. The latter can also be directly compared to CBCT. Right: Optical visualization of the same anatomical location with an overlayed virtual illustration of the implant. Source: HUM00140205

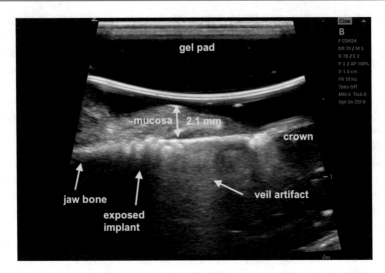

Fig. 12.6 Example of tissue recession after implant placement. The ultrasonic image shows a maximum mucosal thickness of 2.1 mm. Source: HUM00140205

12.4.1 Tissue Recession

Tissue thickness can be assessed with CBCT, though the soft-tissue contrast is low. It can also be assessed by poking with a needle into the soft tissue and reading the depth at which the needle comes to a rest when it impacts the underlying bone or implant. Ultrasound on the other side can visualize the soft tissue in section as shown in Fig. 12.6. Absolute tissue thickness can be immediately assessed using caliper tools on the ultrasound scanner. In this example the mucosa is 2.1 mm thick. A much thicker mucosal tissue can be seen in Fig. 12.7 (6 mm). Repeated thickness measurements can be performed without penetrating the soft tissue mechanically or accumulating radiation dose (CBCT).

12.4.2 Bone Recession

Jaw bone recession is usually diagnosed by means of CBCT if the bone is visually covered by soft tissue. For cases where CBCT is impaired, i.e. those that include nearby implants, bone recession may go undiagnosed or not be reliable. Ultrasound penetrates any overlying soft tissue and can directly visualize the jaw bone surface as well as the implant if it is not fully covered by hard tissue. Figure 12.7 gives an example for this case. The implant threads are seen as the periodic structure in the ultrasound image. In addition, the implant also creates an image artifact, here a veil artifact, i.e. an internal reverberation of the incident sound field inside the metallic implant. Also seen is a horizontal reverberation artifact of the gel coupling pad. Two-dimensional ultrasonic imaging may be lacking an absolute spatial reference.

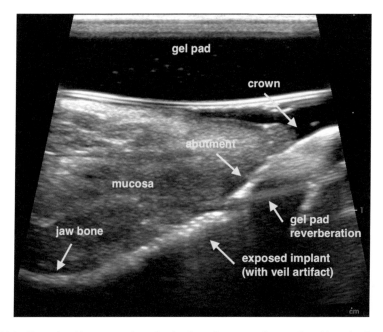

Fig. 12.7 Example of bone recession after implant placement. Current dental imaging based on CBCT cannot yield diagnostic information due to scattering artifacts of CBCT surrounding the implant. This reduces spatial resolution and contrast to a degree that implant delineation versus the jaw bone is not warranted. Source: HUM00140205

Similar to 2D X-ray, there is only one frame within which spatial coordinates can be compared to each other. In other words, directly measuring bone recession from a 2D ultrasound image may be impossible since the absolute location of the image is not known a priori. CBCT encompasses the entire oral anatomy and thus allows for referencing relative to other spatial structures. However, experience and confidence need to be established to understand if referencing a crown, for example, is clinically sufficient for observing spatial bone changes and to what degree they can be quantified.

Reference

1. Prager RW, et al. Three-dimensional ultrasound imaging. Proc Inst Mech Eng H 2010;224(2):193–223. ISSN:0954-4119 (Print); 0954-4119 (Linking). https://doi.org/10.1243/09544119JEIM586. https://www.ncbi.nlm.nih.gov/pubmed/20349815.

Printed in the United States
by Baker & Taylor Publisher Services